RESEARCH METHODS
for Undergraduate Students in Nursing

Second Edition

RESEARCH METHODS

for Undergraduate Students in Nursing

Catherine H.C. Seaman

Associate Professor of Nursing, School of Nursing
University of Virginia, Charlottesville, Virginia
and Associate Professor and Chairman
Department of Anthropology and Sociology
Sweet Briar College, Virginia

Phyllis J. Verhonick

Formerly Director of Research, School of Nursing
University of Virginia, Charlottesville, Virginia
(deceased)

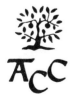 APPLETON-CENTURY-CROFTS/Norwalk, Connecticut

83 84 85 86 / 10 9 8 7 6 5 4 3

Prentice-Hall International, Inc., London
Prentice-Hall of Australia, Pty. Ltd., Sydney
Prentice-Hall of India Private Limited, New Delhi
Prentice-Hall of Japan, Inc., Tokyo
Prentice-Hall of Southeast Asia (Pte.) Ltd., Singapore
Whitehall Books Ltd., Wellington, New Zealand

Library of Congress Cataloging in Publication Data

Seaman, Catherine
    Research methods for undergraduate students in nursing.

    Authors' names in reverse order in 1st ed.
    Includes bibliographies and index.
    1. Nursing—Research.   I. Verhonick, Phyllis J.
II. Title.
RT81.5.S4 1982   610.73'072   81-20530
ISBN 0-8385-8409-8   AACR2

Text and cover design: Jean M. Sabato
Production Editor: Steve Bedney

PRINTED IN THE UNITED STATES OF AMERICA

This book is affectionately dedicated to my family:
John; Cathy, Dick, Kitty, Rick, Jack;
Gwendolyn, Jim, Jamie, Elizabeth; Tony, Diana, and Andrew; Mama;
and all of my kin.

CONTENTS

PART 3: Theory and Sampling

PART 4: Research Designs

PART 5: Collecting the Data

PREFACE

The second edition of this book endeavors to meet the expanding interest of nurses in research. The primary goal is to organize the research process into a simple framework that not only provides a step-by-step introduction to the construction of research projects, but answers questions such as: What makes nursing research scientific? How does scientific reasoning enter into research? How are nursing observations and theory related? What are the various designs and methods used in nursing research? How does the student obtain study subjects? Collect and measure the data? Summarize the findings?

The book is written for both the undergraduate nurse, and for the graduate student who has not had an undergraduate research course. The aim of the book is to assist the student to understand the research process well enough to read the publications in nursing research with a critical perspective; propose and carry out a circumscribed research project; and integrate the reasoning and observations that make nursing research scientific.

Because of the growth of nursing research, the revision of the book has been a sweeping one. Every chapter has been rewritten although occasional portions of the first edition remain. Every page was written with the image of Phyllis Verhonick in mind. Consultation with her was sorely missed.

My thanks go to my colleagues who read and commented on the book as it was being revised, and to Charles Bollinger who encouraged and stimulated the publication.

PART 1

Introduction to the Research Process

CHAPTER 1
Scientific Research in Nursing

CHAPTER 2
Theory, Hypothesis, Concept, and Related Research Terms

CHAPTER 3
Phases and Steps in the Research Process

SCIENTIFIC RESEARCH IN NURSING

Scientific research is a process in which observable, verifiable data are systematically collected from the empirical world—the world we know through our senses—in order to describe, explain, or predict events. Scientific research differs from nonscientific research undertaken by scholars such as theologians, whose work may be careful and systematic, but concerned with unseen phenomena such as supernatural spirits. In contrast, scientific research deals only with what can be observed by one scientist and verified by another. The objectives of scientific research are to answer questions, to discover or revise facts or theories, and/or to solve problems. Scientific research as Notter notes (1963, p. 49) is every nurse's business.

Upon completion of this chapter, the student will be able to: 1) define basic and applied research; 2) state the purposes of research in nursing; 3) trace the rise of scientific research in the ancient art of nursing; 4) describe the place of research in the emergent profession of nursing; and 5) identify trends in the future of nursing research.

APPLIED AND BASIC RESEARCH IN NURSING

Applied research is a process whereby the researcher collects nursing data to be used—that is, *applied*—in the clinical, administrative, or instructional areas. Applied research is designed to: 1) find solutions to nursing problems; 2) evaluate nursing practices, procedures, policies, or curricula; 3) assess the needs of patients, staff, or students; and/or 4) make decisions to change or continue various aspects of nursing.

Chapman's (1977) study is one example of applied research. Chapman conducted a clinical study to determine whether measures of patient stress and welfare differed when various approaches to nursing care—individualized, informative, and routine—were used in the perioperative period. She found that the individualized and the informative approaches to nursing care were more effective than routine nursing care to reduce both the patient's requirement for postoperative analgesics and the length of hospitalization. Her findings suggest solutions to nursing problems concerned with using postoperative analgesics and with length of hospital stay. The study also evaluates nursing approaches and provides data upon which to base decisions to change the approach to nursing care.

Another example of applied research is that of Hain and Chen (1976), who assessed the health needs of the elderly who were living in high-rise apartments. After identifying various health problems, the researchers recommended a number of solutions, including screening and also employing health personnel.

McGillicuddy's research (1977) on the relationship between mothers' rooming-in with their child during the child's hospitalization and the change in the child's behavior enabled her to recommend both administrative changes, such as changes in visiting regulations, and changes in nursing education, for example, experience for the nursing student in caring for a family.

Each of the studies above centers upon the practical application of research, clearly relating research to problem solving, evaluation, assessment, and intervention.

In contrast, basic research undertakes to advance scientific knowledge, whether or not this knowledge is immediately usable in nursing. One example of basic research by nurse scientists is that of Parsons et al (1981), who examined the extent of nerve fiber degeneration in rats' brains following a single cerebral concussion. Since such experimental research is impossible using human subjects, findings from lower mammals may cast some light upon concussion in general. However, using the research findings in nursing practice is not the immediate objective of such basic research. Similar research is that of Raff (1977), who studied the relationship between prenatal exercise and postnatal growth and development in the offspring of albino rats. Basic research adds to the pool of scientific knowledge, but the implementation of this knowledge in nursing is left to others.

Many nursing studies contain elements of both basic and applied research. Often, the distinction between the two has more to do with administrative decisions about financial support than with study content. In this sense, basic research may only imply that the researcher was free to work in the area of choice without justifying the work by immediate practical advantage.

THE PURPOSE OF NURSING RESEARCH

The purpose of nursing research may be summarized as follows: to observe in order to know; to know in order to predict; to predict in order to control; to control in order to practice and prescribe in a professional manner. Each of these purposes will be briefly examined.

To observe in order to know is the aim of all nursing research. The nurse who observes, verifies, and documents her observations works at a crucial level of research. These studies are often called *descriptive* or *exploratory*. They begin when the nurse asks the question "What?" "What are bedsores?" Verhonick (1961) asks, "What are the objective criteria to use to measure bedsores? What causes skin to break down in the first place?" Williams (1972) asks, "What factors contribute to skin breakdown?" Once the factors are discovered and named, the nurse can then explore how they are related to one another. For example, are the factors of age, skin thickness, and diagnosis interrelated to the occurrence of bed sores? Thus, descriptive studies are closely oriented to observation. Yet, the very perception of nursing data is often structured by the scientist's background and education. That is, the nurse observes, or "sees," data from a viewpoint that differs from that of a psychologist or geneticist. For example, the nurse mid-wife wants to describe, or "know," the physiological, psychological, social, and cultural factors associated with maternal and child care. She wants to know how the procedures are alike for all patients and how they differ for some, such as the rural or urban woman, the lower class or middle class, and women of various ethnic origins. However, all scientists ultimately use their observations to try to explain how concepts are interrelated to one another. Such explanations lead to the second purpose of nursing research—to predict.

To predict, the nurse begins with an explanation, predicts what should be found on observation, and tests these predictions in nursing research. The researcher may either predict causality or she may predict that correlations will be found between specified factors. Causality means that one variable such as germ X causes a change in another variable, such as the state of health. Causality is established if the events under specific conditions may be related in such a way that event Y (such as syphilis) will always be observed to follow event X (exposure to the spirochete). However, because many complex factors influence human health and welfare, it is not always possible to establish causality as neatly as the germ theory allows. For example, scientists cannot yet say exactly what causes lung cancer. However, they can say that lung cancer increases as pollution of the inhaled air increases. Predictions can be made that certain factors appear to be associated with a rise in lung cancer.

Correlations, or concomitant variations and associations as these are also called, state that a change in the amount of one variable is related to a change in the amount of another. Correlations may either be positive or negative: As one increases, the other also increases; or, as one increases, the other decreases.

Once such interrelations are made, the nurse can predict that certain populations are at risk to get lung cancer, for example, those who smoke. Predictions such as these can be tested further in research; if the research findings support the predictions, steps can be taken to control harmful factors.

To control is a major purpose of applied nursing research. It means that the nurse has the ability to check, regulate, and exercise directing power over factors that influence the health and comfort of patients or clients. To control pain, discomfort, sickness, anxiety, or fear is an objective of patient care; to control ignorance and superstition is an objective of nursing teaching; and to control the proper flow of information and communication is a goal of nursing administration. A revolutionary approach in nursing is to return control of the patient's body and mind to the patient, with as little recourse to drugs and dependence upon health personnel as possible.

When nursing is able to describe, understand, and explain nursing phenomena; when we can predict what will happen each time we intervene; and if our ability to predict allows us to control the harmful factors and promote the positive, then nursing can fulfill the final purpose—to prescribe.

To prescribe requires a deep involvement in research and practice. In addition it involves a conception of what is good and desirable—the values of the profession and society. A prescription is based on the fact that the goal to be achieved is a desirable one, and the way to achieve the goal is to follow the prescription. To bring about and maintain good health, the prescription states, one must comply with the prescribed regimen of treatment, diet, and/or medication.

Nurses have long practiced and prescribed intuitively. Experience often told them to do one thing rather than another. However, the research process helps nurses put experience and intuition into a statement that summarizes or predicts relationships among concepts and variables. It helps them test the statement in research, and then share the findings with the profession as a whole. In this way, research adds to the accumulating body of nursing science and enables nurses to solve problems and recommend changes.

THE RISE OF SCIENTIFIC RESEARCH IN THE ART OF NURSING

Long before nursing was a science, it was an art. Many aspects of contemporary nursing are rooted in the thousands of years during which nurses attempted to care for and cure the sick with tender, loving care rather than with science. Nursing helped others do what they could not do for themselves—deliver a baby, feed the wounded, or bathe the helpless.

Scanty evidence exists from the archeological record to indicate who were the nurses of antiquity. The work of Solecki (1971) in an ancient cave in Iraq suggests that about 60,000 years ago, women, children, and occasionally an old man remained close to the hearth fires of home. Perhaps they were the first nurses. Evidence from ancient bones found near the hearth suggests the early patients were the handicapped and the injured. The cave dwellers of Shanidar, called the *flower people* by Solecki because they placed clusters of flowers in the graves of their dead, may have utilized local plants as poultices or herbal remedies. Elsewhere in the ancient world, Marshack (1972) found finely made figurines that, he suggests, may have been used in magical rites to assist women in childbirth.

Nursing care moved out of the home when priests established a causal link in the minds of their followers between evil spirits and sickness. For example, in Greece by 1200 B.C., the sick were being treated in temples, where the priests prescribed rest, diet, and bathing.

Among early Christians, both women and men cared for the sick and aged, this practice continuing as the Church gained control over society. However, the dirty and unpleasant work associated with the art of nursing was often left to the lower levels of nurses, who performed disagreeable tasks in hope of a later reward in heaven. The well-to-do and educated tended to supervise rather than deliver direct care. During the Crusades men and women from high statuses served as nurses. In fact, the association of nursing with war and the military left its mark on the character of nurses' training, as well as on the military-like stratification that has long been a part of nursing practice. In the

West, nursing tended to become a task of women, while research tended to be exclusively in the hands of men.

Following the Protestant Reformation, the status of nursing, now based on wage labor supported by taxes, declined. Low wages, lack of education, and the servant-like status of women who were nurses soon brought nursing to a position of disrespect and contempt. The art of nursing fell to untrained, uneducated women, some of whom were inmates of work houses or penal institutions. However, humanitarian reform arose in reaction to the industrial revolution with its accompanying exploitation of the poor and the sick. In Germany, Pastor Fliedner established a five-year program to train nurses. Among those who examined the functioning of the school was Florence Nightingale who, in 1860, founded a school of nursing at St. Thomas's Hospital in England. Nightingale approached nursing primarily as an art but was likewise the first nurse scientist. Her *Notes on Nursing* (1859) not only stresses the use of observation but also contains a wealth of material inviting research.

The most important practical lesson that can be given to nurses, Nightingale writes (*Ibid,* p. 65), is to teach them how to observe and what to observe. In Nightingale's view, devotion is useless without ready and correct observations. While statistics inform us what percent of the population may die, she writes, observation tells us which one will die.

Nightingale was a firm believer in applied research, noting that observations are for the sake of saving lives and increasing comfort rather than for piling up miscellaneous information or curious facts (Nightingale, 1859, p. 70).

Nightingale's approach to nurses' training assisted in the rise of the modern hospital, which came into being along with the improvement of bedside nursing, hospital management, the science of bacteriology, and the introduction of aseptic surgery. At that time, nurses' training included the mastery of scientific techniques and procedures, if not scientific theory. The rise of science and research in nursing was nonetheless underway.

The Development of Nursing Research

Following Nightingale's era, research in nursing practice declined for nearly a century. It was replaced in the United States by research in nursing education and administration, such as that conducted by Nutting (1907), and by research on the function of nurses, such as that reported by Hughes et al (1958).

During the decade of the 1950s, more and more nurses entered the universities to complete undergraduate or graduate education. Research was required to complete the graduate degree. In the universities, many nurses began to form intellectual alliances with those in the social and behavioral sciences (Benne and Bennis, 1959, p. 381), with several consequences First, nurses became researchers in the domain of social and behavioral sciences neglected by many medical doctors. Second, the profession of nursing began to integrate a holistic approach to patients, family, and community, which supplemented the former "organ" or "disease" orientation. Third, the conceptual and theoretical frameworks of the social sciences and behavioral sciences began to make their way into nursing to supplement the theory of the natural sciences. For example, the integrated approach enabled nursing to treat mental illness, rapidly becoming the most prevalent disease in the Western world, with a considerable level of sophistication. Moreover, the appearance of the journal *Nursing Research* also provided nursing during the 1950s with both a forum and a stimulus for research.

During the 1960s, research concerned with patient care and nursing practice began to appear in the literature once more. *Patient Centered Approaches to Nursing*, by Abdellah et al (1960), ushered in the new era. Orlando's *The Dynamic Nurse–Patient Relationship* (1961) focused attention on interaction between nurse and patient. Brown's *Newer Dimensions for Patient Care* (1961–1962) integrated the scientific approach of anthropology and nursing. *Better Patient Care Through Nursing Research*, by Abdellah and Levine (1965), exemplified the rise of the importance of research in nursing.

From this time forward, publications that dealt with nursing research began to accelerate. The National Commission for the Study of Nursing and Nursing Education reinforced the importance of science and research in nursing in its 1970 report, *An Abstract for Action*, which established research as one of the four priorities in the future of nursing. In *Research in Nursing: Toward a Science of Health Care* (1976), the American Nursing Association reported contemporary trends in nursing research, and suggested that nursing was moving toward becoming the science of health care. During the 1970s, edited studies in nursing research included the series *Communicating Nursing Research*, edited by Majorie V. Batey (1968–1978, 11 vol.); Downs and Newman (1973; 1977); Verhonick (1975; 1977); and Downs and Fleming (1979).

During the 1970s, publications concerned with theory in nursing also began to appear: Rogers (1970); Murphy (1971); King (1971); Hardy (1973); Hardy and Conway (1978): and Stevens (1979). The decade of the 1980s promises to produce more. Basic and applied clinical nursing research has shown a similar growth. At first, clinical studies centered upon particular diseases, such as tuberculosis, then studies focused on maternal and child care. Recent clinical research includes a wide variety of topics and designs, such as Lindeman's reports on patient education (1971); Cleland et al's (1971) concern with the prevention of bacteriuria in female patients with indwelling catheters; and Jacox's (1973) work on pain. Diers (1979) combined research in the clinical area with a theoretical orientation developed by Dickoff and James (1968; 1975).

The Importance of Research
to the Nursing Profession

Research is of vital importance to nursing today, as it has never been in the past. The rapid advance of knowledge in the fields of health maintenance, health promotion, and disease prevention, together with the public's demand for the quality of life that good physical and mental health bring, have moved nursing quickly forward. To meet new challenges, investigate unsolved problems, and scrutinize the changes underway in nursing, the individual nurse must actively seek to understand and apply the basic principles of research.

Likewise, research provides the abstract knowledge that is the foundation for establishing nursing as a profession. According to Carr-Saunders and Wilson (1933) the distinguishing mark of a profession is the combination of knowledge and technique. Caplow (1971) more recently includes a knowledge base, autonomy and monopoly in practice, and serious consequences of practice to society. A code of ethics is another distinguishing feature of the professional. Each of these five criteria will be examined briefly, in order to assess the place of research in the rising profession of nursing.

1. *The possession of a large body of abstract knowledge is directly related to research and theory.* Upon what pool of abstract knowledge does nursing draw to make decisions? What theory explains the reasoning behind a decision to intervene in practice, change a curriculum, or reverse an administrative decision? Writing over twenty years ago, Johnson (1959, p. 292) suggests that professional nursing draws its knowledge from the basic sciences. Nurses then apply this knowledge in practice to achieve carefully defined goals. Research findings useful to nursing include those of physics, chemistry, microbiology, physiology, psychology, anthropology, sociology, law, and economics. Nursing research designed to test the findings from these disciplines will expand nursing's body of knowledge.

2. *The achievement of autonomy in nursing is underway.* Bullough (1975) notes the autonomy of the clinical specialists, while Foster and Anderson (1978, p. 199) relate the autonomy gained by nurse practitioners to their willingness to assume major responsibilities. However, further re-

search is needed to establish the nature and permanence of autonomy in nursing. Is nursing autonomy related to the supply of doctors? Will nurses achieve true autonomy only in ghettos or sparsely populated areas where medical doctors do not choose to practice? Does federal funding of the health care of the poor enable nurses to be autonomous? How will the curtailment of federal funds to health and welfare currently underway affect nursing? Answers to such questions are crucial to the establishment and survival of autonomy in nursing.

3. *Monopoly of nursing practice is a legal question, contingent upon both a definition of nursing and support at the legislative level.* As Hinsvark notes (1974), only a few states such as Washington have a law that gives the nurse the right to expanded practice. Research is needed not only to keep abreast of legal questions but also to determine the most effective way to promote the profession and protect the image of nursing.

4. *The social consequences that follow autonomy and monopoly of nursing practice are serious.* This is evident in the report of the National Commission for the Study of Nursing and Nursing Education (1970, p. 163):

> We have become intimately acquainted with the history and the disappointments, as well as the great joys of nursing. Out of this has come the recognition that nursing is not only important, but critical to the future of health care in America.

The social consequences if all nurses withdrew from hospitals, clinics, nursing homes, and public health agencies indicate the seriousness of the social consequences of nursing practice.

5. *The nursing code of ethics is concerned with moral and ethical questions for which the nurse is responsible.* The nursing profession must continually review its code to reflect the changing status of nursing, as well as societal demands. A comparison of the Florence Nightingale Code with the current American Nurses' Association Code (1976), for example, reveals changes in the relationship between nursing and medicine.

There are virtually no formal teaching structures for nursing ethics, either in schools of nursing or other health professional schools, Gortner notes (1979:13). Greater attention must be given to ethics, she suggests, in both research and practice.

Future Directions of Nursing Research

Nowhere is the importance of research in the future of nursing better demonstrated than in the statement of The National League for Nursing (1978), which includes research as one of the ten characteristics of bac-

TABLE 1–1. FUTURE DIRECTIONS OF NURSING RESEARCH SUGGESTED BY LINDEMAN'S 1975 SURVEY

Research *to determine:*
1. How to use research in practice
2. Valid and reliable indicators of quality nursing care
3. Interventions by nurses most effective in reducing patients' psychological stress
4. Valid and reliable methods for staffing that reflect patients' needs and contain costs
5. Effective means of communicating and implementing change in practice
6. The nursing behavior and setting most likely to produce positive effects in a crisis

Research *to evaluate:*
1. Effects of nurses' expanding role in patient care
2. Functions and clinical parameters of nurse practitioners
3. Processes used to provide nursing care in terms of patient outcomes
4. Nurses' role in preventive health service in terms of patient outcomes
5. Effectiveness of various approaches to peer review
6. Nurses' interventions that are most effective in reducing the psychological stress of patients
7. Change in nursing practice

Research *to establish* the relationship between clinical nursing research and quality care.

Reserach *to develop* a set of physical and psychological procedures to assess and improve patient care and nursing intervention.

Research *to explore* means of enhancing nurses' ability to cope with stress.

Research *to clarify* concepts such as the expanding role of the nurse.

Research *to delimit* the functions and clinical parameters of nurse practitioners.

Research *to assess* the relationship between quality of nursing leadership and quality of nursing practice in institutions.

calaureate education in nursing. Emphasis upon research in the undergraduate curriculum assures the profession that a new generation of nurses will possess research skills. What areas of research will nurses pursue in the future? Lindeman (1975) reports the findings of a nationwide survey of nurses, the Delphi survey, which identified the most important areas needing research (see Table 1–1). Evaluation, nursing practice, nursing interventions, and nursing roles were considered to be important areas for research. Fleming (1979) suggests that research in the future should focus on preventive health measures, nursing care, and persistent nursing problems (see Table 1–2). In Fleming's view nursing researchers must find ways to incorporate research findings

TABLE 1-2. RESEARCH NEEDS IDENTIFIED BY FLEMING (1979)

Preventive Health

Research to understand behaviors detrimental to health:
1. Excess use of alcohol and mood-altering drugs
2. Cigarette smoking
3. Poor nutritional practices
4. Carelessness that results in accidental injury
5. Sedentary lifestyles and improper exercise
6. Improper care and supervision of children
7. Lack of knowledge to carry out the parenting role

Research to understand preventive health problems for age groups:
1. Health care of the young
2. Lack of immunization among children
3. Quality of life for city children
4. Child neglect and child abuse
5. Psychosocial disability from poor bonding between mother and infant
6. Incidence that the disabling condition can be decreased
7. Rate and consequences of teenage pregnancies
8. Preventive mental health services to families and youth
9. Health education to improve access to comprehensive care
10. The economics of maintaining and caring for the aged
11. Aspects of leisure time, retirement, coping abilities, and health status of the elderly
12. Demand for health care and hospitalization of the aged

Types of Care

Research related to primary health care:
1. Clarification of the role of the nurse who is practicing primary care
2. Changes in the delivery system of primary care
3. Planning, delivery, assessment, and monitoring of primary care for all ages and socioeconomic statuses

Research related to long-term health care:
1. Identification and resolution for long-term care of chronic conditions such as: diabetes, urological conditions, arthritis, cardiac conditions, glaucoma, cataracts, cancer, cerebral vascular accidents, and mental aberrations

Current Conditions Likely to be Prevalent in the Future

Research related to:
1. Drug abuse: narcotics; alcohol; cigarette smoking; effect on user and, in case of women, on the fetus
2. Stress: identifying, assessing, measuring, and implementing intervention plans to alter loneliness, pain, fear, and adjustment problems
3. Venereal disease; cancer; nutrition problems; and cultural diversity

Problems Identified by Nurses

Research to reduce complications of hospitalization and surgery; to improve outlook for high-risk parents and infants; to improve health care of the elderly; to study life-threatening situations; to study adaptation to chronic illness; to study self-care systems; to study new technological development.*

See Priorities for Research in Nursing. Kansas City: ANA Commission on Nursing Research, 1975.

into nursing practice. Yet Stetler and Marram (1976) warn that research findings must first be evaluated before they are applied to nursing problems. Nurses should be able to predict and assess outcomes of applied research findings.

The American Nurses' Association Commission of Nursing Research has identified a number of questions it hopes will be answered in future nursing research (A.N.A., 1976): 1) How are individuals persuaded to use available measures to prevent illness? 2) How are individuals helped to maintain health? 3) How are people helped to cope with illness? 4) How are complications reduced among those hospitalized or chronically ill? 5) How is illness prevented for those subject to health risks, such as the premature and the elderly? Each question represents a fruitful area to explore in research. Forthcoming answers will not only prevent suffering but will save countless time and money and reduce the investment of energy.

In Leninger's (1976) view, future research in doctoral programs will focus on four areas: the identification of cultural influences on health practices and values; definition of the ways to achieve new levels of health care; invention of systems to classify nursing phenomena; and the formulation of systems to evaluate major components of health care.

In the view of Abdellah (1971), Gortner (1975), and Barnard and Neal (1977), the profession will direct future attention to theory development, conceptual clarification and research.

SUMMARY

Scientific research is a process in which observable data are systematically collected from the empirical world by one scientist and verified by another. Research is commonly divided into basic and applied. *Basic research* advances scientific knowledge, regardless of whether the knowledge is immediately usable or not. *Applied research* is used in nursing practice, teaching, or administration. Most research projects contain elements of both basic and applied research.

The purpose of research is to observe in order to know; know in order to predict; predict in order to control; and control in order to practice and prescribe in a professional manner. Descriptive or exploratory studies help the nurse know what the subject matter of nursing is and what should be studied. Prediction allows the nurse to identify associated factors in order to control other factors such as pain. Once nursing attains the knowledge necessary to understand and predict, it will be more able to control harmful elements, and nurses will move into practice and prescription with greater assurance.

The art of nursing—helping others do what they cannot do for themselves—is an ancient tradition rooted first in the home and then in religious institutions. The decline of nursing as a service to God put nursing practice in a low-status, wage-earning position. Nightingale, scientist and scholar, raised the status of nursing and stressed that observation should be applied for the sake of saving lives and increasing the comfort of the sick. Following Nightingale's era, nearly a century elapsed before research focused on the patient rather than on the nurse or nursing. In the universities, alliances between nursing and the social and behavioral sciences influenced the direction of nursing research.

In order to provide a body of knowledge that allows the nurse discretion and autonomy in practice, research is crucial to the emergent profession of nursing. Research is becoming the focus of many teachers, and behavioral sciences influenced the direction of nursing research.

STUDY QUESTIONS

1. Define the kind of research that has application in the clinical area. Can you propose such a research project?
2. State the four purposes of nursing research.
3. Describe a descriptive or exploratory project you would like to conduct and identify which of the four purposes of nursing research it would fulfill.
4. Write a statement that predicts a causal relationship between germs and disease.
5. Can you use any knowledge gained in nursing to make a prediction about nursing care?
6. Describe some of the factors in patient care you have tried to control, and describe the factors that enabled you to control.
7. Write a nursing prescription. How is it similar to nursing intervention?
8. Write a nursing prescription that the patient can use to intervene in a process that is not good for his or her health.
9. Which purpose of nursing research did Nightingale stress? Explain whether or not it is relevant today.
10. At times, nurses give patients backrubs. Is this an art or a science? Why?
11. To what do you attribute the rise of research in nursing?
12. What are the trends you can identify in future nursing research?
13. Examine Tables 1–1 and 1–2. Which of these research needs most interests you? Which would you like to study or examine in research?

REFERENCES AND SUGGESTED READINGS

Abdellah, F. (1971): Foreward. In Murphy, F. (ed.), Theoretical Issues in Professional Nursing. New York: Appleton, pp. xi–xii.

Abdellah, F. et al. (1960): Patient-Centered Approaches to Nursing. New York: Macmillan. *Abdellah et al change the focus of research from nurses to patients.*

Abdellah, F. and Levine, E. (1979): Better Patient Care Through Nursing Research (2nd ed.). New York: Macmillan. *The second edition of a comprehensive book that integrates research with patient care. Part 4 looks at contemporary status of nursing research.*

American Nurses's Association (1976): Research in Nursing: Toward a Science of Health Care. Kansas City: The American Nurses's Association. Preparation of Nurses for Participation in Research. Code No. D-54 2500. Kansas City: The American Nurses's Association. Priorities for Research in Nursing. Kansas City: The American Nurses's Association. *Publications of the association which reflect the rising emphasis on research.*

Batey, M. (ed.) (1968–1978): Communicating Nursing Research. Boulder: Western Interstate Commission on Higher Education (WICHE). *Eleven volumes of report papers delivered in a conference on research held yearly since 1968. Each research paper is followed by a critique from another nurse scientist.*

Barnard, K. and Neal, M. (1977): Maternal-child nursing research: review of the past and strategies for the future. *Nursing Research 26,* 193–200. *The authors call for the development of classificatory systems of concepts used in practice.*

Benne, D. and Bennis, W. (1959): The role of the professional nurse. *American Journal of Nursing,* May, 837–882. *The authors discuss the problems of the drive for professionalism in nursing and note the alliances formed in universities between nursing and the social and behavioral sciences.*

Brown, E. (1948): Nursing for the Future. New York: Russell Sage. (1961): Newer Dimensions of Patient Care I. New York: Russell Sage. (1962): Newer Dimensions of Patient Care II. New York: Russell Sage. *An anthropologist interested in nursing published the three books above that provided insight into the nursing profession.*

Bullough, B. (1975): Factors contributing to role expansion for registered nurses. In Bullough, B. (ed.), The Law and the Expanding Nursing Role. New York: Appleton, pp. 53–61.

Bullough, B. (ed.) (1980): The Law and the Expanding Nursing Role (2nd ed.). New York: Appleton. *A collection of papers that examine the use of law, perspectives on the expanding role of nurses, and other topics.*

Caplow, T. (1971): Elementary Sociology. Englewood Cliffs, New Jersey: Prentice-Hall. *Chapter VIII contains discussion on professions and occupations.*

Carr-Saunders, A. and Wilson, P. (1933): Professions. In Seligman, E. (ed.), Encyclopaedia of the Social Sciences. New York: Macmillan. *Nearly fifty years old, this article still provides insight and understanding.*

Cleland, V. (1977): Investigations in the clinical setting. In Verhonick, P. (ed.), Nursing Research II. Boston: Little, Brown, pp. 33–75. *Discusses two studies: the effect of situational stressors on the cognitive performance of general nurses, and a study to assess the relative effectiveness of different types of perineal care in preventing bacteriuria in female patients with indwelling catheters.*

Diers, D. (1979): Research in Nursing Practice. Philadelphia: J. B. Lippincott. *Uses ideas generated by Dickoff and James and others to develop chapters on clinical judgment, and studies of factor-searching, relation-searching, association and causal hypotheses testing, and prescription testing.*

Dickoff, J. et al. (1968): Theory in a practice discipline. Practice oriented theory (Part I). Practice oriented research (Part II). *Nursing Research 17,* 415–435; 545–554. *Develops theory related to practice.*

Downs, F. and Newman, M. (eds.) (1977): A Source Book of Nursing Research (2nd ed.). Philadelphia: F. A. Davis. *Sixteen articles deal with research in nursing.*

Downs, F. and Fleming, J. (eds.) (1979): Issues in Nursing Research. New York: Appleton. *Seven articles cover particular problem areas in research.*

Fleming, J. (1979): The future of nursing research. In Downs, F. and Fleming, J. (eds.) Issues in Nursing Research. New York: Appleton. *Reports on the acceptance and scope of research in nursing, research needs, and other issues.*

Foster, F. and Anderson, B. (1978): Medical Anthropology. New York: Wiley. *Chapter 11 deals with "Professionals in Medicine, Nursing."*

Gortner, S. (1975): Research for a practice profession. *Nursing Research 24,* 193–197. *Notes a trend in nursing to integrate theory and research to provide knowledge base.*

Hain, M. and Chen, S. (1976): Health needs of the elderly. *Nursing Research 25,* 433–439. *A study of the elderly living in high-rise apartments.*

Hall, V. (1975): Statutory Regulation of the Scope of Nursing Practice—A Critical Survey. Chicago: National Joint Practice Commission. *Author comments on various definitions found in Nurse Practice Act.*

Hardy, M. (ed.) (1973): Theoretical Foundations for Nursing. New York: MSS Information Corp. *Editor brings together a number of articles contributing to theory.*

Hardy, M. and Conway, M. (1978): Role Theory: Perspectives for Health Professionals. New York: Appleton. *Twelve articles deal with role.*

Henderson, V., Nite, G. et al (1978): Principles and Practices of Nursing (6th ed.). New York: Macmillan. *Part I: Place of nursing in health services.*

Hinsvark, I. (1974): Implications for action in the expanded role of the nurse. In *Nursing Clinics of North America 9,* 411–423. *Effect of nursing and medical practice acts on work activity of nurses.*

Hughes, E. et al. (1958): Twenty Thousand Nurses Tell Their Story. Philadelphia: J. B. Lippincott. *Five-year study on nurses initiated by the A.N.A.*

Jacox, A. and Steward, M. (1973): Psychosocial Contingencies of the Pain Experience. Iowa City, Iowa: University of Iowa College of Nursing. *A study of pain as a biopsyschosocial phenomenon.*

Johnson, D. (1959): The nature of a science of nursing. *Nursing Outlook 7,* 291–294. *The emergence of nursing as a science.*

Leininger, M. (1976): Doctoral programs for nurses: Trends, questions and projected plans. *Nursing Research 24,* 434–441. *Ideas of cultural influences on health.*

Lindeman, C. and Van Aernam, V. (1971): Nursing intervention with the presurgical patient—the effects of structured and unstructured preoperative teaching. *Nursing Research 20,* 196–209. *Authors examine effect of preoperative teaching on postoperative behavior.*

Lindeman, C. (1975): Delphi survey of priorities in clinical nursing research. *Nursing Research 24,* 434–441. *Priorities for nursing research.*

Marshack, A. (1972): The Roots of Civilization. New York: McGraw-Hill. *An examination of the prehistory of people.*

McGillicuddy, M. (1977): A study of the relationship between mother's rooming in during their children's hospitalization and changes in selected areas of children's behavior. *In* Downs, F. and Newman, M. (eds.), A Sourcebook of Nursing Research. Philadelphia: F. A. Davis, pp. 64–77. *Author recommends changes in practice area from research findings.*

Murphy, F. (1971): Theoretical Issues in Professional Nursing. New York: Appleton. *Collection of articles dealing with theories useful in nursing.*

National Commission for the Study of Nursing and Nursing Education (1970): An Abstract for Action. New York: McGraw-Hill. *A national study of nursing.*

National League for Nursing (1978): Characteristics of Baccalaureate Education in Nursing. *A revision of the 1974 statement.*

Nightingale, F. (1859): Notes on Nursing (1970 ed.). London: Gerald Duckworth. *A small book everyone interested in nursing should read.*

Notter, L. (1963): Nursing research in every nurses's business. *Nursing Outlook 11,* 49–51. *Notter's view of research.*

Nutting, M. (1907): The Educational and Professional Position of Nurses. U.S. Gov. Printing. *An early study of nurses in the United States.*

Orlando, I. (1961): The Dynamic Nurse-Patient Relationship. New York: G. P. Putnam's Sons. *Communication between nurse-patient.*

Parsons, C. et al (1981): Nerve fiber degeneration following a single experimental cerebral concussion in the rat. *Neuroscience Letter 24,* 199–204.

Raff, B. (1977): The relationship of planned prenatal exercise to postnatal growth and development in the offspring of albino rats. In Downs, F. and Newman, M., A Sourcebook of Nursing Research (2nd ed.). Philadelphia: F. A. Davis, pp. 78–85. *Example of basic research.*

Rogers, M. (1970): Introduction to the Theoretical Basis of Nursing. Philadelphia: F. A. Davis. *Uses principle of reciprocity to relate man to environment.*

Seligman, E. (ed.) (1933): Encyclopedia of the Social Sciences. New York: Macmillan. *Old, but still relevant.*

Solecki, R. (1971): Shanidar: The First Flower People. New York: Knopf. *Excavations in Iraq reveal prehistoric health conditions.*

Stevens, B. (1979): Nursing Theory. Boston: Little, Brown. *An analysis and evaluation of nursing theory in its present state.*

CHAPTER 2

THEORY, HYPOTHESIS, CONCEPT, AND RELATED RESEARCH TERMS

The words *theory, hypothesis, concept, variable,* and *observation* are among the basic terms of research. Such expressions are a part of the language of science—those words whose meaning is shared by members of the scientific community. Each nurse must learn the language of science, not only to be able to read and understand the publications in nursing and in allied sciences, but to be able to think and write in such terms. However, scientific language often includes words used in everyday conversation without exact meaning. Therefore, the use of such terms in research not only requires that students define each term precisely, but that they understand how each term functions in the research process, as well as how each term is related to others.

Upon completion of this chapter, the student should be able to: 1) identify and define basic terms used in research; 2) state how observation and reasoning function to formulate and test theories; 3) describe the nature of hypotheses; 4) define terms such as *concept, variable,* and *operational definition;* and 5) describe the meaning of concepts such as *assumption, paradigm,* and *model.*

A MODEL OF THE BASIC ELEMENTS
AND METHODS OF RESEARCH

The interrelations among elements of research are shown in Figure 2–1. The model includes: 1) basic concepts of research, such as *theory, proposition,* and *fact;* and 2) methods of theory construction and theory testing. Each concept and method will be examined in turn.

1. Basic concepts of research include fact, proposition, and theory. Figure 2–1 shows the definition of each basic term and the relationships among each. A *fact* is defined as empirically verifiable observations which the mind orders into a concept. The relationship between *fact, concept, proposition,* and *theory* is well illustrated by the following example that Charter (1975, p. 2) draws from a specific nursing care situation:

> The nurse caring for a patient admitted to the hospital following an automobile accident would obtain certain factual information from the patient and family. The recording of *facts* might include: 40 year old male, conscious, no external bleeding; vital signs—blood pressure 90/40, pulse 100, respiratory rate 20. She immediately thinks of shock *(concept)* as she studies the relationship between blood pressure and pulse *(facts).* She knows that gravity will return the blood to the heart and aid circulation (principle), and she is prepared to elevate the foot of the bed. (Note the principle here suggests the nursing action). Thus, the principle used for nursing care is also supported by theories from physiology and physics.

The nurse described above collects *data*—facts that can be observed and agreed upon by others—and orders these facts in her mind into *concepts*—general ideas or abstractions invented from particular observable events, or facts that fit together in a meaningful way. The nurse's ability to make a statement of the interrelationships among the facts, to arrive at the concept of shock, and to understand the theories of circulation and gravity enables her to take nursing action. The nurse utilized the research findings of others that she had learned in the course of education and experience, but she likewise collected her own scientific data in the course of nursing practice, in order to make a decision to intervene.

2. Basic methods of theory construction and theory testing involve reasoning. Theory construction usually begins with inductive reasoning that moves from specific facts to the more general theory. Theory testing begins with deductive reasoning, creating from a general statement or theory a specific hypothesis to be tested in research. Intimately involved with

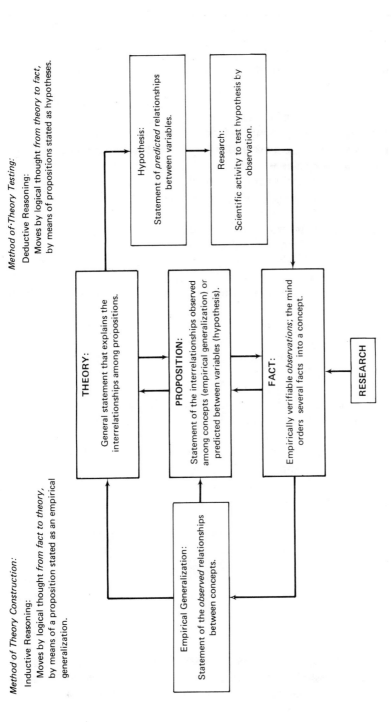

Method of Theory Construction:

Inductive Reasoning:
Moves by logical thought *from fact to theory,*
by means of a proposition stated as an empirical
generalization.

Method of·Theory Testing:

Deductive Reasoning:
Moves by logical thought *from theory to fact,*
by means of propositions stated as hypotheses.

Hypothesis:
Statement of *predicted* relationships
between variables.

Research:
Scientific activity to test hypothesis by
observation.

THEORY:
General statement that explains the
interrelationships among propositions.

PROPOSITION:
Statement of the interrelationships observed
among concepts (empirical generalization) or
predicted between variables (hypothesis).

FACT:
Empirically verifiable *observations*; the mind
orders several facts into a concept.

RESEARCH

Empirical Generalization:
Statement of the *observed* relationships
between concepts.

Figure 2–1. A model of theory construction and theory testing, using
elements and methods of the scientific research process.

both processes is the scientific research process. We will now examine each element of research and the basic methods of theory construction and testing.

Theory: Scientific Explanations of Relationships Among Propositions

Theory is a scientific explanation for the interrelationships among facts, concepts, and propositions. The key words are *explanation* and *interrelationships*. An explanation for interrelated phenomena is a goal of all science, but the practicing professions such as medicine, nursing, law, applied anthropology, clinical sociology, and engineering go one step beyond explanation to application. One of their goals is to use theory in practice to control, to prescribe, or as Diers (1979, p. 33) notes, to change the world for the "better." However, care must be taken to recognize that not everyone may agree on what constitutes "better." The values of one segment of society may not always coincide with all segments.

Nonetheless, people tend to agree that it is better to be well than to be sick. Theories that explain health and sickness are sought everywhere, in order to control sickness and to prescribe measures to recover and maintain good health. For example, the germ theory explains why and how germs and disease are interrelated. The explanation allows practitioners to control disease caused by germs by prescribing vaccination or medication. Few would argue that such change is not for the better.

Theories abound in human cultures, but not all of these theories are scientific. For example, in the past, philosophy and religion provided explanations of events in this world and the next. The medieval view that the world was flat arose from the theory that angels held up the four corners of the earth. Proceeding from this premise or theory, deductive reasoning led to predictions that, if one sailed toward the horizon, one would eventually fall off the edge of the earth. No provision was made for testing such hypotheses, because religious explanations were considered to be eternal truths. Those with inquisitive minds were hampered in testing alternative hypotheses by a lack of instruments and by convention that frowned upon such ventures. Armchair philosophers of the time believed general principles to be self-evident and not in need of empirical testing and observation.

In contrast, scientific theory deals with the empirical world we know directly through our senses, or through inventions that extend our senses, such as the sphygmomanometer or the microscope. Scientific theory is the symbolic dimension of our experiences and observations, a mental invention that systematically orders the things we observe. If the theory is a fruitful one, we can derive statements (propositions, hypotheses) that predict from the theory, and we can then test the predictions in research. However, the theory itself cannot be proved. All theories are tentative: they tentatively explain what we *have* observed in research, and these explanations can be used to predict what we *will* observe in research. Thus, research, observation, and theory are intimately related to one another.

Nursing Theory and Theory in Nursing. There are several views about the construction and use of theory in nursing. One view is that of Mathwig (1971), who believes the theoretical knowledge of nursing must evolve from nursing and nursing alone. She seems to reject the idea of using theory developed in other disciplines. The problem with this approach is that knowledge unique to nursing and nursing alone may be difficult to find, and should such a unique body of knowledge develop, nursing may find it difficult to communicate its meaning to other health disciplines (Stevens, 1979, p. 9).

Johnson (1968), Henderson (1978, p. 22), and others suggest that it is hazardous to attempt to differentiate between borrowed and unique theory, because knowledge does not belong innately to any field of science; thus, what is borrowed and what is unique has no permanence or real meaning.

A view that integrates in some measure both of these views is that of Wald and Leonard (1964), most recently adopted by Diers (1979). This view suggests that the development of *nursing practice theory* is distinct from the theory of practice in any other health field. However, theory and research from other disciplines are readily used, although Diers (p. 65) suggests that a careful evaluation is necessary to fit theory to the problems at hand. Relying heavily on the ideas generated by philosophers Dickoff and James (1968), Diers defines a *theory* as a mental invention whose purpose is to describe, explain, predict, or prescribe (Diers, 1979, p. 69). She examines four levels of theoretical inquiry: 1) naming theory; 2) theory that suggests the connection among concepts; 3) theory that explains and predicts; and 4) theory that both states the goals to be achieved in nursing practice and prescribes activities to achieve the goals (Diers, 1979, chap. 2).

The construction of nursing theories often begins with observations and inductive reasoning, while the testing of theories begins with theory or assumptions and deduces hypotheses to be tested. Induction and deduction alternate in the development and testing of theory. Each of these will be examined.

Inductive Reasoning: Constructing Nursing Theory from Observation. Inductive reasoning is the means by which we explain the things we have observed. It begins with specific observations and moves to construct a general explanation or theory. The first step in the inductive process is to collect data that is significant to the nursing problem under investigation. The second step is to summarize the collected data, using scales, measurements, graphs, and tables. The third step is to synthesize the summarized data into a single statement or observation—the empirical generalization—that states a proposed relationship between concepts. The fourth step is to use the relationships expressed to initiate, reformulate, or clarify theory.

The proposed steps are fluid rather than fixed: the researcher tends to move back and forth between inductive and deductive reasoning, testing and probing as necessary, seldom moving in a straight line. The inductive process may be illustrated with an example that will help clarify the steps usually taken.

As nurses in practice, we may have observed that a number of persons in the local area are committing suicide. Therefore, we wish to observe and study the phenomenon scientifically in order to arrive at an explanation of suicide that will enable us to intervene in the process. We may begin by reading the literature, paying particular attention to a classic nineteenth-century European study of suicide from which we take the definition of *suicide* as "cases of death resulting directly or indirectly from a positive or negative act of the victim himself, which he knows will produce this result" (Durkheim, trans. 1951, p. 44).

Next, we must decide which data about suicide we should collect—work data, personal data, family data, or other. And we must decide how to collect the data. We decide to collect data about the characteristics of the persons who commit suicide—the sex, religion, occupation, and marital status—using a broad review of all of the official documents available.

Once we collect the data, we summarize the observations. We count the frequency of suicide by category, such as sex and religion, summarizing the data in tables or graphs. In analyzing the summaries, we find that certain categories of persons in the population—males of the Protestant faith—are committing suicide with greater frequency than others. We can now make a statement, the empirical generalization, that summarizes the uniformities between two or more variables: Protestant males commit suicide more frequently than others in the population; that is, suicide varies by sex and religion. From such an empirical generalization, inductively reached, we may now use deduction (reasoning from a *premise* rather than from observations) to formulate a working hypothesis that predicts future findings: if one is a Protestant male, then he is in a population at risk for suicide. Induction and deduction alternate in the process of rational thought. Once we state the hypothesis, we may collect further data to test the hypothesis or to develop another empirical generalization.

Yet, we still cannot explain why male Protestants kill themselves more often than others in the population. At this point, the creative ability of the mind enters the process. Drawing on material in the literature, we may attempt a biological explanation: it is the genetic endowment of the individual that explains suicide; that is, males are more susceptible to suicide because of a genetic disposition toward depression that leads to suicide. Or, we may develop a psychological explanation: males committing suicide have a death wish. However, these explanations do not account for the variable of religion. Why are Protestants committing suicide more frequently than Catholics or Jews? To deal with all the variables, we need a social explanation that relates the value system of Protestantism, internalized by males of the faith, with a later vulnerability to commit suicide. Reared to be self-reliant and independent of his family and other primary groups, the Protestant male cannot depend upon the group to sustain him during periods of deep, unrelieved anxiety and distress. Therefore, he is at risk to commit suicide because of his individualistic approach to life. We invent a new concept, "individualism," or "egoism," to stand for the constellation of observations and ideas that arise. Personal disorganization in individuals who are egoistic or individualistic, and thus not strongly integrated into a primary group, may lead to suicide (Durkheim, 1951). We ponder such explanations, explore possibilities of others, and search for ways to test the explanation in research. Theories close to observed data and empirical generalizations, such as the theory above, are called *theories of the middle-range* to distinguish them from *grand theories* that intend to explain universal relationships (such as Einstein's theory of relativity). Middle-range theories (Merton, 1968) are used by the newer sciences, such as sociology and nursing, and deal with *delimited* aspects of phenomena. Since nurses are close to observations of health and disease in daily practice, they may find the inductive method useful to explain carefully delimited aspects of nursing. It is less formidable a task to look for observed regularities between two or more variables, and to build a number of empirical generalizations from which nursing concepts and theory may be developed, than to hope for the creative leap that will produce a grand theory of nursing, explaining all the facts observed in nursing.

The steps in the scientific inquiry may appear to be distinct but in actual fact may shade into one another, making it difficult to tell exactly when observations become empirical generalization and when empirical generalizations become theory (Wallace, 1969, p. vii). As we examine the deductive process that creates hypotheses for testing, we should note that it is likewise difficult to ascertain when theories become propositions, when propositions become hypotheses, and when hypotheses become observations.

Deductive Reasoning: Creating Propositions to Test Explanations and Predictions. Deductive reasoning commonly begins with a theory, or general premise, and moves toward specific observations: it explains and predicts the data we will observe. Deduction is the method used to convert theory into interrelated propositions and hypotheses that can be tested by observations. A simple example will illustrate the system.

First, a theoretical statement—called the *premise, proposition, postulate,* or *axiom*—is formulated or found in the literature. For example, a broad statement held to be true is, "All living things eventually die." This is a major premise. A second proposition, the minor premise, now states, "Man is a living thing." From proposition one and proposition two, a third proposition is deduced: "Therefore, all men must die." Put together in a system, the propositions are seen to be interrelated and to descend from the general proposition or premise to a specific proposition.

1. All living things eventually die.
2. Man is a living thing.
3. Therefore, all men must die.

Such a syllogism, or system of deductive reasoning, produces an hypothesis that we may test: if one is human, then one must die. We may test this hypothesis in several ways. For example, we can observe to see if humans do indeed die. Since we, too, are human, such direct observations are limited in time and space. To extend our observations, we can use other research methods to collect data. We can interview other persons directly or by questionnaire indirectly, to determine if they have observed humans die. Or, we can draw a random sample from a population of humans, to see retrospectively which persons have died in the past, when, where, and of what. If the observations include even one person who has lived for centuries and appears to be immortal, then the theory must be revised to account for this fact. Thus, deductive reasoning begins with a theory and develops a system of interrelated propositions or hypotheses that predict what will be observed. These hypotheses may be tested by using scientific research methods.

Hypotheses: Statements Constructed for
Prediction and Testing

Hypotheses are statements that predict a relationship between two or more variables. Hypotheses are forward looking, guiding the researcher in collecting and analyzing data. Sources of hypotheses include theory, assumptions, observations, working experiences, and the literature. The formulation of hypotheses and the definition of its variables come early in the planning phase. Formulation requires painstaking work. Testing hypotheses requires a judgment: Does the data warrant the support of the hypotheses? The sources of hypotheses and the formulation and testing of each hypothesis are now examined.

1. Sources of hypotheses include: 1) theory; 2) assumptions; 3) observations; 4) working experiences; and 5) the literature. To derive hypotheses from theory, we proceed in the classic manner by means of a formal deductive system. However, such systems appear more frequently in the older sciences, which have had a longer period of development than nursing. But, nursing can use these systems to develop hypotheses related to nursing. For example, behavior modification proposes that behavior is a direct function of the environment. Using such a proposition, the student may predict a relationship between rewards and punishments and a change in behavior detrimental to health, such as drug use, cigarette smoking, or poor eating habits. Rottkamp (1976) developed the hypothesis that "spinal cord–injured patients with impairment in body-positioning behaviors who receive an intervention that incorporates behavior-modification techniques. . .will improve in their body-positioning performance to a measurable degree. . . ."

To derive hypotheses from assumptions, the researcher first states the assumption and then predicts what will be found in research. For example, Robischon (1977) became interested in pica, the habitual ingestion of nonedible substances, because she was concerned over the poisoning of children from eating lead paint. She believed hand-to-mouth behavior associated with eating in general was related to development. Her assumptions included the following: child development proceeds as an integrated system in interaction with the environment; development proceeds in orderly, patterned, identifiable and measurable sequences. Based on these assumptions, Robischon's hypothesis was: children who practice pica have a lower developmental level than children who do not exhibit these behaviors.

To derive hypotheses from observation, the researcher makes a statement about the relationships between the observed regularities, that is, the facts or concepts, called the *empirical generalization*. From this statement, then, the researcher deduces an hypothesis. For example, Alderson (1974) observed that patients who had high fevers seemed to experience time differently, and thought that a possible relationship existed between the concepts *high fever* and *perception of time*. To predict a relationship, Alderson derived the following hypothesis: if body temperature rises a specified number of degrees above normal, then the patient will experience time differently.

Deriving hypotheses from working experiences is similar to the process described for observation. Such hypotheses that arise during the experiences and observations of everyday life are called *working hypotheses*, or predictions that lie close to observed data (Conant, 1947, p. 137). As the nurse encounters certain facts or observations in the course of nursing practice, the nurse thinks of alternative explanations which she or he then tests. For example, if a nurse sees a patient with hypertension collapse on the floor, some explanations flash through the nurse's mind: the patient has had a cerebral accident; the patient has had a heart attack. To test these working hypotheses, the nurse observes signs and, if possible, questions the patient. If the first hypothesis seems wrong, the nurse may test others in rapid succession. A *nursing diagnosis* is defined as a statement of the probable relationships between an identified negative health behavior and the factors contributing to its occurrence (Brill and Kilts, 1980, p. 154). It is a predictive state that refers to a possible relationship between factors. Such working hypotheses must be tested in research.

To derive hypotheses from the literature, the student may begin with any of the points above: the theory stated in research reports, the assumptions, or the documented observations and working experiences.

2. *Formulation of hypotheses requires the student first to identify what relationship she or he is predicting.* For example, a nurse familiar with Alderson's (1974) work on the relationship between high fever and the perception of the passage of time may wonder if homebound patients with fevers who take their own medication can accurately perceive the passage of time in order to take medication on schedule. To state the relationship, the nurse must link the abstract idea of perception to the actual fact of taking medications on time. In addition, the nurse must predict what he or she expects to find in research and define the variables in such a manner that each is observable and measurable: if a patient's temperature rises three degrees above normal, then the patient will take medications off schedule. Once the initial statement is written, the student must ask the following questions to judge its usefulness: Is

the statement concise and unambiguous? Are the concepts and variables stated in a clear and specific manner? Do the variables refer to data that are observable and measurable? Do instruments exist to measure the variables, or can the variables be easily developed and tested? Are the sources from which the hypothesis was formulated clearly identified and stated? Careful work, self-criticism, and assistance from experts are essential in the development of the art and science of hypothesis formulation.

3. *In many ways, testing hypotheses is similar to a trial by a jury.* The jury is comprised of ourselves and our fellow scientists, who examine all aspects of the research, beginning with the research hypothesis and including a scrutiny of research design, sampling methods, research methods, and data analysis. In cases where the hypothesis and findings can be expressed and analyzed in quantitative form, statistical tests are likewise helpful.

The research hypothesis is formulated to test either for association or causality. Establishing causality is a difficult task when the research involves the complex behavior of persons, because causal factors are often multiplex rather than single. Associations, or correlations, indicate how specified factors occur or vary together: as one increases the other may increase (positive correlation), or as one increases the other may decrease (negative correlation). For example, Olgas (1974) was interested in the association between the health status of a parent and the way the children perceive their own bodies. She sought to predict whether children of handicapped parents have a different body image than do children of nonhandicapped parents: Is there an association between the body image of the child and the health status of the parent, whether handicapped or not? In such cases, the difficulty of establishing causality is obvious—many factors contribute to the body image of a child. But, if it can be demonstrated that the body image of a child is associated with the handicap of the parent, nursing intervention may be considered on the basis of this information.

Causal hypotheses state that the cause X must occur in time before the effect Y. The experiment that includes before and after tests, as well as an experimental and a control group, is the most effective method for establishing a cause–effect relationship. For example, Van Ort and Gerber (1976) hypothesized that the topical application of insulin (the cause) would cause decubitus ulcers to heal faster (the effect). However, to test this hypothesis, two groups of patients who are alike in every way (sex, age, race, diagnosis, kind of decubitus ulcer) would have to be tested. One group would receive topical applications of insulin while one would not. If the experimental group who received the insulin healed faster than the group who did not receive the insulin, the insulin may be said to have "caused" faster healing. However, other variables may have intervened. The genetic factor may have influenced the results, or undetected factors may have been responsible. For example, what causes the toxic shock syndrome? Tampons have been implicated, but a cause–effect relationship has not been established beyond doubt.

Concepts

Concepts are the words or symbols that stand for the mental images we form from reality. Concepts get their precise meaning from the formal definitions assigned by scholars and scientists in a particular field. Unfortunately, the definitions of terms and concepts may differ among scholars, and meanings may change over time. When disparities in definition exist, the researcher must be careful to clarify precisely how to define the concept, noting the scholarly sources. *Nursing care* is one of the oldest concepts of nursing, used by Nightingale and many scholars since that time. *Patient-centered care* was suggested nearly two decades ago (Abdellah and Levine, 1965, p. 84), while *self-care* is even older (Orem, 1959).

Nursing diagnosis is a concept that has undergone considerable change (Gordon, 1979). Currently accepted diagnostic nomenclature has thirty-seven concepts, including *anxiety, comfort, coping, fear, grieving, spirituality,* and *verbal communication* (Gebbie, 1976). Concepts exist at varying levels of abstraction. They may be close to observations, such as *verbal communication,* or highly abstract and removed, such as *spirituality.*

To transform an abstract, unobservable concept into a measurable, observable variable, an operational definition is used. An *operational definition* is a step-by-step set of directions that specify what the researcher must do, in order to observe and measure the concept under study. The first step is to clearly define the concept; the second step is to describe the procedures by which the concept is converted into an observable and measurable variable. Operational definitions are constructed before data are collected (see Chapter 10, "Research Methods").

Variables

Variables are concepts that have been defined by operational definition in such a way that changes or variations can be observed and measured. Variables are classified in several ways: independent variables; dependent variables; extraneous variables; and attribute variables.

An *independent variable,* also called the *experimental, causal, stimulus,* or *treatment variable,* is manipulated by the researcher to study its effect upon the dependent variable. Manipulation refers to the fact that the researcher does something with the independent variable. If the independent variable is a nursing treatment, the researcher manipulates it by giving it to some study subjects and withholding it from others.

The *dependent variable*, also called the *effect*, the *response*, and at times, the *criterion measure*, is the behavior or outcome the researcher wishes to predict and explain. The change in the dependent variable is presumed to be caused or associated with the independent variable. Lindeman and Van Aernam (1977) were interested in the effect of preoperative teaching (the independent variable) on the length of stay and the need for analgesics in the postoperative patient (the dependent variables). They wanted to predict or explain what caused one patient to need less analgesics and to stay in the hospital fewer days. Did preoperative instruction make a difference?

Extraneous variables are those which are present in large numbers in any research involving human subjects and may interfere with the research findings. Extraneous variables may act as unwanted independent variables and confuse the results of the research. Common extraneous variables are attribute variables.

Attribute variables are preexisting characteristics of the study subjects, such as education, occupation, income, age, weight, medical diagnosis, or any other characteristic that varies from one individual to another. Such characteristics may be studied themselves as independent variables. For example, race may be studied to see how it is associated with hypertension. However, race becomes an extraneous variable when another factor, such as a drug, is being studied to determine its effect on high blood pressure. Then, the race of the person may be a factor that acts upon the blood pressure and confuses whether the drug caused the effect or not.

Assumptions, Paradigms, and Models

Assumptions are basic principles assumed to be true. They are statements whose correctness or validity is taken for granted (Abdellah and Levine, 1965, p. 698). At times, a number of assumptions are used to deduce hypotheses in the absence of formal deductive systems. Researchers are forced to make assumptions when the state of knowledge does not allow them to prove or disprove certain statements. Assumptions are found in a number of research studies, and these studies are helpful in identifying sound assumptions.

Paradigms bring assumptions into the open, along with the concepts employed in a study. Paradigms include theory, applications, and instrumentation used in a study (Kuhn, 1964, p. 10). Paradigms not only define what is to be studied, but how. Natural sciences, such as biology, have the paradigm, evolution, upon which most agree. However, the social and behavioral sciences have many competing paradigms. Nursing uses the paradigms of other sciences when these are helpful, modifying each for use in the nursing milieu.

A *model* is the symbolic or physical representation of an abstract idea, an analogy of the actual phenomenon. For example, physical models include lifelike constructions, such as the model ship, abstract physical representations such as the DNA model, or abstract diagrams and blueprints. Conceptual models for nursing practice include the Peplau model, the Orem self-care model, the Roy adaptation model, and many others (Riehl and Roy, 1980).

SUMMARY

The identification and definition of basic terms in research is a necessary component for all professional nurses who wish to undertake a research project of their own or to read the research publication in nursing with understanding.

The interrelations among some of the basic terms in research may be shown in a model that includes the elements of research—*theories, propositions,* and *facts*—and the methods of reasoning—*induction* or *deduction*—that lead to constructing and testing theories.

Hypotheses are propositions formulated to predict a relationship between two or more variables that can be tested in research. Sources of hypotheses include theory, assumptions, observation, working experiences, and the literature. The formulation of hypotheses is a precise task that requires careful, critical work from the researcher. Testing hypotheses is done by collecting and analyzing data, either for causality, a difficult task if human subjects are used, or for correlation, which indicates how factors vary. *Concepts* are the words or symbols that stand for the mental images we form from reality. Nursing concepts include nursing care and many other ideas at varying levels of complexity. To transform an abstract concept into an observable, measurable variable, an operational definition is used.

An *operational definition* is a step-by-step set of directions that specify what the researcher must do in order to observe and measure the concept under study. The operational definition enables scientists to test or replicate the work of one another, and to specify precisely what they intend to observe and measure during the data-collection phase.

Variables are concepts that have been defined by operational definition in such a way that changes or variations can be observed and measured. Variables include the *independent variable;* the *dependent variable;* the *extraneous variable;* and the *attribute variable.* The independent variable is that manipulated by the researcher to study its effect on the dependent variable. The independent variable is also known as the *experimental, causal, stimulus,* or *treatment variable,* while the dependent variable is known as that which is affected by or responds to the independent variable. The change in behavior or outcome in the dependent variable that the researcher hopes to explain or predict is presumed to be caused by or associated with the independent variable. Extraneous variables are present in large numbers and may interfere with the action of the independent variable or be mistaken for its action. Attribute variables are characteristics of the study subjects, such as age, race, or medical diagnosis, that pre-exist and may act as extraneous variables.

Assumptions are basic principles often documented in the literature and assumed to be true, although not proven. *Paradigms* bring assumptions into the open, and include theory, applications, and instrumentation used in a study. Nursing uses the paradigms of both the natural and social sciences, modifying them for use in the nursing milieu. *Models* are physical or symbolic representations of abstract ideas. Conceptual models for nursing practice include those of Peplau, Orem, Roy, and many others.

STUDY QUESTIONS

1. Draw a diagram that shows the relationships between theory, propositions, and facts. What is the place of research in this model?
2. Find an article in *Nursing Research* or in another research journal. Does the author refer to a theory or a set of assumptions? Are concepts defined? Are operational definitions used? Does the researcher seek to establish and define correlation or causality? What nursing concepts can you identify? Does the researcher begin with observations or theory? Are hypotheses stated? Is inductive or deductive reasoning used?
3. Think of an observation you have made in the course of nursing practice. Can you identify one or two concepts associated with the observation?
4. List all the new terms you have encountered in this chapter and define each.
5. Describe how observation and reasoning function to formulate or test theory.
6. Write an operational definition of some aspect of nursing care that you would like to study. What factors make it measurable and observable?

7. A paradigm upon which biology is based is that of evolution. Two concepts used in the paradigm are adaptation and natural selection. Applications include investigating how people adapt to the environment. Can you use such a paradigm in nursing to explain how disease, environment, and nursing relate to each other? Can research assist in gathering data to answer this question?

8. In nursing practice, you notice that seriously ill patients tend to respond to nurses' touching them. Formulate an hypothesis that predicts the effect of touching on a seriously ill patient.

9. Edward Jenner (1897) observed that dairy maids generally had good complexions, seldom showing the pock marks of those who survived small pox. Summarize Jenner's observations into an empirical generalization. Write an hypothesis deduced from the empirical generalization. How could the hypothesis be tested?

REFERENCES AND SUGGESTED READING

Abdellah, F. and Levine, E. (1965): Better Patient Care Through Nursing Research. New York: Macmillan, chap. 5.

Alderson, M. (1974): Effects of increased body temperature on the perception of time. *Nursing Research 23. Clinical study of perception.*

Brill, E. and Kilts, D. (1980): Foundations for Nursing. New York: Appleton. *Textbook.*

Charter, S. (1975): Understanding Research in Nursing. Geneva: W.H.O. Offset Pub. No. 14. *Relationship between concepts and principles is discussed.*

Coleman, L. (1980): Oren's self-care concept of nursing. In Riehl, J. and Roy, C., Conceptual Models for Nursing Practice (2nd ed.). New York: Appleton, pp. 315–328. *Oren's self-care concept summarized and applied.*

Code for Nurses (1977): *American Journal of Nursing,* 2581–2585. *Standards of practice.*

Conant, J. (1947): On Understanding Science. New Haven: Yale University Press. *Definition of working hypothesis.*

Dickoff, J. and James, P. (1968): Researching research's role in theory development. *Nursing Research 17,* 204–206.

Diers, D. (1979): Research in Nursing Practice. New York: J. B. Lippincott. *Clinical research emphasized.*

Downs, F. (1967): Ethical inquiry in nursing research. *Nursing Forum 6,* 12–20. *The problem of ethics in research is discussed.*

Downs, F. and Newman, M. (eds.) (1977): A Sourcebook of Nursing Research (2nd ed.). Philadelphia: F. A. Davis. *Eight nursing studies evaluate nursing intervention; seven explore indices of health.*

Downs, F. and Fleming, J. (eds.) (1979): Issues in Nursing Research. New York: Appleton. *Seven articles; trends, issues and future of nursing research are discussed.*

Durkheim, E. (1951): Suicide. Spaulding and Simpson (Trans.). Glencoe, Ill.: The Free Press. *A classic study in research.*

Gebbie, K. (1976): Summary of the Second National Conference on Classification of Nursing Diagnoses. St. Louis: St. Louis University. *Currently accepted diagnostic nomenclature is discussed.*

Goode, W. and Hatt, P. (1952): Methods in Social Research. New York: McGraw-Hill. *Chapters 3–7 deal with science, values, concepts, and hypotheses.*

Gordon, M. (1979): The concept of nursing diagnosis. In The Nursing Clinics of North America. Philadelphia: W. B. Saunders. *Conceptualization of nursing diagnosis is discussed.*

Hardy, M. (ed.) (1973): Theoretical Foundations for Nursing. New York: MSS Information Corp. *Theories and concepts, including stress, crises, adaptation, and general systems theory.*

Johnson, D. (1968): Theory in nursing: borrowed and unique. In *Nursing Research 17. Johnson discusses theory, noting that knowledge does not belong to any field of science exclusively.*

Kuhn, T. (1962): The Structure of Scientific Revolutions. Chicago: University of Chicago Press. *Discusses how scientific knowledge accrues and changes.*

Lindeman, C. and Van Aernam, B. (1971): Nursing intervention with the presurgical patient—the effects of structured and unstructured preoperative teaching. In Downs, F. and Newman, M., A Sourcebook of Nursing Research (2nd ed.). (1977): Philadelphia: F. A. Davis, pp. 45–63. *Clinical study reported.*

Mathwig, G. (1970): Nursing science—the theoretical core of nursing knowledge. *Image, 4, 20–23. Presents the view that nursing theory should evolve from nursing rather than from other disciplines.*

McCorkle, R. (1981): Effects of touch on seriously ill patients. In Fox, D., Readings on the Research Process in Nursing. New York: Appleton, pp. 114–125. *Clinical study; defines touch.*

Merton, R. (1968): Social Theory and Social Structure. New York: The Free Press. *Part I discusses theories of the middle range.*

Olgas, M. (1974): Relationship between parents' health status and body image of their children. *Nursing Research 23, 319–324. Olgas predicts a relationship between parents' health status and body image of child.*

Orem, D. (1971): Nursing: Concepts of Practice. New York: McGraw-Hill. *Framework for model of self-care.*

Riehl, J. and Roy, C. (eds.) (1980): Conceptual Models for Nursing Practice (2nd ed.). New York: Appleton. *Includes a number of theoretical models for nursing practice, such as Peplau, Neuman, Roy, Johnson, and Orem.*

Robischon, P. (1971): Pica practice and other hand-mouth behavior and children's developmental level. In Downs, F. and Newman, M. (eds.), A Sourcebook of Nursing Research (2nd ed.). Philadelphia: F. A. Davis. *States assumptions.*

Rottkamp, B. (1981): A behavior modification approach to nursing therapeutics in body positioning of spinal-cord-injured patients. In Fox, D., Readings on the Research Process in Nursing. New York: Appleton, pp. 107–113. *Develops hypothesis for her research study.*

Stevens, B. (1979): Nursing Theory: Analysis, Application, Evaluation. Boston: Little, Brown. *Specific theorists examined to familiarize reader with nursing theory.*

Van Ort, S. and Gerber, R. (1976): Topical application of insulin in the treatment of decubitus ulcers. *Nursing Research 25,* 9–12. *Suggests causality.*

Wald, F. and Leonard, R. (1964): Toward development of nursing practice theory. *Nursing Research 13,* 309–313. *Discusses the development of theory in practice.*

Wallace, W. (1969): The Logic of Science in Sociology. Chicago: Aldine. *Brief book examines theories, empirical generalizations, hypotheses, and observations; emphasizes their interrelations.*

CHAPTER 3

PHASES AND STEPS IN THE RESEARCH PROCESS

The student who seeks to initiate a research project for the first time often wonders where to begin. This chapter provides a simple model to help answer that question (see Figure 3–1). The model is a calendar wheel, a diagram of the phases and steps of research placed in a temporal framework. However, the particular time framework of each project must be individually determined. The circular design of the model suggests the unending process of research: the communication of research findings that concludes one project provides the springboard for further research.

Upon completion of this chapter, the student should be able to: 1) depict and explain a model of the phases and steps of the research process; 2) state briefly what occurs in each phase and step; 3) identify chapters in this book that deal with each step; and 4) construct a model that includes the time framework of his or her own research.

THE MODEL

The model provides at a glance the phases of the research project. The student should understand the model for several reasons: 1) to gain an overview of the project from beginning to end; 2) to learn to prepare a timetable that allocates the time reasonably spent at each phase; 3) to

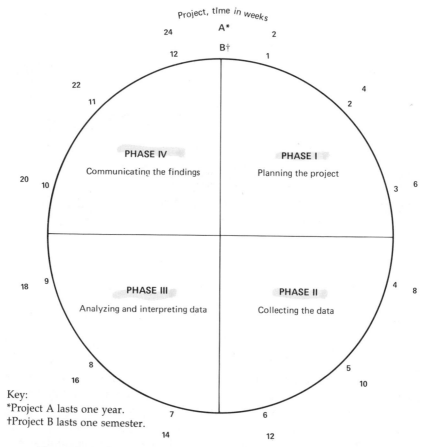

Figure 3–1. Calendar Wheel: Four phases of the research process in a temporal framework.

anticipate what must be done in early steps in order to be prepared for later ones; 4) to examine the research literature more effectively by comparing the research reports of others; 5) to write a rough draft of the research paper step-by-step by documenting the work in each phase of the model. In addition, the model provides a guide to the organization of this book—reference to pertinent chapters is made at each step.

As each phase is discussed, the steps within individual phases of the model are added. However, every research project is unique. The sequence and number of steps within each phase and the time spent at each step may vary according to the individual research project. But the four phases of research remain stable. The student always begins with Phase I, planning. Then, in Phase II, the student collects the data and, in Phase III, the student describes, analyzes, and interprets it. Finally, in Phase IV, the student presents findings in written or oral form, communicating the results of the research.

The student must carefully calculate the time to be spent in each of the phases. A project to be completed in one year or in one semester requires a rigorous division of the time available. Phases of approximately six weeks each (three weeks for semester projects) may be realistic, but this depends upon whether the study is descriptive or explanatory. Descriptive studies may require more time for collecting data, while explanatory projects may require more time for planning. However, both of these phases must come to an end in time to analyze and interpret the data, and to write (and rewrite) the research report. Projects that take place in the summer or have longer periods for the research require their own timetable. Using the model as a guide, each researcher should construct a calendar wheel and check off each step as it is completed and documented. Each of the four phases and the steps that usually occur in each phase will now be examined briefly. Later chapters will explore each of the steps in greater detail.

PHASE I: PLANNING THE
RESEARCH PROJECT

During Phase I, the student completes most if not all of the following steps: 1) identify a researchable problem; 2) formulate the research proposal; 3) define concepts and variables; 4) state objectives or hypotheses; 5) examine possible ethical implications of the research proposal; 6) review pertinent literature; 7) identify theory, assumptions, and limitations of the proposal; 8) describe the research design; 9) describe the methods of research, including sampling, data collection, instruments to be used, and method of data analysis; 10) obtain informed consent from subjects to be studied in the pilot study; 11) conduct pilot study and revise proposal in the light of findings; and 12) plan how to communicate findings (see Figure 3–2). Each of these steps will now be examined.

Step 1. Identify a Researchable
Problem in Nursing

The first step is to select an area of interest to the student and importance to nursing, and then to delimit this to a specific circumscribed problem that is researchable and identifies exactly what the student plans to study (see Chapter 4). The student who is uncertain about what to do, or would like to replicate a good study if possible, may begin

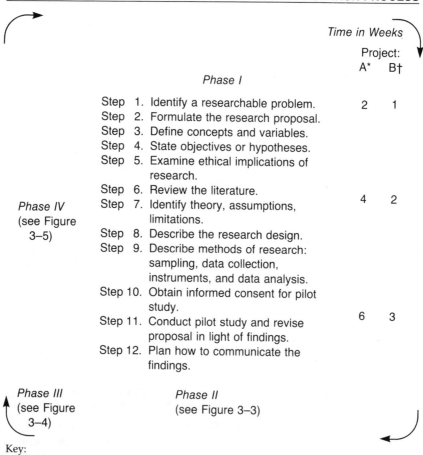

Time in Weeks

Project:

A*   B†

Phase I

		A*	B†
Step 1.	Identify a researchable problem.	2	1
Step 2.	Formulate the research proposal.		
Step 3.	Define concepts and variables.		
Step 4.	State objectives or hypotheses.		
Step 5.	Examine ethical implications of research.		
Step 6.	Review the literature.	4	2
Step 7.	Identify theory, assumptions, limitations.		
Step 8.	Describe the research design.		
Step 9.	Describe methods of research: sampling, data collection, instruments, and data analysis.		
Step 10.	Obtain informed consent for pilot study.		
Step 11.	Conduct pilot study and revise proposal in light of findings.	6	3
Step 12.	Plan how to communicate the findings.		

Phase IV
(see Figure
3–5)

Phase III
(see Figure
3–4)

Phase II
(see Figure 3–3)

Key:
*Project A lasts one year.
†Project B lasts one semester.

Figure 3–2. Phase I: Steps in planning the research project.

immediately with an initial review of the literature. Good research reports state the general importance of the study early in the report and follow this immediately with a statement of the specific problem that was studied. For example, in her report of maternal stress and neonatal pathology, Downs (1977) states in the opening paragraph why the study is important for nursing: the former steep decline in perinatal mortality has decreased, and nursing needs to study factors such as stress that may contribute to this undesirable state. Johnson (1975) identifies a potential nursing problem: pulmonary complications following general anesthesia. She then specifies what she plans to study: the outcome criteria that evaluate respiratory function during the postoperative period. Such studies formulate and delimit a significant research problem, narrowing the general question down to a manageable form.

Step 2. Formulate the Research Proposal

The research proposal is a written summary of steps one through nine, stating what the student intends to do, how he or she plans to do it, who or what comprises the study sample, when and where the study is to be done, and the timetable for the study. The proposal is often written for the approval of a professor or committee, but it assists the student as well. The proposal begins with the identification of the problem and moves step-by-step through all elements of the planning stage, which are pretested in the pilot project. As the student moves through the steps, the research proposal is often written and rewritten many times to refine the proposal (see Chap. 4). The final writing is usually done after the pilot study, when changes may be incorporated in the light of weaknesses and strengths identified at that time.

Step 3. Define the Concepts and Variables

The student must define each concept or variable early in the study, not only to understand what is to be examined but to communicate this information to others. This is not always an easy task. Bloch (1974) expresses her frustration in the search for definitions, coming face to face with a "semantic jungle." Where definitions are confused, the student must spend time to define and communicate with clarity the meaning of each concept. In particular, operational definitions require careful work, as these describe how the variable under study is to be observed and measured. Definitions found in the literature that have already been developed and tested in research should be used whenever possible.

Step 4. State Objectives or Hypotheses

Objectives are what the student proposes to accomplish in the research, the specific short-term measurable goals to be met. For example, a specific objective may be to describe a phenomenon such as child abuse. The student may plan to develop, or find in the literature, an operational definition that defines how to observe and measure child abuse. At the conclusion of the study, both the reader and the researcher can determine whether the objectives of the study were met.

Hypotheses are statements formulated to predict a relationship between two or more variables. The student who has defined a researchable problem and formulated the research proposal has identified a relationship between nursing concepts or variables to be tested in research. For example, Schmitt and Wooldridge (1981) tested the hypothesis that extra preparation for surgery would decrease the stress and anxiety of patients and would lead to a more rapid postoperative recovery. McCorkle (1981) predicted that "touching and verbally stimulating a seriously ill patient [would] produce an increase in the number of positive acceptance responses." The student who wishes to use an hypothesis may examine the literature to find a similar study whose hypothesis is stated and whose variables are defined.

Step 5. Examine the Ethical Implications of the Research

At this point, the student is wise to examine the ethical implications of the study. Should the research proposal deal with problems too complex to solve in the time available, it is possible to modify the research proposal without losing too much time and effort. An ethical study is one that does not harm the study subjects. All subjects are carefully informed concerning the following: the purpose of the study; their part in it; any possible discomfort; how privacy will be guarded; their right to refuse to participate or to stop participating without penalty; and the manner in which data will be used. The student must also gain the approval of committees that investigate studies using human subjects, and must receive the written informed consent of each study subject (see Chapter 5).

Step 6. Review the Literature

An initial review of the research publications often takes place early in the project, as soon as the general area of interest is defined. Such an early review helps identify a researchable problem and formulate the research proposal. However, the initial review must be followed by a more critical review that concentrates on the strengths and weaknesses of each study (see Chapter 6). The review should be as complete as time allows. The student should examine definitions of concepts, objectives, and hypotheses; identify competing theoretical frameworks and research studies that support or refute these; and compare research designs. The student should also examine how the sample for study was selected, how the data were collected, and what instruments and methods of data analysis were used. The student may find a study to replicate, or a well written study to use as a guide.

Step 7. Identify Theory, Assumptions, and Limitations

All research benefits from a clear statement of the theory or assumptions to which the research proposal is related. The goal of all research is to provide scientific explanations for what is observed, and to predict what will be observed under given circumstances. Nursing has drawn on a broad range of theories from the natural, behavioral, and social sciences. Currently, nurses are seeking to produce theory peculiar to nursing practice (see Chapter 7). Theories of stress, behavior, transcultural nursing, learning, development, and systems are often found in basic nursing textbooks. Research articles usually specify the theory or assumptions upon which the study is based. *Limitations* are aspects of the research that were not studied. For example, a study of the behavior of hospitalized children may be limited to a particular age group or to those children having a common diagnosis. The student may summarize the use of theory, assumptions and limitations as he or she examines the research literature.

Step 8. Describe the Selected Research Design

Research designs include the experiment, the survey, and the documentary design (see Chapter 9). An experiment often examines how a treatment or stimulus (the independent variable) affects subjects exposed to the treatment (the dependent variable). The experimental design describes, step-by-step, how the research will be conducted. Crucial elements of the experiment include how the research subjects are selected and how controls are used (see Chapter 8). A survey is a research design that uses questionnaires and interviews. Important elements of the survey include not only how the subjects are selected, but also their willingness to answer the questionnaire or interview. The number of returns from a questionnaire and the ability of the respondent to answer the questions determine the extent to which the design is successful. The proper development of the questionnaire form and interview schedule are also crucial.

The documentary design uses material already in existence, such as public and private records. Getting access to the material, finding records that are complete and legible, and discovering whether or not the writer recorded material accurately are important.

Other research designs include "field studies," in which the researcher investigates the phenomenon in its natural setting. The researcher may live and work on the site, collecting data in a community, mental hospital, or health clinic. The descriptive case-study design centers upon an in-depth investigation of one unit—a patient, a disease, a group, or an institution.

The student selects the research design that is ethically appropriate and describes the design carefully, using a step-by-step plan to act as a guide.

Step 9. Describe the Research Methods

The methods of sampling, data collection, and analysis and interpretation are the heart of every research project. *Sampling* is the selection of study subjects from the target population under study (see Chapter 8). Precise methods must be used to be able to apply research findings from a small sample to the population from which it was drawn.

Methods of data collection include observing, questioning, and measuring, or a combination of these (see Chapters 10, 11, and 12). Observation is a basic method of collecting data. When the phenomenon under study cannot be observed, the researcher asks questions, either face-to-face in an interview or by using questionnaires. *Measuring* is the set of rules that assign numbers or values to objects to represent the variation of some attribute. For example, to measure weight, the rules designate that the object be placed on a scale that records pounds, ounces, or grams. To measure height, other rules are used. To measure attitudes, quality of patient care, degree of pain, or condition of a patient is more difficult. Qualitative scales have been developed to approximate quantitative measures.

To collect data using a specific method requires careful description of the instrument being used. At times, several methods may be used simultaneously. For example, to measure the effect of touch on seriously ill patients, McCorkle (1974) used observation, questioning, tape recorders, and electrocardiographs. In addition, she developed a special work sheet to record nonverbal responses.

To analyze data, descriptive statistics must be used to summarize findings (see Chapters 12 and 13). If specific sampling techniques are used, inferential statistics are used to infer from the sample to the population from which the sample was drawn (see Chapter 14).

Step 10. Obtain Informed Consent from Study Subjects to be Used in the Pilot Study

As we saw in Step 5 above, *informed consent* is the voluntary consent given by the study subjects, after they are fully informed of every detail of the proposed research, including the rights to participate or not and to withdraw from the study at any time without penalty. Thorough comprehension of the proposed participation is a crucial factor of informed consent (see Chapter 5). Informed consent must be obtained from subjects in both the pilot study and the "real" study. Permission for both may be sought at the same time by using identical forms.

Step 11. Conduct the Pilot Study

The pilot study is a small-scale dress rehearsal that proceeds as if it were the actual study, except for the fact that subjects who will participate in the actual study are not used. However, they may be selected at this point. The primary objective of the pilot study is to test as many elements of the research proposal as possible, in order to correct any part that does not work well. For example, the pilot study tests whether the variables defined by operational definition are actually observable and measurable. Instruments and scales are likewise tested to determine if each actually measures what the researcher intends it to measure. If a questionnaire is used, the pilot study reveals any problems the respondents have with either the instructions or the wording. If an interview schedule is used, the pilot study answers many questions, including the following: Is a proper place available for the interview? How much time is needed to ask all the questions? Is more than one interviewer needed? Are they properly trained? Do the subjects understand the wording of the questions?

The time and effort to conduct a pilot study is well worth it. Pitfalls and errors that may prove costly in the actual study may be identified and avoided.

Step 12. Plan How to Communicate the Research Findings

Although the communication of research findings may seem far away at this point, it is helpful to spend a few hours to consider how the research findings will be communicated. Research reports are often required as a part of course work. The written report and oral presentation may be the first step in reaching a broader audience. The student may wish to investigate the possibility of presenting the paper at a professional meeting or locating a journal that publishes student papers. Whether it is published or not, the well-prepared research paper may be useful to the student to communicate the experience as a researcher to graduate schools or to prospective employees. Careful work in research makes a contribution to the profession, and experience in certain areas of research are reflected in the scientific practice of nursing. Chapter 16 discusses more fully the communication of research.

PHASE II: THE COLLECTION OF DATA

Phase II implements all of the plans made in Phase I to collect the data. If the study subjects have not been selected from the target population, this is the first step, as Figure 3–3 indicates. The second step is to contact the subjects, as well as any agencies involved, to explain the study and obtain their informed consent. The sampling process is a crucial element of the research design. It determines from whom or what the data are

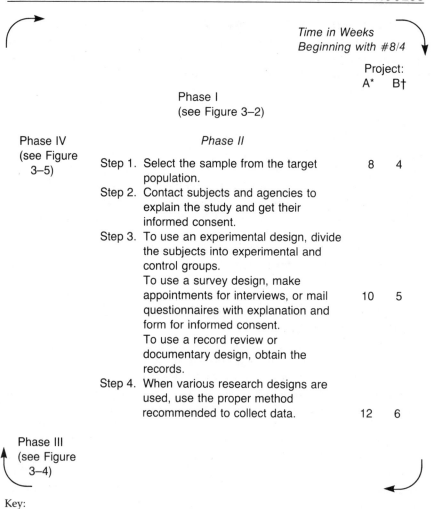

Time in Weeks
Beginning with #8/4

Project:
A* B†

Phase I
(see Figure 3–2)

Phase IV
(see Figure
3–5)

Phase II

	A*	B†
Step 1. Select the sample from the target population.	8	4
Step 2. Contact subjects and agencies to explain the study and get their informed consent.		
Step 3. To use an experimental design, divide the subjects into experimental and control groups.		
To use a survey design, make appointments for interviews, or mail questionnaires with explanation and form for informed consent.	10	5
To use a record review or documentary design, obtain the records.		
Step 4. When various research designs are used, use the proper method recommended to collect data.	12	6

Phase III
(see Figure
3–4)

Key:
*Project A lasts one year.
†Project B lasts one semester.

Figure 3–3. Phase II: Steps in collecting the research data.

to be collected, which in turn influences the method of data analysis that can be used. If sampling uses a process that affords each unit in the target population an equal chance of being chosen for study, then many methods of data analysis may be used. Any other kind of sampling limits the type of analysis but may be useful in descriptive or exploratory studies. The method by which data are collected varies by research design. An experiment observes and measures two groups (experimental and control); the survey involves questioning and measurement; and the record review requires asking questions of data. The student may observe, question, or measure—the most frequently used methods—and he or she may use instruments to help perform these methods. In addition, classification is a means of data collection that may be useful. This method requires that the student develop categories into which observations will fall. For example, if the student is studying high blood pressure, she or he may construct categories such as age, race, sex, residence, and socioeconomic status. A data sheet containing these categories enables the student to fill in the information quickly and efficiently.

Once the data collection phase is finished, or is stopped for practical reasons, the phase of data analysis and interpretation begins.

PHASE III: ANALYZING AND INTERPRETING THE DATA

The task in Phase III is to summarize, analyze, and interpret facts and observations (see Figure 3–4). The first step is to examine raw data for completeness and accuracy. An incomplete or inaccurately completed questionnaire must be discarded. Next, the raw data must be transferred to a general tally table or work sheet, in order to bring categories of data together. The categories may be male/female; categories of ages; or public patients/private patients, depending entirely on what information was collected. The tally marks are then counted, and the counts are summarized. In addition, special purpose tables help summarize data (see Chapter 13).

Rates, ratios, and percentages are used to summarize data such as occupation, marital status, or type of illness. For quantitative data, summary measures such as mean, median, and mode are used. These are descriptive summaries and may be used to compare and interpret data from descriptive or exploratory studies.

If the sample has been drawn randomly, a process that affords each unit in the population an equal chance of being chosen, inferential statistics may be used to analyze data, estimate parameters, and test null hypotheses (see Chapters 14 and 15).

The student examines the research findings and applies these to the research proposal to interpret in the light of objectives or hypotheses. Then the student summarizes the research findings and

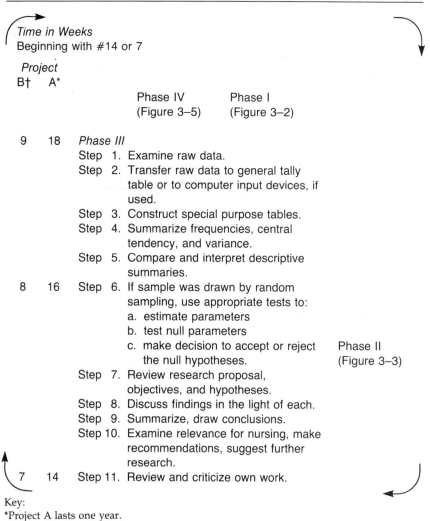

Time in Weeks
Beginning with #14 or 7

Project
B†   A*

		Phase IV (Figure 3–5)	Phase I (Figure 3–2)

9   18   *Phase III*
          Step 1. Examine raw data.
          Step 2. Transfer raw data to general tally
                   table or to computer input devices, if
                   used.
          Step 3. Construct special purpose tables.
          Step 4. Summarize frequencies, central
                   tendency, and variance.
          Step 5. Compare and interpret descriptive
                   summaries.
8   16   Step 6. If sample was drawn by random
                   sampling, use appropriate tests to:
                   a. estimate parameters
                   b. test null parameters
                   c. make decision to accept or reject   Phase II
                      the null hypotheses.   (Figure 3–3)
          Step 7. Review research proposal,
                   objectives, and hypotheses.
          Step 8. Discuss findings in the light of each.
          Step 9. Summarize, draw conclusions.
          Step 10. Examine relevance for nursing, make
                   recommendations, suggest further
                   research.
7   14   Step 11. Review and criticize own work.

Key:
*Project A lasts one year.
†Project B lasts one semester.

Figure 3–4. Phase III: Steps in analyzing and interpreting data.

draws conclusions from the summaries. Next, the student discusses the importance of the research findings for nursing, states recommendations, and makes suggestions for further research. The student should now carefully review and criticize the work, noting any weaknesses that may be corrected by future research.

Time in Weeks

Project		Phase IV
B†	A*	Communicating Findings‡

12	24	Step 1. Select method and means of communications.
		Step 2. Complete tables and graphs in finished form.
		Step 3. Write introduction, including problem statement, definitions, objectives, hypotheses, assumptions, and limitations.
		Step 4. Write review of literature, summarizing polar theories and research findings.
		Step 5. Designate the theoretical framework or findings of previous research to which study is addressed.
		Step 6. Relate theory or former research to problem statement or hypotheses.
		Step 7. Discuss research methods, with particular attention to sampling methods, how instruments were judged to be reliable and valid, and problems.
11	22	Step 8. Present findings.
		Step 9. Relate findings to problem statement and hypotheses.
		Step 10. Summarize research project.
		Step 11. Criticize research project.
		Step 12. Draw conclusions: relation to theory or prior research; relevance for nursing.
		Step 13. Complete bibliography, abstract, and give title to paper.
		Step 14. Submit final draft to colleague for criticism.
		Step 15. Present paper or submit for publication.
10	20	Step 16. Revise and resubmit, if necessary.

Key:
*Project A lasts one year.
†Project B lasts one semester.
‡Please note that Step 1 begins with either Week 20 (year project) or Week 10 (semester). The steps are listed from top to bottom for sake of convenience in reading.

Figure 3–5. Phase IV: Steps in communicating findings of the research project.

PHASE IV: COMMUNICATING THE RESEARCH FINDINGS

The final phase of the research process is the communication of findings. The research report, either written or oral, must communicate each step (see Figure 3–5). It is usually wise to complete tables and graphs, since these aid in the process of communication. The structure of the report may follow Figure 3–5. Chapter 16 is also devoted to writing the research report. The report should be well organized and in enough detail to inform, but at the same time it should be succinct. Whether professors, other scientists, or laymen, the audience to be reached determines how the report is presented. The student should also become familiar with the publication policies of various journals, since each has its own guidelines. The goal of the report should be kept in mind, together with appropriate writing style. The confidentiality of subjects and agencies should also be protected.

SUMMARY

A model may be devised that depicts the phases and steps of the research process. The Calendar Wheel is a model that divides the process into phases and steps, and assists the student to prepare a timetable that allocates the time to be spent in each phase. The model also suggests the unending process of scientific research: the conclusion of one project provides the data upon which another may be based.

The four phases of research include planning, collecting data, analyzing and interpreting data, and communicating the findings of the research. Each phase may be divided into various steps that may differ in some ways from project to project. Common steps in Phase I require the researcher to: 1) identify a researchable problem; 2) formulate the research proposal; 3) define concepts and variables; 4) state objectives and hypotheses; 5) examine ethical implications of research; 6) review the literature; 7) identify theory, assumptions, and limitations; 8) describe the research design; 9) describe the methods of sampling, data collection, instrumentation, and data analysis; 10) obtain informed consent for a pilot study from agencies and study subjects; 11) conduct a pilot study and revise the research proposal in light of the findings; and 12) plan how to communicate the findings.

Phase II, the collection of data, relies heavily on two central processes: 1) selecting the sample from which the data are to be collected and obtaining informed consent from study subjects and involved agencies; and 2) selecting the method that is suitable to collect data in light of the research design being used. Both the sampling process and the methods are complex issues intimately related to research designs, as well as to the ability to generalize from the small sample under study to the larger population from which the sample was drawn. The student needs to think carefully about these matters in terms of all the factors involved, including time. Specific chapters in the book deal with each of these elements of the research process.

Phase III, the summarization, analysis, and interpretation of data, begins with an examination of raw data and transforms it into summaries, including frequencies, measures of central tendency and variance, and tables or graphs. Studies that have used random sampling can use inferential statistics to estimate parameters and test null hypotheses. Once data summaries and estimates are concluded, the student can analyze these in the light of the research proposal, including objectives. The student draws conclusions from the analysis and discusses what these mean to nursing in general. Next, the student may make recommendations that are relevent for practice, administration, or teaching, or the student may suggest further research. Finally, the student carefully reviews and criticizes the research project, in preparation for communicating the findings.

Phase IV is concerned with communicating the research by oral presentation or written report. The organization and substantive approach depends in part upon the audience. The student re-examines the goals of the research and organizes the content in the proper format, using a writing style that is appropriate for the prospective readers, whether scientists or laymen.

The temporal model presented is an idealized paradigm of the research process, which the student modifies with assistance from pertinent chapters of the book.

STUDY QUESTIONS

1. If you were to study any nursing problem you could, what would it be?
2. Identify the central concepts of your problem above.
3. Examine the following problem: Radical mastectomy in women is an instance of the general phenomenon of changes in body image.

This problem offers an opportunity to investigate the process of adjustment that takes place when a women is faced with a loss of the breast, a symbol of femininity and motherhood (Benoliel, 1975, p. 194). What are the concepts in the problem that need definition? Is this a researchable problem?

4. Do you foresee any ethical implications of the proposed research problem?
5. If you were to undertake the study of such a problem, what objective would you plan to meet?
6. Given the information in question three above, where would you begin a review of the literature?
7. Have you encountered any theory that would be helpful in such a study?
8. Beginning with the assumption that surgical disfigurement alters a woman's self-concept, what could you predict you would find if you observed or questioned a woman who had had a mastectomy two weeks previously?
9. If you were to develop a research design or plan to study patients with mastectomies, what would be the four phases of the research design?
10. What is a pilot project?

REFERENCES AND SUGGESTED READINGS

Abdellah, F. and Levine, E. (1965): Better Patient Care Through Nursing Research. New York: Macmillan, ch. 5. *The steps in the research process.*

Bloch, D. (1974): Some crucial terms in nursing: what do they really mean? *Nursing Outlook 22, 689–694. Cites the difficulty of finding consensus on the definition of concepts.*

Brink, P. and Wood, M. (1978): Basic Steps in Planning Nursing Research: From Question to Proposal. North Scituate, Mass: Duxbury Press. *Each chapter explains a step in research.*

Fox, D. (1976): Fundamentals of Research in Nursing (3rd ed.). New York: Appleton. *Chapter 3 includes nineteen stages in a three-part plan of research.*

Johnson, M. (1975): Outcome criteria to evaluate postoperative respiratory status. *American Journal of Nursing 75, 1474–1475. Formulation of a significant problem for nursing.*

Lin, N. (1976): Foundations of Social Research. New York: McGraw-Hill. *Chapter One includes eight phases of research.*

McCorkle, R. (1981): Effects of touch on seriously ill patients. In Fox, D., Readings on the Research Process in Nursing. New York: Appleton. *Instruments used include observation, questionnaire, tape recorder, etc.*

Polit, D. and Hungler, B. (1978): Nursing Research: Principles and Methods. New York: J. B. Lippincott. *Chapter 3 includes 15 steps in the research process.*

Selltiz, C. et al (1976): *Methods in Social Relations* (3rd ed.). New York: Holt, Rinehart, and Winston, pp. 12–14. *Brief treatment of the major steps in research.*

Simon, J. (1976): Basic Research Methods in Social Science. New York: Random House, ch. 7. *Includes the steps in an empirical research study.*

PART 2

The Research Proposal, Ethical Issues, and Review of Literature

CHAPTER 4
The Research Proposal

CHAPTER 5
Ethical Issues in Nursing Research

CHAPTER 6
A Critical Review of the Literature

THE RESEARCH PROPOSAL

A research proposal is a written summary of what the researcher intends to do, how, and why. The research proposal is forward looking. It describes the anticipated plan of research for the approval of the supervising professor, committee, or funding agency. A well written proposal is a valuable tool for the student, well worth the time and effort put into its development. The proposal anticipates as many of the elements of the research process as possible and provides a model that helps the student write the research report. The research proposal is written during the planning phase of research, implemented during the phases of data collection and analysis, and described in the communication phase.

This chapter is designed to help the student identify a researchable problem and write a research proposal. Upon completion of the chapter, the student should be able to: 1) identify a significant problem in nursing; 2) state the characteristics of a researchable problem; and 3) write a research proposal that includes what the researcher intends to study and why, objectives and hypotheses, ethical considerations, theoretical viewpoints, design, and methods.

SOURCES OF SIGNIFICANT RESEARCHABLE PROBLEMS IN NURSING

Nursing problems become research problems when the researcher can identify what to observe, what questions to ask, or what to measure. Sources of significant problems in nursing are the clinical area, the literature, experienced professionals, and the student's own interest. The researcher may observe a problem in the clinical area and then examine pertinent research reports for further information. Or, the researcher may begin with the literature. Advice from professors and practitioners of nursing may point the way to a stimulating research project already underway that the student can join. However, the interest of the student is the most fruitful source of nursing problems. The student's curiosity and energy light the fire necessary for sustained commitment throughout the project.

The Clinical Area

The clinical area of nursing is one in which patients or clients are observed, treated, cared for, advised, and/or taught. It is a fertile area for identifying problems in practice, teaching, or administration. To identify problems in the clinical area, Diers (1979) suggests that we begin by asking a series of questions: 1) "I wonder why. . ."; 2) "What is this?"; 3) "What is happening here?"; and 4) "What happens if. . .?"

1. The nurse who wonders why she observes certain events in nursing may be noting a discrepancy: things are not the way the nurse thinks they should be. Or else, what the nurse knows varies from what she or he needs to know. For example, Dee et al (1965) noticed that certain patients were receiving excellent nursing care, while others seemed uncomfortable and unattended. She wondered why this was so. Upon investigation, she found that patient care seemed related to the way nurses felt about the patients: those regarded favorably received good care, while those regarded unfavorably did not, a discrepancy in the way things were and the way they should be. Noting discrepancies is a major step in the identification of a clinical nursing problem, which then may be described or explored.

2. The nurse who wonders what it is that he or she is observing is searching for the name of the problem. For example, what is the name of the needs of a grieving spouse in the hospital setting (Hampe, 1974)? What is the name of the feeling that families have when a psychiatric patient is returning home? What are the names of the various processes associated with dying in a hospital (Glaser and Strauss, 1966–1968)? Searching for

a name leads the nurse to describe, classify, and name nursing phenomena. Nursing diagnoses are the names given to the descriptions
and classification of nursing observations. The nurse who isolates specific factors from observations in order to describe and name these factors is using *naming theory,* an explanation for the classification of nursing data.

3. *The nurse who wonders what is happening here is searching for relationships
between named variables.* In this case, the names of the concepts or variables are known, but the relationship between them is not. For example,
Brown et al (1977) wondered about the relationship between drug interactions and the consequences of these interactions for elderly patients
in nursing homes who were prescribed these drugs. Williams (1972)
wondered what factors were related to the incidence of decubitus ulcers
among hospitalized patients; and Amborn (1976) was interested in
which of twenty-two clinical signs were most related to the need for
tracheo-bronchial suctioning. Beginning with observation, all such problems lead inductively to the formulation of factor-relating theory.

4. *The nurse who wonders what would happen if . . . seeks to predict a relationship between variables.* He or she may wonder how factors vary in
terms of one another (correlation), or if one factor causes the other
(causation). For example, what happens if a person smokes? Is the person at risk to get cancer? Is smoking correlated with cancer? What happens if there is a rise in fever, and is it associated with changes in the
perception of time passage (Alderson, 1974)? What is the effect of nursing on the incidence of postoperative vomiting (Dumas and Leonard,
1963)? What happens when the nurse prepares a patient for surgery by
precise teaching methods? Will the patient be able to deep breathe and
cough more effectively? Will the patient stay in the hospital less time
and need analgesics less frequently (Lindeman and Van Aernam, 1977)?

The nurse can find significant problems in the clinical area by asking
the right questions or by reviewing the literature.

The Nursing Literature

Nursing literature is a readily available source of important research
problems in nursing (see Chapter 6). Abdellah et al (1960) over two
decades ago identified twenty-one areas of patient needs from which
problems may be identified. More recently, Abbey (1980) developed the
acronym *FANCAP* (Fluids, Aeration, Nutrition, Communication, Activity, Pain) to provide a mnemonic device for reminding nurses of possible
problem areas. Roy (1980) identifies problems of adaptation, including
physiologic needs of patients, self-concept, and role and relations of

interdependence. Roy's model reveals the kind of problems found when deviations from the desired state occur. Lindeman (1975) published a list of areas that nurses themselves identified as problem areas needing research: patient care and education; alleviation of stress and pain; indicators to measure quality nursing care; and the nursing process. Each of these defines sources of problems in the clinical area, in teaching, or in administration.

Fox (1976, p. 214) suggests a significant problem for both nursing service and education: to delineate *what* needs to be measured and to devise instruments to measure the phenomenon. For example, what characteristics should nurses measure to define good nursing care? What can be measured to predict the reaction of patient X when nurse Y enters the room? What identifies the freshman student who will be a functioning nurse of the future? These are challenging questions.

Stress is a problem area that received considerable attention following Selye's (1965) publication *The Stress of Life*. Recently, Kjervik and Martinson (1979) examined a number of areas stressful to women that should be the concern of nursing: child bearing, poverty, pain, and the loss associated with divorce, widowhood, or death. Many books contain articles specifically related to nursing problems: Downs and Newman (1977); Downs and Fleming (1979); and Verhonick (1977, 1979). The journal *Nursing Research* is a fertile source of problems. For example, a series of articles (1977, p. 26) is concerned with research in nursing specialties, such as maternal-child nursing, community health, and psychiatric nursing. Each article suggests significant areas for research.

Suggestions of Experienced Professionals
Professors, clinical specialists, and experienced nurses are important resources to aid the student in identifying significant nursing problems. It is a rare professional that does not welcome the interest of a student in his or her area of research or clinical speciality. At times, it is possible for the professional to invite the student to participate in on-going research. Such participation provides the student with an exceptional opportunity to examine the research proposal, instruments, recording processes, and ethical implications of a sophisticated research project.

Student Interest
Student interest is often the best source of a problem for study. A burning interest in a particular area of nursing practice, education, or administration is vital to make the research come alive. It transforms what could be a routine and demanding chore into a stimulating and rewarding experience. The student's fresh approach to nursing enables her or him to identify nursing procedures that often are ritualistic and useless at best, and may be costly and traumatic. The student views the

profession from a new and vital perspective—a resource of considerable importance to nursing.

CHARACTERISTICS OF A RESEARCHABLE PROBLEM

Several characteristics define a researchable problem for study: 1) availability of data, 2) feasibility, 3) importance, and 4) general applicability. A research proposal is no better than the problem it proposes. Therefore, the problem must be not only sound, it must be researchable.

Availability of Data

Not all data are equally accessible to all researchers. For example, an undergraduate student may have difficulty getting access to certain subjects such as rape victims, patients undergoing sex change, or patients involved with child abuse. The subjects may object, or the hospital or supervising personnel may protest the study of sensitive areas such as these. If reliable and valid instruments are not available, data may also be difficult to collect. In addition, the collection of cultural data may require more hours of observation than the researcher can afford. If the researcher plans to obtain data by asking questions in interviews or by questionnaire, the willingness and the ability of the respondent to answer the questions must be assessed. To obtain data from records, the records must be available and complete, and the data must have been accurately and legibly recorded. To obtain data from an experiment involving human subjects, ethical questions must be answered and permission obtained from various committees concerned with the protection of human rights.

Therefore, a good research question that does not have a dependable and available source of data may begin and end with the question itself.

Feasibility of the Research

The second characteristic of a good research proposal is its suitability or practicality. What is practical for one researcher may not be appropriate for another. Nevertheless, certain criteria apply to nearly all projects. Those of special concern include time, money, space, equipment, cooperation of agencies and personnel, and the personality of the researcher. Each of these will be examined briefly.

Time. Every study needs a timetable, although this may vary in terms of the researcher's status and the project's funding. Undergraduate nurses must integrate research with other courses and course work with the number of weeks in the academic semester or year. Graduate students have a similar problem, which may be complicated if a supporting grant has deadlines of its own. The nurse in practice must consider time for research, in addition to the regular schedule for work. Therefore, it is expedient to examine the research problem and proposal in terms of the length of time necessary to complete each step of the study. It may be necessary to reduce the scope of the problem, or reduce the number of variables under study. A second dilemma arises from the times that data must be collected. For example, a study of pain during childbirth must consider not only when the patient may go into labor, day or night, but likewise the changing rhythms of labor. Another problem is observing several women simultaneously in labor. A good research proposal allows for a practical timetable in terms of both the researcher's program of study or work and the time necessary for proper data collection.

Money. The simplest research project costs money. Costs of small items such as index cards, paper, pencils and pens, typewriter ribbons, paper clips, rubber bands, and file folders soon add up. It is a rare study that does not also include the purchase of books and journals or the reproduction of articles. If a questionnaire is to be used, postage both to send and to return the questionnaire must be calculated, as well as the cost of envelopes and paper. An interview may call for transportation and, at times, long distance phone calls. If the use of a computer is necessary to analyze data, these service charges must be calculated, including the costs of keypunching and coding. A good research question is one that falls within the financial ability of the researcher to pay and produces results that reimburse the researcher or the granting agency.

Space and Equipment. Certain research projects, such as a survey or questionnaire, need little space or equipment beyond a desk, paper, and pencil. Others may require instruments to measure physiological functioning and special rooms for conducting experiments. A simple interview needs privacy and quiet, in order for the interviewer and respondent to communicate with one another freely. Audio-visual aids of various types, such as recorders, cameras, and projectors, offer considerable assistance but may be beyond the resources of the neophyte researcher. A sound research question involves no more need for space and equipment than can be met within the limits of time and money available to the investigator.

Cooperation of Agencies and Personnel. Cooperation of others may often depend upon legal and ethical consideration, as well as availability of unrestricted data. For the undergraduate nurse, the length of time required to obtain permission to collect data in schools, industries, nursing homes, or hospitals may exceed the time available. And permission may be denied. A letter or phone call by a high official or influential person in the field may help, but these persons must be available to the researcher. The nurse in practice is in an enviable position—the collection of data may occur in the course of practice. However, consent of supervisors and subjects is necessary and ethical. In order to test whether a research question is feasible in terms of cooperation of crucial agencies or persons, permission should be obtained as early in the research process as possible.

Personality of the Researcher. Certain nurses seem better suited for certain kinds of research than others, although difficulties in this area are not always easily foreseen. An experienced investigator in the same field may be able to predict the success of a particular nurse. Often, a pilot project may point up difficulties that otherwise would be unpredictable. An aggressive personality may do better with a questionnaire survey than with an interview, although a timid nurse may find it difficult to knock on doors and interact with strange persons. A good research proposal must take into account both the personality of the researcher and the variables examined above.

Importance of the Research Proposal
The most important nursing questions deal with the nursing care of the sick, maintenance of the health of the well, and evaluation of health care. Moreover, the frequency with which problems in health care are occurring is important. For example, how often do hospitalized patients get bedsores? How frequently are illegitimate children born prematurely? How often are clinic appointments broken? How frequently do patients know the side effects of the drugs they take? The frequency of a problem affects not only the health of the population but also increases the cost of health services. For example, frequent infection of surgical wounds means a longer and more costly stay in the hospital for the patient.

General Applicability of the Findings
Research proposals are generally applicable when they can be related to theory and when the subjects to be studied are selected from the target population by a method of random sampling (see Chapter 8). Some theories used in nursing research are the systems theory, theories of human development, the stress theory, and theories of adaptation (see Chapter 7). The theoretical framework helps the researcher explain

the relationships among the facts observed during the phase of data collection.

FORMULATING THE RESEARCH PROPOSAL

The research proposal is intimately related to the research problem. Research problems become research proposals when the student can precisely state the following: 1) what is to be studied and why; 2) the objectives and/or hypotheses of the study; 3) the ethical implications, if any; 4) the theoretical viewpoints, assumptions, and limitations; 5) the research design, sampling, and methods. As the student reviews the literature related to the problem and attempts to obtain a proper sample of study subjects from a target population, a research proposal may go through many revisions. A well formulated research proposal repays the researcher for the time and effort it takes and informs the reviewers. The anticipated plan of research is summarized, the extent to which the findings may be generalized to other times and places is made apparent, and the potential for application in the clinical area becomes evident.

What the Researcher Intends to Study

The researcher states the problem to be studied in the opening paragraph of the research proposal. The general area of study is first introduced, the importance to nursing is indicated, and then the exact problem is specified. The following example illustrates these points:

> The general effect of hospitalization upon the emotional and mental health of children is a question of importance to nurses who must daily assess the condition of their patients. The relationship between hospitalization and the emotional and mental status of children has been well studied by Bowlby (1952, 1956, 1969) and others. Nurses such as McGillicuddy (1977) have investigated the effect of hospitalization on the child, if the mother stays in the room with him. Does the mother's rooming-in with her child make a difference in the child's subsequent behavior? This research proposes to study that question, to examine the effect of the mother's rooming-in with her child on his subsequent behavior after he has left the hospital.

The brief introductory paragraph above has identified the general problem area, suggested its importance to nursing, referred the reader to examples in the general literature and the nursing literature, and specified exactly what the researcher is proposing to study.

What the researcher intends to study must now be explained further by defining each major concept by operational definition, which clarifies what is to be observed and measured. Definitions should be drawn from the literature to strive for consensus in the meaning of nursing concepts and variables. Drawing on a similar but more extensive study by McGillicuddy, the student defines the concepts as follows:

1. *Rooming-in.* The mother remains with the child 24 hours a day during the first two days and at least ten hours daily thereafter until discharge.
2. *Child.* Those children who are 14 months or older but not yet 49 months old; who are hospitalized for minor surgery, including eye surgery and tonsillectomy.
3. *Behavior.* Selected ways of behaving by the child, including eating, sleeping, and toilet behaviors.
4. *Effect.* The effect of the mother's rooming-in with her child on the child's subsequent behavior, as measured by the mother's response to a questionnaire answered after the child has been home for a month and compared with the mother's response to a questionnaire answered on the day of her child's admission to the hospital.

The researcher who uses hypotheses not only specifies what is to be studied, but also predicts a relationship between the variables:

If the mother rooms-in with her child during hospitalization for minor surgery, then the child will manifest increased maturity in selected areas of behavior compared with the child whose mother does not room-in.

Objectives

An *objective* is an intent, a statement of what the student proposes to accomplish in the research. It denotes observable measurable attributes that make it possible to determine whether the objective has been met. To be meaningful, the stated objective must communicate to the reader the exact intent of the researcher. The most important characteristic of an objective is to identify the tasks the researcher plans to perform during the study. As the following examples drawn from different research reports demonstrate, each objective expresses only one intended outcome:

- An objective of this research is to compare the communication patterns of elderly male and female patients.

- An objective of this study is to record the words that various patients use to describe the functions of their bodily organs.
- An objective of this study is to state factors that increase the opportunities for mothers of hospitalized children to participate in their care.

When a number of objectives are developed, these should be stated in the order of importance. Each objective should be related to the research design and methods. Descriptive or exploratory studies rely on objectives more often than explanatory studies, which tend to rely on hypothesis.

Ethical Implications

At some point in the research proposal, the researcher must inform the reviewer of the ethical implications of the study and how these will be handled. Forms for informed consent may be attached to the proposal, and forms indicating the protocol for research on human subjects may be included, together with any other information required by the human investigations committee that a particular school may have. Both agencies and subjects must be considered in the plan to obtain informed consent.

Review of the Literature

The review of the literature may either be interwoven into the identification of the problem, the definition of concepts, the theoretical section, the research design and methods; or it may be presented in a section of its own. The review should identify pertinent studies about what is known and what remains to be learned. It should provide a background of the problem to be studied and convince the reviewer that the researcher has explored significant studies and has a grasp of the theory and research findings relevant to the proposed research. The preliminary proposal that the student submits for the first tentative approval may not include all citations, but the finished proposal should demonstrate a thorough grasp of the studies documented in the literature.

Theory, Assumptions and Limitations

A theory provides the explanation for observed facts and relationships, predicts what the researcher will observe, and summarizes what is known about the topic under study. The researcher states the theory used to deduce the hypotheses and refers the reader to any previous research relevant to his or her proposal. In the absence of well developed theory, the researcher states the assumptions that underlie the proposal. Assumptions are statements whose validity can be found in the literature or are considered to be self-evident. Some examples of assumptions are:

- Child development proceeds as an integrated system in interaction with the environment (Robischon, 1977, p. 155).
- The development of mothering ability is determined by the mother's previous experience, her current life situation, and the inborn behavior of the infant (Durand, 1975, p. 152).

Limitations establish the parameters, i.e., the boundaries, of the research. Ability to include limitations in the proposal enhances the quality of the proposal. Some examples of limitations are:

1. The sample for this study will be limited to one child with Down's syndrome.
2. This investigation will be limited to children between 19 and 24 months.
3. The sample will be limited to children living in intact family units.

Limitations should not stop with the statement of the population sampled but should include the researcher's opinion about the ability to generalize or apply the study's results beyond the study sample. In addition, the researcher should assess the ability of any instruments to be used to measure what the researcher intends to measure. If an instrument is not valid, the researcher should delay the proposal until an instrument of demonstrated validity is found (Fox, 1976, p. 292).

Research Design

The research design is often described in a single paragraph that indicates whether the design is experimental, partially experimental, a survey, or a historical documentary:

- This experimental study will determine whether a causal relationship exists between the amount of touching a seriously ill patient receives and the number of positive responses that the patient makes.
- A three-group experimental design will be used to test the hypothesis.
- Two of the groups will be control groups and one will be experimental.
- The researcher intends to use a record review to collect data on

the birth weights of babies born to primiparas who smoke and those who do not smoke.

- The design of research is a descriptive survey that uses a questionnaire to measure the tendency of operating-room nurses to desire friendly interaction with others.
- The research design is an exploratory survey (interview) to determine whether poor women perceive health workers as threatening.

Research Methods

The researcher reports the method to be used to collect data, whether by observation, questioning, measuring, or a combination of the three. The following examples suggest a few of the various combinations.

1. Data will be collected by direct observation of two observers.
2. A questionnaire will be administered by an observer. A tape recorder will record any verbal interactions.
3. Data will be collected using measures of blood pressure, pulse rates, and temperature readings.
4. Data will be collected by interviewing patients to determine how much they know about the side effects of medications they are taking.

Instruments. The instruments used to collect data may be described in a manner similar to the following:

1. The instrument to be used to measure psychological stress response is the Zuckerman's Affect Adjective Check List consisting of 61 adjectives that have emotional overtones. The subjects will check every word that describes their present feelings.
2. Heart-rate measurement instruments include a two-channel direct writer that will record ECG.
3. A questionnaire of 27 items will be used to assess behavioral changes.

Sampling

An important part of the research proposal is how the sample is to be selected. The following examples illustrate some of the sampling methods used in research:

1. A sample of 100 seriously ill patients will be selected from a 1000-bed general hospital in Central City. An alphabetical list of seriously ill patients in intensive care and coronary care will be

obtained weekly. Those patients who are oriented to their surroundings, who can hear well and do not have speech problems, and who are between 20 and 60 years of age will be included in the sample. These patients will be alternately assigned to an experimental or control group, beginning with a flip of a coin to designate the initial assignment.

2. A random sample of 800 nurses will be chosen from a list of nurses registered with the West Virginia State Board of Nurse Examiners at the time of the survey.
3. Data will be collected during the intensive study of one case of Down's syndrome.
4. The sample will be comprised of patients admitted for surgery in which general anesthesia will be used. Patients admitted during one month will serve as the control group, while patients admitted during the next month will serve as the experimental group.

Methods of Data Analysis

Numerous methods of data analysis may be selected, including the plan to develop various categories for descriptive data; to use descriptive statistics appropriate to the scale used to summarize and compare data; or to use inferential statistics to test hypotheses. If the use of a computer is planned, this should be noted in the proposal.

SUMMARY

A research proposal summarizes what the researcher intends to do, how it will be done, and why it is important for nursing. The proposal anticipates as many elements of the research process as possible. It is written during the planning phase, implemented during the data collection phase, and described during the communication phase.

To write a sound research proposal, the student must be able to identify a significant problem in nursing, state the characteristics that are researchable, and use this information to write that portion of the research proposal that specifies the general area of study and the specific problem to be studied.

Sources of significant researchable problems in nursing include the clinical area, the literature, experienced professionals, and the student's own interest. Problems in the clinical area can be identified by asking questions such as, "I wonder why?"; "What is this?"; "What is happening here?" and "What happens if. . . ?" A number of books and journals in the nursing literature, such as *Nursing Research*, include helpful information about nursing problems. Experienced professional nurses may be engaged in on-going research that the student may be invited to join. However, the best source of a research problem is often the student herself.

Characteristics of researchable problems include available data and feasible or practical research, in terms of time, money, space, equipment, cooperation of others, and the personality of the researcher. All of these should be carefully weighed before selecting a problem for study. The importance of the proposed research to nursing must be examined, such as nursing care of the sick, maintenance of good health in the well, evaluation of health care, and the frequency with which the problem occurs.

Once the problem is selected, the student is launched. The formulation of the research proposal begins with a brief paragraph that describes what the researcher intends to study and its importance to nursing. This is followed by a definition of the major concepts used in the study. Operational definitions then clarify what is to be observed and measured.

The objective of the study defines what the student intends to accomplish in the research project. The most important characteristic of the objective is to identify the tasks the student will perform during the research. Hypotheses are used in explanatory research to predict what will be found in research.

A section of the proposal must be devoted to a thorough description of the research design, whether it will be an experiment, a survey, or an historical documentary review of records. The research methods and instruments that will be used to select a sample and collect data receive particular scrutiny from the reader and require a careful exposition by the student.

The assumptions of the study—statements documented in the literature, or ideas considered to be correct—should be clearly stated to demonstrate the student's grasp of theory and research. The limitations of the study, or those aspects of research that will not be studied, should be noted to enhance the quality of the research proposal.

A brief but significant review of the literature provides a background for the study and helps convince the reader that the student understands what has been discovered and what remains to be learned.

Ethical implications must be anticipated and dealt with in a professional manner. Proper forms should be processed, and the student should be ready to proceed, once permission is obtained from all necessary agencies and subjects.

STUDY QUESTIONS

1. You have just received a large grant to study a nursing problem of your own choosing. What will you study?
2. If you are uncertain about what to study, name three sources of significant nursing problems.
3. In your own case, what identifies a problem that is researchable and one that is not?
4. What ethical consideration must be given to nursing research in general?
5. What are the ethical implications of the nursing problem you selected in Question 1?
6. Name and discuss four characteristics of a good nursing problem and research proposal.
7. Identify the what, who, how, when, and where of your proposal.
8. Define the central concepts of your problem.
9. Establish four or five clear objectives for your study proposed above.

REFERENCES AND SUGGESTED READINGS

Abbey, J. (1980): FANCAP: what is it? In Riehl, J. and Roy, C. (eds.), Conceptual Models for Nursing Practice (2nd ed.). New York: Appleton, pp. 107–118. *Mnemonic device to identify possible patient problems.*

Abdellah, Fay et al (1960): Patient-Centered Approaches to Nursing. New York: Macmillan. *The identification of patient needs suggests problem areas for research.*

Alderson, M. (1974): Effect of increased body temperature on the perception of time. *Nursing Research 23*, 43–49. *An example of a clinical problem.*

Ambron, S. (1976): Clinical signs associated with amount of tracheo-bronchial secretions. *Nursing Research 25*, 121–216. *A problem in the clinical area.*

Bowlby, J. (1956): Maternal-child separation. In Soddy, K., Mental Health and Infant Development. New York: Basic Books. *Maternal bonding is discussed.*

Brown, M. et al (1977): Drug–drug interactions among residents in homes for the elderly. *Nursing Research 26*, 47–52. *A problem in health care of the elderly.*

Dee, F. et al (1965): Self-acceptance of nurses and acceptance of patients: An exploratory investigation. *Nursing Research 14*, 345–350. *Observation detects a problem in the clinical carea.*

Diers, D. (1979): Research in Nursing Practice. New York: J. B. Lippincott. *Nursing problems in the clinical area identified.*

Downs, F. and Fleming, J. (eds.) 1979: Issues in Nursing Research. New York: Appleton. *Seven articles examine research issues.*

Downs, F. and Newman, M. (eds.) (1977): A Sourcebook of Nursing Research (2nd ed.). Philadelphia: F. A. Davis. *Fifteen articles evaluate nursing intervention and explore indices of health.*

Dumas, R. and Leonard, R. (1963): The effect of nursing on the incidence of postoperative vomiting. *Nursing Research 12,* 12–15. *Seeks to predict a relation between variables; the problem: patient anxiety.*

Durand, B. (1975): Failure to thrive in a child with Down's syndrome. *Nursing Research 24,* 272–286. *Assumptions stated.*

Fox, D. (1976): Fundamentals of Research in Nursing (3rd ed.). New York: Appleton, pp. 25–26. *Problem areas discussed.*

Glaser, B. and Strauss, A. (1966): Awareness of Dying. Chicago: Aldine. (1967): The Discovery of Grounded Theory. Chicago: Aldine. (1968): A Time for Dying. Chicago: Aldine. *A variety of problems associated with dying.*

Hampe, S. (1974): Needs of the grieving spouse in a hospital setting. *Nursing Research 24,* pp. 113–120. *Problems identified from needs.*

Kjervik, D. and Martinson, I. (eds.) (1979): Women in Stress: A Nursing Perspective. New York: Appleton. *Twenty articles examine stress in various situations.*

Lindeman, C. and Van Aernam, B. (1977): Nursing intervention with the presurgical patient—the effects of structured and unstructured preoperative teaching. In Downs, F. and Newman, M., A Sourcebook of Nursing Research. Philadelphia: F. A. Davis, pp. 45–63. *Identifies problems in the clinical area.*

Lindeman, C. (1975): Delphi survey of priorities in clinical nursing research. *Nursing Research 24,* 434–441. *Problems given priorities in nursing.*

McGillicuddy, M. (1977): A study of the relationship between mothers' rooming-in during their children's hospitalization and changes in selected areas of children's behavior. In Downs, F. and Newman, M. (eds.), A Sourcebook of Nursing Research. Philadelphia: F. A. Davis, pp. 64–77. *Includes definition of concepts.*

Robischon, P. (1977): Pica practice and other hand-mouth behavior and children's developmental level. In Downs, F. and Newman, M. (eds.), A Sourcebook of Nursing Research. Philadelphia: F. A. Davis, pp. 152–170. *States assumptions.*

Roy, C. (1980): The Roy adaptation model. In Riehl, J. and Roy, C. (eds.), Conceptual Models for Nursing Practice. New York: Appleton, pp. 179–188. *Problems of adaptation.*

Selye, H. (1965): The Stress of Life. New York: McGraw-Hill. *Problems of stress.*

Verhonick, P. (ed.) (1975): Nursing Research I. Boston: Little, Brown. *Articles on the problems that nurses study.*

Verhonick, P. (ed.) (1977): Nursing Research II. Boston: Little, Brown. *Articles on problems in the clinical setting.*

Williams, A. (1972): Study of factors contributing to skin breakdown. *Nursing Research 21,* pp. 238–243. *Problem factors in the clinical area.*

CHAPTER **5**

ETHICAL ISSUES IN NURSING RESEARCH

A good research problem conforms to moral, ethical, and legal standards of scientific inquiry. A researcher should have deep concern for human welfare and sensitivity for the rights of research subjects. Any research that may be harmful violates the ethical code of nursing and may be illegal.

This chapter is designed to help the student become aware of the issues related to the use of human subjects in research. Upon completion of this chapter, the student should be able to: 1) describe the relationship between values and ethics; 2) state the rights of human subjects; 3) identify subjects who are vulnerable and need to have their rights protected; 4) describe problems concerned with the researcher's withholding information or with fully disclosing research plans to subjects; 5) identify the steps to take to secure informed consent; and 6) discuss the nurse's role in research.

VALUES AND ETHICS

Values are the ideas that members of a society share about what is important, worthwhile, good, and bad. Values underlie standards and are the criteria by which means and ends are judged. *Ethics* refers to the study and evalution of human conduct. *Applied ethics* examines actual human conduct in real situations. Research involves both values and ethics. For example, it is a basic scientific value that it is better to know than not to know. The behavior associated with this value is to seek knowledge through research. This applied ethic may come into conflict with the right of human beings to determine for themselves what will be done to them. A tension exists, therefore, between human rights that restrict the freedom of inquiry and the injunction to seek knowledge, which promotes research.

The need to protect human rights is amply demonstrated by research in which potentially harmful experiments were performed on elderly patients, children, and sick persons. Aged and infirm hospital patients were injected with live cancer cells without being informed that cancer was in any way involved (Lear, 1966; Langer, 1966). Mentally retarded children were deliberately exposed to infectious hepatitis, which could have resulted in considerable physical harm to them (Capron, 1973). Treatment was withheld from a group of men with venereal disease during the 1930s, because they were part of an experiment (Dempsey, 1981).

When the research designs of these experiments became public, the resulting outcry led to the development of guidelines to protect human subjects at both the governmental and professional levels. For example, the federal government, through the Department of Health, Education, and Welfare, developed policies that mandated informed consent (1974) and privacy (1976). The American Nurses' Association developed *Human Rights Guidelines for Nurses in Clinical and Other Research,* which were first adopted in 1967, and updated in 1975.

THE RIGHTS OF HUMAN SUBJECTS

The first right of human subjects is not to be harmed physically, psychologically, or emotionally. Other rights include self-determination, privacy, confidentiality, the right to maintain self-respect, the right to refuse to participate in research or to withdraw from participation without any penalty, and the right for services. Each of these will be examined.

1. The right not to be harmed has received little consideration in the past. It is reported that Edward Jenner deliberately exposed an eight-year-old child to cowpox, in order to try a new vaccine (Hayter, 1979). The good that Jenner did is remembered, while the possibility that the child may have been harmed has been forgotten. Unforgotten in the Western world, however, are the Nazi experiments that were conducted by highly qualified scholars with a flagrant disregard for the well-being of the captive human subjects.

The best known example of psychologically harmful research is that of Milgram's (1963) study of obedience to authority. The test was designed to determine how many persons would continue to obey the commands of an authority figure, even when they thought they were endangering the life of another. The procedure required that the subjects give what they thought were increasingly powerful electric shocks to another person (who was actually a stooge). Of the forty subjects, 65 percent continued to give shocks to the end of the series, even though there was a question of harming what they thought was a powerless person. Urged on to give the shocks by the researcher, the subjects were clearly anguished and tense: sweating, stuttering, and trembling. One subject had a violently convulsive seizure. The right of the subject not to be harmed had been brought into serious question.

2. *The right of self-determination includes informed voluntary consent.* Subjects who give voluntary consent are free from constraint and coercion of any kind. *Informed consent* means that the subjects have full knowledge and understanding about the research project in which they are being asked to participate. The volunteers should be free to decide to participate or not after they have been fully informed about the research. Informed consent includes providing the subjects with a full description of:

1. The purpose of the project and its general value;
2. All procedures used in the research and why;
3. The subject's part in the research, including the amount of time and energy the research will take;
4. Any possible pain, discomfort, stress, or loss of autonomy or dignity;
5. How privacy, confidentiality, and anonymity will be guarded;
6. The manner in which data will be used.

Informed consent implies that promises will be kept, no deception will be practiced, the self-respect of subjects will be protected, and ethical guidelines will be carefully followed. The manner in which data will be used should be explained, and the subject should give permission for such use. To allow the data to be put to any other use or to fail to describe all the uses is unethical.

3. *The right to privacy in our society is a tradition of considerable importance.* In some cases, the idea of being watched is illegal—the "peeping Tom" is liable for prosecution. Any intimation that "big brother" is watching in the privacy of the home, or that anyone else is observing private behavior is repugnant. Privacy enables a person to behave and think without interference or the possibility that private behavior or thoughts may be used to embarrass or demean the person later. Therefore, research methods that observe or question may invade privacy.

Participant observation is a method of collecting data in the field, or "natural" setting, by direct observation. This method may invade the privacy of individuals who do not realize they are being studied. Degrees of the researcher's participation range from total participation by living and working with the research subjects to nonparticipating observation by merely observing. The degree of disclosure to subjects also varies—from no disclosure, to partial concealment, to full disclosure. Participant observation is considered a powerful method for exploratory research, but there is a serious question of an invasion of the subject's privacy. Since the research setting is a part of everyday activity, little effort is made by the subject to conceal behavior. In particular, disguised participant observation is viewed as unethical.

The Privacy Act of 1974 (NIH Guide, 1976) raises questions concerning data collection techniques that use drugs, tests, or other processes that may invade privacy. Tests such as the "F scale" (fascistic scale) may reveal aspects of a person's personality, such as antidemocratic or authoritarian characteristics, that could prove embarrassing. The use of instruments such as tape recorders, cameras, or one-way mirrors to collect data without a subject's knowledge or permission is an invasion of privacy. Questioning sedated persons or giving mind-altering drugs without the full knowledge of the subject is unethical and may be illegal.

Personal activities, opinions, attitudes, beliefs, letters, diaries, and records are private property and are not subject to study without permission. The researcher must ascertain the extent to which each subject is willing to share privacy. Even if the researcher promises to maintain privacy of research data, data may fall into other hands if records are stored. The records may be subpoenaed or stolen, or crucial material may be copied by someone with temporary access to the records.

Data stored in computers are a potential threat to privacy since individuals often do not know what is stored or even if it is accurate. The use of such data is not only unethical, it may mislead the research. Records of patients to which the nurse has full access in practice requires the patient's permission, if the nurse wishes to use the records for research.

4. *Confidentiality and anonymity are two processes that protect the subject best. Confidentiality* is the researcher's ability to keep data sources protected.

Anonymity is the researcher's ability to keep subjects nameless. Anonymity is potentially handicapping to the researcher, because it prevents the researcher from contacting subjects in a survey who do not return questionnaires. Rather than sending reminders to the few who do not respond, the entire sample would have to be sent reminders, sometimes a rather expensive undertaking. Anonymity also prevents any longitudinal or follow-up studies. Confidentiality may be the best means of protecting subjects without damaging the research. To maintain confidentiality, the data is coded with numbers instead of names, and the records that note which names go with which numbers are kept under lock and key. Name and code numbers are kept in different locations entirely. The data may then be kept for further study long after the names are needed and have been destroyed. If a loss of confidentiality is threatened, all records should be destroyed. Subjects should be informed of all measures used to maintain confidentiality and anonymity.

To maintain confidentiality and anonymity in published reports, pseudonyms are useful for subjects, agencies, and geographical settings. The key to the pseudonyms, like the names associated with the numbers, are kept locked and in different locations. Any other information that can reveal the identity of persons or places is carefully handled, being burned or shredded rather than thrown into wastebaskets, where retrieval is possible.

5. *The right to maintain self-respect and dignity is associated with the right not to be harmed in any way.* This includes the right not to be deceived or led into doing things that may later distress or cause injury to the subject's self-concept. The Milgram experiments are a good example of the use of deceit. The use of "stooges" and the experimenter's prestige and power to urge the subject to do things caused distress during the experiment and later. *Debriefing* is a process of disclosing to the subject all information previously withheld and explaining why the information was withheld. This is an attempt to undo any harm that was done, either by withholding information or by deceit. Debriefing is more effective if the subject is told in advance of the research that it is not possible to reveal every aspect of the research ahead of time, but that the subject will be fully informed later. The information allows the subject to consider this aspect of the research before giving consent. The subject should be informed of all that was withheld and should decide whether or not the data should be published.

6. *The right to refuse to participate or to withdraw from participation without fear or recrimination is the subject's right, even though withdrawal may damage the research project.* The researcher must make the subject aware of this

right and allay any fears the subject may have that refusal to participate or withdrawal from the project will in some way hurt him or her. Patients have been known to believe health care would be withdrawn if they either refused to participate or wished to withdraw. Any promises of reward, such as money, free nursing care, or better nursing care, should not be used, since these may be coercive. The cooperation of patients or subjects is better achieved by explaining what the research is about and the importance the findings may have. Altruistic motives or the possibility of making a contribution to scientific knowledge is often enough to encourage participation. Should the subject decide to stop participating, the researcher must be prepared to accept the decision.

7. *The right for services is a concern of the researcher, if the patient who comes for service is involved in research at the same time.* Some patients may be denied services or may be exposed to an approach that is experimental rather than traditional (Walizer and Wienir, 1978, p. 159). The solution to this problem is to let everyone get both the experimental and the traditional treatment, but at different times. However, this is not always possible. A patient dying of cancer may insist upon the new experimental drug and is not likely to have the time for both the traditional and the experimental treatments. To evaluate traditional services and to provide the best possible service requires research and sometimes experimentation. However, the rights of the subjects as persons require that they exercise informed consent and be allowed to volunteer in an experiment.

VULNERABLE SUBJECTS WHO NEED
SPECIAL PROTECTION

Vulnerable subjects either are unable to give informed consent or are captive subjects. The less able a person is to protect himself or herself, the more vigilant the reseacher must be. Vulnerable subjects include children, the mentally ill or retarded, the aged, captive persons, the poor, the dying, and the sedated or unconscious.

1. *Children are believed to be incapable of weighing the risks and benefits of a research project and should not even be asked to give informed consent.* However, the question arises of the definition of a *child*. At what age does a person leave childhood and become capable of making a decision regarding research? Various criteria are applied: marriage, military service, economic independence by working, living away from home, grad-

uating from high school, or being of a certain age, such as 18 or 21. Minors have been allowed to make a number of crucial decisions by court order. One judge allowed a 14-year-old to make the decision to be a kidney donor. In the past, parents were able to give consent for their children, but this is now being questioned. Hayter (1979, p. 125–126) cites a number of studies that deal with this issue. Certain circumstances, such as being chronically ill, emotionally disturbed, or alienated from the family, tend to increase the child's risk of being harmed by participation in research. Children may also be damaged by being put in a position of informing on parents or conditions in the home.

2. *The mentally ill or mentally retarded are vulnerable subjects because they may be unable to comprehend the implications of the research.* In such instances, informed consent may have to come from both the subject and a relative or guardian. Some agencies appoint responsible persons as patients' advocates to assess the risk-benefit ratio.

3. *The aged need special consideration.* Some cannot comprehend and, in this way, resemble children or the mentally incompetent. Others comprehend well, but feel a pressure to comply, especially if they are not in a good position to make all their own choices. The dependent, those in nursing homes, or the incapacitated may feel they should please those in authority. This requires the researcher to exercise special care.

4. *Captive persons, such as prisoners, men and women in the armed forces, students, the dependent poor, friends and family of researchers, and employees all are vulnerable (Hayter, 1979).* In the past, prisoners have been used for research and are vulnerable to promises of early parole, money, special privileges, or prestige. Soldiers, sailors, and others in the armed services are trained to obey superior officers and may be rather helpless. Students too are under the authority of professors or are subject to peer pressure. Without being fully aware of the pressure, the researcher may ask family and friends to participate in a study. The love and trust of friends and family may over-ride their concern. This puts the burden on the researcher to be aware of the dangers and risks.

5. *The poor who are dependent on certain facilities for health care may believe they must comply with a request for research.* At times, money is forthcoming to study an aspect of health care in a poverty-stricken area. However, money may not be available to maintain services once the research is complete. The ethical issues involved in these cases must be carefully weighed by the researcher, who must be concerned about the rights of human subjects.

6. The dying, sedated, or unconscious person is vulnerable. At best, the dying are under stress and may be incapable of dealing with research issues. At the same time, however, some may gain satisfaction from the help they are able to provide others. Each case is unique, requiring the researcher to deal with it differently. The sedated person is seldom able to handle implications of the research. For example, a student who wishes to study the various methods of childbirth should obtain informed consent before the time of labor. The unconscious or anesthetized should only be subjects of research if they have given informed consent when totally conscious.

The key to research on vulnerable subjects who need special protection is to eliminate all subjects who cannot give informed consent freely and with understanding. The less able a subject is to protect himself or herself, the greater is the burden on the researcher to protect the subject.

WITHHOLDING INFORMATION

A major problem with informed consent is that disclosure of the details of a study may change the nature of the subject's response. Some researchers believe that informed consent may be avoided or misleading explanations may be given if there is a very low risk to the subjects. The "cover story" for example, satisfies the curiosity of the paticipants without revealing the true nature of the research. In such cases, the subjects' right of free choice has been sharply diminished, thereby raising ethical questions. Deception, the willful use of false information, is unethical, even if the subjects are later apprised of the deception. The Milgram study described above is a classic case of deception: the subjects were deceived about the true nature of the experiment and about the fact that stooges were being used. Debriefing, a complete disclosure of all information previously withheld, does not always reverse the harm that is done. If information will be withheld, the subject should be advised of this before he or she gives informed consent.

STEPS TO TAKE TO SECURE
INFORMED CONSENT

The first step is to locate or construct a proper informed consent form (see Figure 5–1). The form must include all of the information the subject needs to make an informed decision to participate in the research or not. The following information should be included:

1. An invitation to participate in the study, with times, dates, and purpose of the study.
2. An explanation of why the subject was selected.
3. A statement describing all procedures that will be used, the purpose and frequency of each procedure, and how long each will take.
4. An explanation of the subject's part in the procedures, including the amount of time and energy.
5. Any possible discomfort, stress, inconvenience, or loss of dignity and autonomy that may be experienced.
6. The risk/benefit ratio that may be expected.
7. A description of any standard treatment being withheld.
8. A statement explaining the way that confidentiality and anonymity will be maintained.
9. Any compensation to be expected, whether monetary or otherwise.
10. The right of the subject to refuse to participate or to withdraw from participation without fear of recrimination.
11. Assurance that the researcher will answer all questions.
12. A statement noting that the researcher has explained all elements of the study to the subject, and that the subject indicates by signature that he or she has read the information provided and has decided to participate.

Below the informational portion of the form, space must be allowed for the signature of the subject, the researcher, and a witness; and the time and date of the signatures.

Once the consent form is constructed and pretested, the student is ready to secure the approval of the appropriate human rights committees. Many universities that receive federal funding require research to be approved by various supervising committees. Schools of nursing often form their own committees to preview the students' research proposals and to review consent forms. Committees may be both regulator and resource to the student. In the process of review, committee members may advise the student of proper steps to take to improve the research approach.

After the consent form and the proposed research have been approved, the student must identify subjects and agencies and approach them for consent. For example, a study of hospital nurses may require the student to obtain permission from the director of nurses, before

Purpose of the study: _____.
Invitation to participate: _____.
Why subject was selected: _____.
Procedures, purpose, length of time needed, frequency of procedure: _____.
Discomforts, inconveniences expected: _____.
Risks, if any: _____.
Benefits, if any: _____.
Withholding standard treatment, if any: _____.
Time, energy required of subject: _____.
How confidentiality, anonymity, privacy will be maintained: _____.
Compensation to be expected, if any: _____.
Right of subject to refuse to participate or withdraw: _____.
Assurances that researcher will answer all questions: _____.
Concluding statement: "I have read all the information above and have made a
    decision whether or not to participate. My signature indicates that I have been
    informed and have decided to participate."

_____	_____
Date	Signature of subject
_____	_____
Time	Signature of subject advocate, if necessary; note relationship
_____	_____
Signature of witness	Signature of researcher

Figure 5–1. Informed consent guidelines.

contacting the individual nurses. If patients are the subjects of research, the task may be more difficult. Most hospitals have human investigation committees that review all research in which patients are involved. The student must present the proposal to the committee and defend it. Before contact with patients is made, suggested revisions must be incorporated into the study.

THE ROLE OF THE NURSE IN RESEARCH

The nurse may be investigator, participant, or the subject of research. As in other applied sciences, the nurse is also a consumer of research, interested in findings that may point the way to more efficient practice. As an investigator, the nurse must understand the scientific principles associated with empirical research. As a participant in others' research, the nurse has the right and responsibility to be informed and to consent to the role she is designated to play. As the subject of research, the nurse has the right of informed consent and self-determination.

SUMMARY

Ethics is the study and evaluation of human conduct. *Applied ethics* examines actual human conduct in real situations. *Values* are the ideas that members of society share about what is important, worthwhile, good, and bad. Research involves both ethics and values. However, the value held by scientists—that it is better to know than not to know—may come in conflict with the rights of human subjects for self-determination.

Rights of human subjects include the right not to be harmed, the right of self-determination, privacy, and the right for services. Each of these is related to other rights, such as the right to maintain self-respect and dignity, to remain anonymous, and to have confidential material remain confidential.

Vulnerable subjects who need to have their rights protected are of special concern to the researcher. These subjects include children, the mentally ill or retarded, the aged, the poor, the dying or unconscious; and captive persons such as prisoners, those in the armed forces, students, and friends and families of researchers.

A major problem with informed consent is the effect that disclosure may have on the research. Deception is unethical, but the researcher may inform subjects that full disclosure will follow the research. Debriefing informs the subject of all elements of the research after the research but before publication. This allows a subject who has given permission for delayed disclosure to refuse to have the information that concerns him or her published.

A number of steps must be taken to secure consent from study subjects. The researcher must describe all procedures that will be used, including the amount of time and energy subjects will be required to expend. Any discomfort subjects may experience, as well as the risk/benefit ratio, must be described. The subjects must be informed of the manner in which data will be used and why the collection of such data is valuable. The subjects must understand that they may refuse to participate in the study or withdraw without fear of recrimination. The researcher must state how confidentiality and anonymity will be maintained and must assure subjects that all questions will be answered. The informed consent statement must be dated and signed by the researcher, the subject, and at least one witness.

The nurse may be a researcher, a participant, a subject, or a consumer of research. In all cases, the nurse must be alert to all possible ethical questions and speak out against any unethical practice that becomes known.

STUDY QUESTIONS

1. What is the relationship between values and ethics in nursing?
2. You are the chief nurse in a privately supported children's rehabilitation center. A research team has been given permission to conduct research in the clinic. What are the rights of the patients? What are your responsibilities?
3. As a nurse, which persons must you be particularly concerned about when they are potential subjects in research? Why?
4. Discuss how you would feel if you had been a subject in Milgram's experiment and the researcher fully "debriefed" you.
5. You are planning a research project on pain. The project has been approved and the adult subjects have been selected. To give full information about the project—special nursing care and a placebo versus routine nursing care and medication—would damage the validity of the findings. What should you do?
6. You are planning to conduct a study to determine by questionnaire the attitudes of nursing students toward abortion. Write a brief form that is usable for informed consent.
7. What is the role of a nurse who reads a research project that seems to be unethical?

REFERENCES AND SUGGESTED READINGS

Abdellah, F. (1967): Approaches to protecting the rights of human subjects. *Nursing Research 16*, 316–320. *Ethical values in nursing research.*

American Nurses' Association (1968): The nurse in research. ANA Guidelines on Ethical Values. *Nursing Research 17*, 104–107. (1975): Human Rights Guidelines for Nurses in Clinical and Other Research. Kansas City, Mo.: ANA. *Guidelines in nursing research.*

Annas, G. et al (1977): The Subject's Dilemma. Cambridge: Ballinger. *Includes research with children, prisoners, fetus. Describes efforts of legal system to deal with laws of informed consent.*

Arminger, B. (1977): Ethics of nursing research: profile, principles, perspective. *Nursing Research 26*, 330–336. *Research situations.*

Downs, F. (1967): Ethical inquiry in nursing research. *Nursing Forum 6*, 12–20. *Ethical aspects of nursing research.*

Gray, B. (1976): An assessment of institutional review committees in human experimentation. *Nursing Digest 4. The place of the institutional review committee.*

Hayter, J. (1979): Issues related to human subjects. In Downs, F. and Fleming, J., Issues in Nursing Research. New York: Appleton, pp. 107–147. *Examination of informed consent and other ethical issues.*

Jacobson, S. (1973): Ethical issues in experimentation with human subjects. *Nursing Forum 12, 58–71. Ethics in experimental research.*

National Institute of Health (1974): Research projects involving human subjects. *Guides for ethical research.*

Veatch, R. and Branson, R. (eds.) (1976): Ethics and Health Policy. Cambridge: Ballinger. *Examination of ethics, including informed consent bibliography.*

CHAPTER 6

A CRITICAL REVIEW OF THE LITERATURE

Review of the literature refers to an extensive, exhaustive, and systematic examination of publications relevant to the research project. *Critical review* refers to the examination of the strengths and weaknesses of appropriate publications. The review of the literature is usually divided into two parts: first, the student locates as many of the important publications as feasible; then the student reviews critically those publications of particular significance to the project.

Upon completion of this chapter, the student should be able to: 1) state reasons why a review of the literature is an essential part of every research project; 2) describe how to conduct a literature review; 3) state how to identify and summarize pertinent publications; 4) describe how to conduct a critical review of the research literature; and 5) criticize the structure and content of the research report when it is written.

THE LITERATURE REVIEW: AN ESSENTIAL PART OF EVERY RESEARCH PROJECT

The review of the literature is an essential part of every research project for many reasons: First, the student is able to determine the extent to which theory and research are developed in the field under study, the opposing theoretical perspectives, and the research that supports or does not support opposing perspectives. Second, the student can identify the definition of concepts and variables already established in the literature and examine elements of research used by others, such as designs, methods, scales, instruments, measures, and techniques of data analysis that may prove useful in the proposed project. Third, the student can discover what is known and what remains to be learned in the field, and may identify a study that can be replicated or whose findings may be compared and contrasted with the proposed study. Fourth, the student may become aware of difficulties experienced by others, which may save time, money, and error, and may identify ethical problems. Finally, the student may find a research report that is so well structured and easy to read that it will be useful as a guide in writing the research report.

THE PRELIMINARY REVIEW OF THE LITERATURE

The first stage of the review of the literature is a general, preliminary search that attempts to locate all pertinent publications for a quick perusal. The second stage is a more critical review of the major works to identify the merits, strengths, weaknesses, and shortcomings of each. As the researcher gains experience, he or she may conduct a critical review as a part of the preliminary review, and may immediately discard publications that do not meet standards. A review of the literature may precede, accompany, or follow the initial formulation of the research proposal. The student may go to the literature first, write a tentative proposal, and then examine the literature; or the student may have a research report in hand, formulate an initial research proposal, and then conduct a more intensive search of the literature. The two processes work intimately together, each influencing the other.

The preliminary review generally includes three steps: 1) to identify and locate important publications; 2) to summarize and record the content of publications; and 3) to compare related elements, such as the theoretical perspective, definitions, research designs, methods, instruments, and findings. Each of these will be examined.

Identification of Important Publications

The first step in the preliminary review of the literature is to identify what has been published in the field, when, and by whom. The best place to begin is with the most recent publications. These often summarize and criticize earlier work, report contemporary research, and provide bibliographies for further perusal. The most recent publications are found in journals, since articles can be written and published well in advance of books. Such publications may be located in two ways: by a computer search of the literature provided by most health science libraries, and by a manual search of the local library.

The most rapid access to citations from current journals is obtained by a computer search of the literature. *MEDLARS*—medical literature analysis and retrieval system—is designed to achieve rapid access via the computer-based bibliographic processing system to hundreds of thousands of journals in the National Library of Medicine, in Bethesda, Maryland. *MEDLINE*—an "on-line" computer search—provides immediate if limited references, while the more extensive "off-line" searches are more expensive and slower, being sent by mail. Other acronyms designed to refer to specific subject areas include *CATLINE*, which provides a list of books on the proposed topic; *CANCERLINE*, which provides literature on cancer; *SOCIAL SCISEARCH*, corresponding to the publication *Social Science Citations Index*; *SOCABS*, corresponding to *Sociological Abstracts*; *SCISEARCH*, corresponding to *Science Citations Index*; *ERIC*, corresponding to *Current Index to Journals in Education*; and many others that the librarian can explain.

The researcher should begin a computer search by conferring with the librarian designated to work in these areas who will explain how the request for literature review is matched against the citations in a particular data base, and the mechanics involved in making a request for information. The steps are simple but important: First, the researcher states the information completely and accurately, using the terms from *MeSH*, the medical subject headings. Next, the researcher manually searches the *Index Medicus* to identify publications whose bibliographies may be helpful. Third, the researcher carefully completes any further information required by the library.

MEDLARS and *MEDLINE* provide access to journals but not books. A search of journals over the past two to three years is sufficient in most cases, although the data base dates back to 1963. The system is programmed to subjects, not authors. Authors, like books, theses, PhD dissertations, and technical reports, require a manual search. *MEDLARS* is especially useful to coordinate several related subjects and to find citations on a single subject. It is important to note that precise information is required. Due to vague or improperly stated requests, many researchers have obtained long lists of citations not pertinent to their work. Consultation with the librarian in the beginning saves later frustration, especially when the researcher is pressed for time. "Off-line" requests may take more than a week to process and mail.

Manual searches to identify relevant publications include an examination of the card catalog, indexes, abstracts, and various reference sources. It is helpful to begin a manual search by first consulting with the librarian, who will help familiarize the researcher with both the physical plan of the library and the resources available. The librarian will expedite the manual search within the local library and will arrange for an interlibrary loan of materials that the local library does not have.

The card catalog is an alphabetical arrangement of all the publications held by a particular library. The catalog includes authors, subject headings, and publication titles. Authors are filed by surname, in alphabetical order, and by given name, where a number of surnames such as *Smith* are the same. When searching the card catalog, it is wise to have the author's complete name. Titles are filed by the first word, unless the first word is an article such as *the* or *an*, in which case the second word of the title is used. To locate publications by subject, the researcher begins with the broad heading such as *Nursing* and then looks for subcategories under the general term. Information on the card that helps identify pertinent work includes dates and places of publication, publisher, cross-references, number of pages, and call number. The call number is used to locate the book physically in the library. Two systems of call numbers are used: the *Dewey Decimal System* (numbers only), and the *Library of Congress System* (letters and numbers). To find materials not listed in the card catalog, the researcher turns to indexes, abstracts, directories, and bibliographies.

An index is a list of books and articles about topics; likewise, it is the list of authors and subjects commonly found in the back of a book. Nursing indexes include the *Nursing Studies Index*, by Virginia Henderson et al, a four-volume annotated index that lists all studies reported from 1900–1959. *The Cumulative Index to Nursing Literature* reports work from 1956 forward, while the *International Nursing Index* includes worldwide nursing literature from 1966 forward. Other indexes are published by various journals, such as *Nursing Research, Nursing Outlook,* and the *American Journal of Nursing*. The journal indexes are both annual and cumulative, combining subject and author listings. Other useful indexes are the monthly *Index Medicus*, whose January issue lists Medical Subjects Headings by name of article, author, and date; the *Abridged Index Medicus;* the *Science Citation Index,* which lists an author followed by those citing the author; and the *Hospital Literature Index*.

Abstracts are short statements giving the main ideas of an article or book. These have appeared in *Nursing Research* since 1959, the articles being classified by both author and subject headings. "Abstracts of Studies in Public Health Nursing 1924–1965" appears in *Nursing Research* (Spring 1959, p. 45–115), listing monographs and articles from twenty-one periodicals. Other abstracts may be found in *Excerpta Medica, Psychological Abstracts,* and *Sociological Abstracts*.

References sources for nurses are found in *Nursing Outlook* (May 1972, "Reference Sources for Nurses", p. 338–343) and in *Canadian Nursing* (March 1972, "Information Resources for Nursing Research", p. 40–43). Other useful reference works include Blake's and Roos's (eds.), *Medical Reference Works* (1967), and Gates's *Guide to the Use of Books and Libraries* (1969).

Once a list of useful books and articles is in hand, a search is made to locate and scrutinize these. It is always desirable to use primary sources whenever possible. *Primary sources* are first-hand accounts of events, such as diaries, patient charts, letters, eyewitness accounts, journals, autobiographies, research reports, and information collected by interview and questionnaire. *Secondary sources* are second-hand accounts, such as histories, biographies, textbooks, and other materials that give secondary analysis of the data found in primary records. The careful researcher never relies solely on secondary sources, although these often furnish valuable leads to primary work. If possible, the researcher reviews the primary work, in order to judge and analyze the data. The use of primary sources acts as a check against errors that may have crept into a secondary source and been perpetuated by dependence upon these sources alone.

Books and articles not available in the local libraries may often be obtained by interlibrary loan. However, requests should be made early, since the process tends to be slow and the time available to scrutinize these sources is limited.

The amount of time spent in the preliminary search of the literature varies according to the nature of the research study, the amount of material available, and the length of time that may reasonably be allocated to the search. For a circumscribed study of one year, four weeks may be all of the time available for both the preliminary search and the critical review of the literature. Such limitations should be kept clearly in mind, since it is easy to be led into interesting by-paths not strictly related to the research question.

Summarizing and Recording

Once the researcher identifies and locates the pertinent literature, then he or she makes a record of the sources studied and summarizes the pertinent information found in each. A systematic procedure for recording the information pays dividends in the long run, although it is a rare researcher that does not resort to scribbling on scraps of paper from time to time, only to regret it later when the scraps have disappeared.

The most common and useful method for recording bibliographical information is to write the complete information for each publication on a separate 3 × 5 card. Information should include 1) the surname of the author or authors, followed by the complete given name; 2) the complete title and subtitle of the book or article; 3) the date, publisher, place of publication, and edition; 4) the journal in which the article appears, date in detail, and pages of the article; 5) the bibliography or index, whether or not it is present and extensive; and 6) the call number of the local library (a time saver when the book must be checked in and out). The bibliography cards should be kept in alphabetical order, in a permanent file specifically for that purpose. It will then be available as a ready source to cite relevant work in the body of the research report, as well as in the final bibliography. It is also a resource that will grow over the years, as the researcher records new publications.

An orderly system must be devised for recording the substance of an article or book. A number of ways are useful, and individuals often devise their own unique system. The long-term benefits of establishing a concise yet flexible system are considerable. An author of many books and publications suggests the following system.* Obtain a number of 3 × 5 slips of pastel-colored paper and/or mark a number of 3 × 5 cards with a color code in the upper-right-hand corner, such as orange, blue, and green. Use the pale orange slips or cards marked with an orange marker only for direct quotes from the literature. When definitions of concepts are used or specific hypotheses are noted direct quotes are especially necessary. Use blue slips to summarize information directly from an article or book, without criticism or comment. Use green slips to record insight, ideas, or criticism of the publications (such original thoughts are often lost unless immediately documented). Use white slips for other reseachers' criticisms of an article or book. This system is a fool-proof one for avoiding the dangers of plagiarism, for separating the content of the book or article from the reader's opinion, and for preserving the insight and ideas of the reader.

Prepared index cards for literature reviews are also available from commercial sources. These cards have rows of holes around the edges, which may be coded and notched. Together with more complex coding schemes, these may be developed if the project is an extensive one and the publications are numerous and broad. The most important approach is an orderly and systematic one that summarizes an article or book with the same format each time. This enables the researcher to make quick comparisons. The following system may be helpful:

1. To select a pertinent book or article from a general review of the literature, examine the book or article quickly. For a book, examine the title page that gives the author's credentials; then scan

---

*Personal advice from Professor Edgar Thompson of Duke University.

the table of contents, the index, the bibliography, and the charts and tables. Read the preface rapidly to determine the author's purpose; then thumb through the chapters quickly to assess substance. If the book is promising, keep it for a critical review. For an article, examine the author's credentials, quickly scan the problem statement and the hypotheses, and then focus on the methods of research used, especially how the sample was selected and the data analyzed. Read conclusions and summaries, and note the use of theory and other research studies. Retain sound and pertinent literature for summary and critique.

2. To summarize and record information, first note the author, title of article, and year of publication. If further information is needed, this immediately refers the reader to the bibliography card.

3. Record information from a research report in the following order: 1) problem statement; 2) definition of concepts (direct quotes on orange-coded slips or cards); 3) hypotheses, if any; 4) theories or assumptions used; 5) method of research, including how the sample was drawn; 6) instruments and scales used; 7) type of research (descriptive or explanatory); 8) methods and findings of data analysis; 9) interpretation of data, especially whether hypotheses were supported or rejected; and 10) recommendations and suggestions for further research, if any. Make special note of implications for nursing practice or theory.

4. Note data that was *not* included, such as limitations that were not noted, means of establishing the validity and reliability of instruments that was not given; theory that was not used, or former studies that were not examined.

Comparison of Content

Upon completion of the summaries, the student can compare the different approaches of the individual scientists to the same problem. The definition of concepts, for example, not only reveals the degree of consenses among nursing scholars, but at the same time enables the student to document the source of his or her own definitions. A comparison of the theory utilized helps uncover competing theories used to explain the same phenomenon—information the student can include in his or her own review of the literature. Research reports in addition cite previous studies which support (or do not support) the selected theory and derived hypotheses.

A comparison of research designs allows the student to consider whether a survey (questionnaire or interview), a record review (historical or documentary approach) or an experiment is most suitable for the student's proposed project. Comparing the different designs also allows the student to compare the research method used to collect data—observation, questioning, measuring, or a combination of these. In addition the student may find valid instruments and techniques of data analysis helpful in the proposed project. Data summaries from similar studies may provide a basis for the student to compare findings from the proposed research project.

Finally, the student may find a study that seems appropriate to replicate—a considerable saving in time and effort. Replication has the added virtue of increasing the depth of research in a particular area of nursing.

HOW TO CRITICIZE A RESEARCH REPORT

As students complete the preliminary review of the literature, they become aware of differences among the research reports—of both the merits and the shortcomings. Such evaluations, or critical reviews, allow the student to assess the strong and weak elements of others' research, thereby aiding his or her own critical examination.

While expertise in evaluation comes with experience, a number of scholars (Fleming and Hayter 1974; Fox 1976; Downs and Newman 1977; Polit and Hungler 1978) suggest guidelines which assist the beginning researcher's evaluation of research reports.

Evaluation is made of both the structure—how the report is put together and organized—as well as the content, the sum and substance of the research. Both the structure and content of a research report depend to some extent upon the experience and qualifications of the author as well as upon the nature of the research. For example, pioneering research differs from research which replicates an established study.

Evaluating the Qualifications of the Author

Brief biographical material often accompanies research reports and books. This information assists the student in judging the qualifications of the author. It is not realistic to expect the same kind of research from a beginner that one expects from an experienced professional engaged in a long-term research project. The reader, therefore, needs to evaluate both the qualifications of the author as well as the nature of the research reported. A beginning researcher who designs a simple, yet important, project should receive higher marks than one who chooses a problem that is either too large or too complex.

The Structure of the Report

The way the report is organized may vary from one researcher to the next. However, in all cases the organization should be logical. It should begin with a clear identification of what is to be studied and how, and end with a summary or conclusion recommending further study or application. Often the report follows the sequence of steps taken in planning the research, and collecting and analyzing the data. The researcher adds the final steps (summary, conclusions, and recommendations) after interpreting the data analysis in the light of the objectives, theoretical framework selected, and hypotheses. The structure of the report, therefore, is evaluated on the basis of its logical flow. Since the logic of the structure is intimately related in many cases to the content of the report, the content and structure are often evaluated together.

Criticizing the Introduction to the Research Report

The purpose of the introduction is to inform the reader what was studied and why the topic is important to nursing. The general area of study should be focused on a specific problem that is feasible, related to available data, and ethically appropriate. The statement which informs the reader precisely what the researcher had proposed to do (and did) is evaluated on the basis of its clarity, conciseness and comprehensiveness. The statement describes what was studied and how; who was studied—the target population—and how the sample was obtained from the population; and when and where the study took place. The purpose of the study—observation in order to know, predict, control, explain, or practice—often follows.

The introduction may also include the definitions of the concepts used in the research statement, the objectives of the study, the hypotheses, the assumptions, and the limitations of the study. The author may place these separately immediately following the introduction.

The reader evaluates the concepts on the basis of their definition. The definition must be clear and appropriate, and be rooted in the literature. The definition of variables is judged on the basis of the clearly designated dependent and independent variables, and the operational definitions defining the variables by denoting the observable, measurable phenomena which make the variable visible.

The reader evaluates the objectives on the basis of their ability to communicate the intent of the researcher, whether to inform (define, identify, name); to analyze (compare, contrast, distinguish); to classify (organize, systematize); or interpret (differentiate, discriminate, explain). The objectives are judged on the basis of their ability to denote measurable attributes of the study while the author is evaluated on the basis of how well he or she met the objectives.

Hypotheses are evaluated on the basis of: 1) a clear prediction of the relationship between its variables; 2) the clarity and conciseness of each statement; 3) the identification of the independent and dependent variables; 5) the theory or previous research to which it was related; 6) its relationship with the author's research statement; and 7) whether the author reached definite conclusions on each.

The assumptions are evaluated on whether they are based on the opinion of experts, previous research reports, or theory. The reader evaluates the assumptions in terms of their foundations. Limitations, aspects of the research which were not studied, are evaluated on the ability of the author to recognize factors which limit the applicability of the research findings.

Evaluating the Review of the Literature
The review of the literature is judged on the basis of its organization, comprehensiveness, and summary of opposing theory and research findings. The reader should also judge the extent to which the author used primary sources. The author is likewise evaluated on the basis of his or her grasp of the breadth and depth of the literature review pertinent to the problem under study.

Judging the Research Design
The research design is evaluated on the basis of its appropriateness. An experimental design should include methods of sampling, control, and manipulation. The reader evaluates the survey design according to the method used to select the sample, the worth of the instruments used, the ethical implications of the study, and the quantity and quality of response. A study of records and documents (historical design) is evaluated on several bases: 1) the accuracy of the records—whether the recorder was willing and able to write observations accurately; 2) the completeness of the records—whether any records were lost or destroyed; and 3) access to the records—the extent to which the author had full entrance to records. Historical research is open to more interpretation than any other type of research. Therefore the reputation and credentials of the author should be carefully evaluated.

Evaluating Research Methods
The research methods are the means by which the author collects research data from the study sample. Research methods include either observation, measurement, questioning, or all of these. "Sampling" is the method where the study subjects were selected from the target population. Sampling is a critical aspect of research determining the

extent the study sample data may be generalized to the larger population. The data-collection methods and the sample-selection methods must each be carefully evaluated.

Observing. The author should make it clear whether he or she was a participant observer or a nonparticipant observer, and whether or not he or she was the sole observer. The author who relies upon personal observations must be judged on how well he or she defined what was to be observed, made objective rather than subjective observations, and related the observations to his or her research project. The author must reveal whether the subjects being studied were informed or whether concealment was used. The latter suggests ethical implications which must be judged. The author who was assisted by other observers must document how these were trained. The reader must also assess the adequacy of the training. Finally, a judgment of the biases introduced by the human observer must be made including both the selective attention of the observer and the effect of observation on those observed.

Measuring. An evaluation of measurement is often a complex task since the reader must judge whether the correct instrument was used in the measurement and whether the author measured what should have been measured to answer the research question. One group of researchers (Johnson et al, 1977, pp. 33–44), for example, wanted to measure children's distress behavior during orthopedic cast removal. She used pulse rate, verbal and nonverbal behavior as measures of distress. The reader must judge whether these factors do indeed measure distress and if this is what should have been measured.

In addition, the reader must evaluate attitude scales, questionnaires, and interview schedules used by the author. Since these rarely accompany research reports, the reader must rely on the author to report how it was determined that these were good measures. Physiological instruments such as the sphygmomanometer, thermometer, and scales which weigh pounds and ounces are more familiar measures, but the author should report how it was determined such measures were accurate. The reader should expect the author to give a clear description of the instrument, report whether the instrument had been tested, and describe how the instrument was used. The reader should also evaluate the use of the subject's time in conjunction with a particular instrument—both the merits of the instrument and the amount of time required from the subjects should be clearly reported. Failure of the author to describe instruments and explain how and why each was used (and pretested) marks the study as ineffective.

Questioning. Asking questions directly by interview or indirectly by questionnaire is a common way to collect data. Questioning is evaluated in terms of the instruments used (the questionnaire and interview schedule) which should be described by the author if not included with the report. If interviews are used, the author should report how interviewers were trained. If questionnaires were used the author should report the number returned and the extent to which all questions were answered. Subjects who refused to participate should also be noted.

Sampling. These procedures are critical for evaluating the extent the research findings can be applied in general or only in reference to the small sample studied. The author must have chosen the sample by a scientific process such as random sampling (each unit in the target population is given an equal chance of being chosen) in order to be assured that the sample represents the population. Therefore, the procedures for selecting the sample of study subjects should be carefully described, as should the size and characteristics of the sample. Failure to report sampling procedures greatly weakens any research report.

Criticism of the Analysis and Interpretation of Data

The analysis of data is dependent upon all that has gone on before: how the sample was drawn, the use of controls, the type of scale utilized, whether hypotheses were supported and objectives met. The reader judges whether the author has included: 1) a complete discussion of the data; 2) a thorough examination of each hypothesis including the use of appropriate statistical analysis and the decision to accept or reject the hypothesis; 3) an explanation of how missing data were handled; 4) presentation of data in tables and graphs together with a description of each table and graph; and 5) the use of experts where needed to assist in the analysis of data.

The reader must judge whether the author interpreted the data properly. Each hypothesis or objective should be discussed in the light of research findings reported in the review of the literature. The author should make clear whether the findings of their study agree or disagree with previous reports. The author should also state which relationships have been illuminated by the study and report how much their findings can be generalized.

In addition, the reader judges the author on the report's relevance to nursing. The significance of the study should be clear, and the author should likewise suggest what further research needs to be conducted.

Evaluation of the Bibliography, Abstract, and Writing Style

The bibliography reflects the review of the literature, the search for valid and reliable instruments, definitions of concepts, formulation of the research statement, the objectives, the hypotheses, and any other material used in the content. Each reference cited in the body of the report should be included in the bibliography. The bibliography should be presented in a consistent and acceptable form, and if time and space allow, annotations should be included. If appendices are used, these should be concise, complete, and well organized.

The abstract, a brief summary of the research article, is often required for publication. The abstract should clearly describe what was studied, how it was studied, how the sample was drawn, how the data were analyzed, and the findings of the research. The abstract needs to be one concise paragraph.

The reader should also judge the writing style of the author. If the research has considerable merit but the writing style is poor, the labor and care of the project may be all but lost. However, criticism of the writing style should not be confused with criticism of the research itself. Effective communication of research depends upon the author's ability to organize as well as write clearly and objectively.

SUMMARY

Review of the literature refers to an extensive, exhaustive, and systematic examinaton of publications relevant to the research project. Critical review refers to the process by which the student examines the strengths and weaknesses of appropriate publications. The student must first locate important publications and then review these critically.

Review of the literature is necessary for the following reasons: to determine how well theory and research are developed in the field of study; to define concepts; to examine research designs, methods, scales, instruments, measures, and techniques of data analysis used by others; to identify a study for replication or comparison; to examine difficulties reported by others; to define ethical implications of similar studies; and to identify a guide to use in writing the research report.

The preliminary review consists of three steps: 1) to identify and obtain important publications; 2) to summarize and record relevant contents; 3) to compare what is reported in publications.

Identification of important publications begins with the most recent publication in journals. The most rapid access to journal citations is by computer search such as MEDLARS or MEDLINE. Other acronyms such as CATLINE refer to specific subject area in published articles. Manual search of card catalogs, indices, abstracts, and reference sources is necessary to obtain other literature such as books.

The researcher must devise an orderly system to summarize and record contents of the literature. Bibliographical cards are essential and may be supplemented by various systems of color coding to identify direct quotes, the researcher's own words and insights, and criticism of the publications.

Comparison of the recorded summaries of the literature enables the researcher to: contrast definitions of concepts, uncover competing theories used to explain the same phenomenon, consider the various designs that have been utilized to study the same problem, examine different methods of data collection, and find valid instruments already developed.

A criticism of publications entails evaluating the following: the qualification of the author to undertake the research, the logical structure of the report, and the extent to which the introduction informs the reader of what the author has studied—the problem, definition of concepts, objectives, hypotheses, variables, operational definitions, assumptions, and theoretical perspective. Criticism of the publication includes a judgment of how well the author has reviewed the literature—both the comprehensiveness and the types of publications used, whether primary or secondary sources. The criticism of the publication also involves judging the research design, whether it is appropriate for the study; judging the research methods, whether the method of sampling allows the author to generalize his or her findings; and judging whether the method of data collecting was ethical and proper. A criticism of the analysis and interpretation of data includes a judgment of whether the author has completely discussed the data, tested the hypotheses, presented the data in tables and graphs, used experts to assist where necessary, and explained how missing data were handled. An evaluation of the data interpretation involves a judgment of how the author compared his or her findings to others in the literature; generalized from the sample to the target population properly; examined his or her own weaknesses and strengths, and reported limitations; suggested implications for nursing; and recommended application in practice or further research.

A criticism of the bibliography involves an examination of the extent and date of the publications and whether all works cited in the report were included in the bibliography. The reader must likewise judge whether the abstract is clear and succinct, and if the writing style is well organized and objective.

STUDY QUESTIONS

1. Discuss the reasons for beginning a research project with a review of the literature.
2. What is the meaning of a critical review of the literature?
3. What does MEDLARS mean? How is it used? If available, examine library resources.
4. Select two articles related to your research proposal or a nursing problem in which you are interested. Summarize the problem statement, the research proposal, objectives if any, hypotheses if any, methods of data collection, findings of the study, implicatons for nursing, and suggestions for further research. Does the article include a bibliography of current publications?
5. Visit your library and locate the card catalog, indexes and abstracts in nursing, and discuss how to arrange inter-library loans. Find out how to utilize other resources with the librarian.
6. Select an article from *Nursing Research* to criticize, noting both strengths and weaknesses.
7. Begin a bibliography of your own.

SELECTED SOURCES OF RESEARCH IN NURSING AND ALLIED FIELDS

I. **Journals which publish reports of nursing and related research include:**
Administrative Science Quarterly
Advances in Nursing Science
American Journal of Public Health
American Sociological Review
Current Anthropology
Hospitals (Journal of the American Hospital Association)
Hospital Progress
International Nursing Review
Journal of Advanced Nursing
Journal of Gerontologic Nursing
Journal of Nurse-Midwifery
Journal of Nursing Education
Journal of Obstetric Gynecologic and Neonatal Nursing
Medical Care
Modern Hospital
Nursing Clinics of North America

Nursing Dimension
Nursing Forum
Nursing Outlook
Nursing Research
Nursing Science
Public Health Reports
Research in Nursing and Health
The American Journal of Maternal Child Health
The American Journal of Nursing
Western Journal of Nursing Research

II. **Abstracts and excerpts include the following:**
Abstracts on hospital management studies. *Quarterly Index,* University of Michigan. Available on request beginning with Vol. 1, No. 1, Sept. 1964.
Abstracts of studies in public health nursing 1924–1957. *Nursing Research* 8:45–115, Spring 1959.
Basic Reference Aids for Small Medical Libraries

III. **Bibliographies useful in nursing research include:**
Bio-bibliography of Florence Nightingale; Bishop and Goldie, International Council of Nurses, 1962.
Bibliographies of Nursing prepared for and published by the N.L.N. 1957, 14 volumes; now out of print.
Medical Behavioral Science published and distributed by the University of Kentucky Press, Lexington, 1963. Contains a selected bibliography of cultural anthropology, social psychology, and sociology in medicine.
Reference Tools for Nursing is a selected classified list of books, pamphlets, and periodicals prepared by Inter-agency Council for Library Tools for Nursing, 1964.

IV. **Dictionaries:** *American Nurses Dictionary.* Philadelphia: W. B. Saunders, 1949.

V. **Encyclopedias:** *The Encyclopedia of Nursing.* Philadelphia: W. B. Saunders, 1952 prepared under the supervision of Lucile Petry. Terms used in nursing texts analyzed.

VI. **Guides to Library Resources:** Strauch, K. and Brundage, D. *Guide to Library Resources for Nursing,* New York: Appleton, 1980. Includes annotated listings of publications in nursing, and library information.

VII. **Handbooks:** *Library Handbook for Schools of Nursing,* 1953; N.L.N.E. Makes recommendations on organizing and administering a nursing library.

VIII. **Indexes**
American Journal of Nursing: Annual and Cumulative Indexes. Combined subject and author listings since 1900.
Card catalog of the library books.
Cumulative Index to Nursing Literature, subject and author guide to 54 periodicals in nursing and related fields since 1956.

National Library of Medicine: nursing, hospital, books, studies, and technical reports.

Nursing Outlook: Annual and Cumulative Indexes, combined subject and author listing since 1952.

Nursing Research: Annual and cumulative Indexes combined subject and author listing.

Nursing Studies Index, edited by Henderson, V. Philadelphia: J. B. Lippincott, 1963. Annotated guide to reported studies. Four volumes.

Public Health Nursing, an index to ANA and NLN publications, government publications, pamphlets and book reviews.

Research Grants Index, yearly report by the Division of Research Grants describes current research projects being conducted under Public Health Service by subject matter, name and address or principle investigator.

International Nursing Index includes world wide nursing literature from 1966.

IX. **Inventories and Lists**

Clearing House List of Studies in Nursing since 1955 by ANA.

The Nation's Nurses by Marshall and Moses, New York; ANA 1965.

History of Nursing Source Book, New York: G. P. Putnam's Sons, 1957; gives excerpts from writings on nursing from Biblical times.

Nursing Research: A Survey and Assessment by Simmons, L. and Henderson, V. New York: Appleton, 1964. Describes the beginnings of nursing research, directions, and forces impeding or promoting development.

Inventory of Social and Economic Research in Health published annually by Health Information Foundation, Chicago.

X. **Statistical Guides**

Facts About Nursing published annually by the ANA since 1935.

Statistical Abstract of the United States, published annually by the Government Printing Office, Washington, D.C.

XI. **Yearbooks**

The Yearbook of Modern Nursing edited by Conway. New York: G. P. Putnam's Sons, 1959. Reviews literature on nursing trends, education, research, practice.

REFERENCES AND SUGGESTED READINGS

Downs, F. and Newman, M. (1977). Elements of a research critique. In Downs, F. and Newman, M. *A Sourcebook of Nursing Research* (2nd ed.). Philadelphia: F. A. Davis pp. 1–15.

Fleming, J. and Hayter, J. (1974): Reading research reports critically. *Nursing Outlook* 22, 172–176.

Fox, D. (1976): Fundamentals of Research Nursing, (3rd ed.). New York: Appleton pp. 27–30.

Johnson, J. et al (1977): Altering children's distress behavior during orthopedic cast removal. In Downs, F. and Newman, M. *A Sourcebook of Nursing Research* (2nd ed.). Philadelphia: F. A. Davis pp. 33–45.

Leininger, M. (1968): The research critique: nature, function and art. Batey, M. (ed.), *Communication Nursing Research: The Research Critique.* Boulder: WICHE, pp. 21–23.

Polit, D. and Hungler, B. (1978): Nursing Research: Principles and Methods. New York: J. B. Lippincott Co. *Chapter 5 deals with locating and summarizing information.*

Stetler, C. and Marram, G. (1976): Evaluating research findings for applicability in practice. *Nursing Outlook 24,* 559–563.

Treece, E. and Treece, J. (1977): Elements of Research in Nursing (2nd ed.). St. Louis: C. V. Mosby. Chapter 7 "The Library Search."

Walizer, M. and Wienir, P. (1978): Research Methods and Analysis. New York: Harper and Row, pp. 136–150.

PART 3
Theory and Sampling

CHAPTER 7
Theory in Nursing Research

CHAPTER 8
Sampling

CHAPTER 7

THEORY IN NURSING RESEARCH

A *theory* is an explanation for the interrelations among facts, concepts, or propositions. A theory summarizes what is known from past work and predicts what will be found on future observation. The student uses theory in research to provide a framework constructed from past ideas, understandings, and research findings, and to provide a foundation for the proposed research project. The student also uses theory to generate hypotheses that predict what will be found when data are collected and analyzed. The theoretical framework—the set of interrelated concepts and definitions—enables the student to contribute the findings of even a small project to the larger theoretical perspective that uses the same theoretical frame of reference.

The student identifies the theoretical framework to be used in the research project from an early review of the literature. However, the search for pertinent theories soon leads to the discovery that nursing lies at the theoretical crossroads of many disciplines. The challenge to the student is to determine which of these best explains the problem to be studied, and which lends itself to research.

Upon completion of this chapter, the student should be able to: 1) identify some of the major theories reported in the nursing research literature; 2) describe what the theory is explaining or predicting; 3) report nursing research that has used various theories; and 4) describe an approach to the construction of nursing theory.

The primary purposes of the chapter are to enable the student to select a theoretical framework useful in the proposed research project and to help the student identify theoretical frameworks used in published nursing research reports.

MAJOR THEORIES REPORTED IN THE NURSING RESEARCH LITERATURE

Too many theories are reported in the nursing literature to examine in the space of one chapter. However, a number of the theories tend to fall into several categories: 1) learning theory; 2) development theory; 3) theories of adaptation, stress, and homeostasis; 4) systems theory; 5) social theories; and 6) cultural theories.

Learning theory includes theories of conditioning, social learning, and Gestalt, or cognitive, theory. Developmental theory examines changes that occur through time in the physical, mental, psychological, and social structures. Theories of adaptation, stress, and homeostasis examine how individuals or groups survive and function in a particular environment. Systems theory is diverse, focusing at times on behavioral systems and at other times on systems of interaction and communication, or adaptation modes. Social theories examine factors that are external to individuals, such as social class, but that affect their life chances and life-styles. Theories of symbolic interaction, such as role theory, seek to explain how symbols and meanings establish the rules, roles, and images of self and others in daily life. Cultural theories examine how traditional ways of life affect the behavior, values, beliefs, and perceptions of individuals and groups. Each of these will be examined briefly to identify their major concepts and to note nursing research that has used such theories to develop hypotheses or to select what will be observed.

LEARNING THEORY

A major concern of nursing is learning, a process in which past experience or practice results in a lasting change in behavior, motivation, or perception. The predominant sources of learning theory are: 1) behaviorism, rooted in the conditioning theory developed by Pavlov and modified by Skinner and others; and 2) the cognitive theory of learning proposed by *Gestalt* psychologists and modified by Piaget, Festinger, and others.

Conditioning

The theory of classical conditioning was developed by Pavlov (1928), who studied the effect of imposed learning upon innate reflexes. Pavlov used the instinctive behavior of hungry dogs to salivate when presented with food to teach the dogs to salivate when they heard a buzzer. He accomplished this conditioning by introducing the sound of a buzzer together with the presentation of food. Salivation, an unconditioned response, came to be associated with the sound of a buzzer, the conditioned stimulus. Learning took place when the stimulus known to produce a response was presented along with a new stimulus that the researcher wanted the subject to learn to associate with the response. The process was repeated over and over until the response was elicited from the new stimulus alone. Thus, the stimulus-response conditioning theory of learning was launched. *Stimulus* is broadly defined as an external or internal event that brings about an alteration in behavior; *response* is the alteration in the behavior. The theory proposes that behavior can be explained and predicted by examining the relationship between stimuli and response.

Operant Conditioning: Behaviorism

The classical theory of conditioning was modified by Skinner and others, who examined the relationship between learning and the action of the individual upon the environment. *Operant*, or instrumental, conditioning proposes that learning occurs as the individual acts upon the environment to obtain a reward or to reduce tension. The reward increases the likelihood that the desired response will occur. *Behaviorism*, as this approach is called, rejects the unobservable completely and is concerned only with human behavior in terms of observable and measurable responses to stimuli. In this view, all behavior is conditioned by habit and can be learned or unlearned. Behavior results from the association learned when the response to a stimulus is reinforced by rewards or extinguished by punishment or failure to reward.

Derived from operant conditioning and a body of experimental work, behavior modification has been used by O'Neil (1972) and Rottkamp (1976), among others, to study the effect of stimuli on various health problems. O'Neil examined the effect of three types of reinforcement in teaching a child with cerebral palsy to walk. The study consisted of 240 sessions of approximately 30 minutes each. Reinforcement included social reinforcement (saying, "Good, Nancy, good"); material reinforcement (giving Nancy marbles to play with); and food reinforcement (spoonsful of ice cream). Results showed the behavior modification techniques were effective in teaching Nancy to crutchwalk.

Rottkamp studied the effect of demonstration, shaping of body positions, and social reinforcement (attention from the nurse) on patients with spinal cord injuries to improve their performance in body positioning. The experimental group of patients who received the behavior modification techniques showed a greater difference in the frequency of patient-initiated changes of body position than did patients who did not receive the behavior modification techniques. Rottkamp drew on stimulus-response theory to formulate her hypothesis that spinal-cord-injured patients with impairment in body-position behaviors would improve in their body-positioning performance to a measurable degree, after receiving demonstration, shaping, and positive social reinforcement.

Operant conditioning principles have also been used to modify incontinence in neuro-psychiatric geriatric patients (Grosicki, 1968), and to teach self-help activity to the profoundly retarded (Bensberg et al, 1965).

Social Learning

Theories of social learning are closely associated with the stimulus-response-reinforcement theory of learning but place emphasis on the social elements such as the process of imitation and identification, or the "locus of control" concept developed by Rotter (1972). *Locus of control* refers to the extent to which individuals believe that people in general have control over their own destiny and understand why they behave as they do.

Holaday (1974) used Rotter's theory to explain the perception and behavior of twenty-four chronically ill children. She found that the chronically ill children tended to view the success or failure of their achievement efforts as external, that is, as due to luck or to others. Windwer (1977) examined the relationship among locus of control, social desirability, and the psychoprophylaxis method of childbirth. Six hypotheses were formulated for study, none of which were supported. Lowery and DuCette (1976) examined the relationship between locus of control and patients' response to diabetes. Patients who viewed the locus of control as external were found to have less diabetic information but fewer diabetic problems over time, whereas patients who viewed the locus of control as internal had more information but showed no decrease in the number of diabetic problems.

Gestalt and Cognitive Theories of Learning

Gestalt is a German world that means form or pattern. A basic assumption of this approach is that the whole is greater than the sum of its parts. Learning occurs in the process of problem-solving. The learner identifies similar patterns or categories, recognizes the relationship between the categories through insight, and draws conclusions. The brain gives a cognitive structure to sensations and perceptions. The thoughts, attitudes, beliefs, and behaviors of which a person is cognitively aware—that is, *knows*—is a result of active problem-solving and goal-seeking activity. Behavior is not molded by stimuli, responses, and reinforcement alone but includes the process of knowing, learning, and thinking.

Small (1980) used Piaget's theory of sensorimotor cognitive development in her research on visually impaired children to assess the spatial awareness and perceived body image of these children compared with normally sighted children. The relation of objects in space and the development of *object permanence*—searching for lost or hidden objects because the child knows an unseen object is nonetheless permanent—are necessary small states for the development of the child's body image and awareness of the body and objects in the space surrounding the body. Small drew on the theory to develop hypotheses that predicted the relationship between being visually impaired and perceiving body images and spatial awareness. The findings revealed that there are overwhelming differences between the visually impaired child and the normally sighted child, in spatial awareness and in perceived body images.

Festinger (1957) developed a theory of cognitive dissonance that explains how a person may simultaneously possess two cognitions, one the opposite of the other, called *dissonance*. This arises after an attempt to elicit overt behavior that is at variance with private beliefs. The individual tries to establish internal consistency or harmony among personal beliefs and knowledge. Stillman (1977) used the theory to examine the relationship between beliefs and preventive health behavior. Findings indicate that women who believe themselves to be susceptible to breast cancer practice breast self-examination more often than women who do not perceive themselves to be highly susceptible.

DEVELOPMENTAL THEORY

Development theory examines changes that occur through time, first on one level and then on another. Piaget's cognitive theory is a developmental theory that suggests cognition proceeds through five phases, with a number of levels in each phase. The time span for the full development of formal operations is fifteen years. Freud's theory of personality development begins at birth and includes a number of parallel processes that continue over many years. Erikson's neo-Freudian theory of personality development incorporates the entire span of human life, as does Havighurst's tasks of development (see Table 7–1). Therefore, studies of development are constrained by time to examinations of segments of development.

TABLE 7–1. THEORIES OF DEVELOPMENTAL PHASES

Age in Years	Piaget (Cognitive)	Erikson (Personality)	Freud (Personality)		Havighurst's Tasks
0	Sensori-motor	Phase I: Basic	Oral Stage	ID	Learning:
1	Phase	Trust			to walk
					to talk
2			Anal Stage	Ego	to control body
3	Precon-ceptual	Phase II: Sense of	Phallic	Super-ego	sex differences
			Stage		simple concepts
4	Phase	Autonomy			to relate emotionally
					right from wrong
5	Intuitive Thought	Phase III: Sense of	Latency		to play
			Stage		games
6	Phase	Initiative			gender roles
					to read, write, calculate
7					Developing:
					concepts for living
8	Concrete Operations				morality, values
9	Phase	Phase IV: Sense of			attitudes
		Industry			Achieving:
10					personal independence
					peer-relationships with both
11			Genital		sexes
			Stage		sex roles
12	Phase of Formal				emotional independence
13	Operations	Phase V: Sense of			Accepting:
					the physical body
14		Identity			
					Preparing:
15					for a career
					for economic independence
16					for marriage and family
					for civic competence
17					socially responsible
					behavior
18					norms and values
					Selecting a mate
					Marriage and adjustment
		Phase VI:			Expanding a family
		Sense of Intimacy			Rearing a family
Adulthood		Sense of Generativity			Adjusting to middle and old
Late adulthood		Sense of Integrity			age

In order to examine how health habits change and what the child knew and used in everyday life, Aamodt (1972) investigated the perceptual or experiential history of Papago children. She looked for the cognitive cultural patterns of meaning that could be related to health and healing. The 13-month study led Aamodt to identify a number of themes centered upon the meaning of being a Papago and the meaning of sickness.

Although they are used less in research because of the time span necessary for observation, the concepts used in the developmental theory of Freud, Erikson et al have passed into nursing literature and practice.

A developmental theory that encompasses a shorter time span is that of Peplau (1952), who examined the development of interpersonal relations between nurse and patient. The roles of the patient and the nurse develop through four simultaneous but different phases. The patient enters the orientation phase, assessing the new environment. At this point, the nurse is in the assessment phase, listening as the patient expresses needs and feelings. In the second phase, identification, the patient feels a sense of belonging and identifies with the nurse, who is entering her second phase of identifying with the patient, making nursing diagnosis, and formulating nursing care plans.

In the third phase, exploitation, the patient has identified with a nurse and is now able to make use of the services offered, although mixed feelings of dependency and independency may occur. In this phase, the nurse takes steps to intervene to help both patient and nurse reach mutual goals and intended consequences.

In the last phase, resolution, the patient gains independence from the nurse. At this point, the nurse evaluates the growth that has occurred in both people.

The patient assumes various roles through the four phases, such as infant, child, adolescent, and adult. The nurses interacts with the patient by assuming reciprocal roles: mother surrogate, sibling surrogate, counselor, leader, resource person, and in the final phase, adult.

Using the case study method, Nordal and Sato (1980) studied the use of Peplau's model in clinical practice. Three cases were examined to investigate the developmental growth and maturity of both the patient and the nurse. Roy (1980) used the Peplau model to examine the interaction of a patient and nurse. She found both the patient and the nurse to be anxious and to feel threatened, with little development of therapeutic interpersonal relations.

Another developmental perspective was used by Robischon (1977) in her study of *pica*, the habitual ingestion of nonedible substances. The relationship between the development of behavior and the practice of pica was explored. Robischon found that hand-to-mouth behavior scores of motor development were lower among children who practiced pica.

THEORIES OF ADAPTATION, STRESS, AND HOMEOSTASIS

People adapting to the environment is a central theme in the work of nursing theorists such as Roy (1980) and Levine (1967), and is a factor in the work of King (1971), Neuman (1980), and others.

Adaptation is a process in which persons adjust in a particular environment in order to function and survive. Successful adaptors are those who survive and leave offspring to carry on the genetic and social characteristics that enabled survival. However, individuals who would have died in the past now survive and function. Phenylketonuria, an inborn error of metabolism, was formerly severely handicapping. If recognized early, it can now be successfully treated with special diet. The individual adapts to various stressors in the external and internal environment, using compensatory mechanisms in the physiological and psychosocial structures.

Stress, the tension resulting when changes occur in the physical and social environment, is a factor in all states of illness. The relationship between adaptation and stress has been explored by Selye (1956, 1976), who developed a theory to describe and explain the relationship. Selye defines *stress* as a state manifested by the "General Adaptation Syndrome." The syndrome evolves in three stages, as the body attempts to adapt to stressors. The first stage is alarm, arising when agents such as disease or injury call forth an increase in the vital activity of the body to resist. The second stage is resistance, marked by the full adaptation of the body to the stressor. The final stage is exhaustion, arising during the course of lengthy resistance to severe stressors. The body's energy is finite; therefore, if not reversed, this stage leads to death.

Adaptation and homeostasis are related in theories of equilibrium-disequilibrium. *Homeostasis,* a term coined by physiologist Walter Cannon (1939), means "staying the same." The process of homeostatic regulation involves the theory of a system maintained by negative feedback. Every deviation from the normal triggers a response to correct it (see Figure 7–1).

The simple system in the figure is maintained at a normal state through the process of negative feedback, which stimulates processes to remove excesses or deficiencies when these arise. Negative feedback systems are at work, both inside and outside the individual.

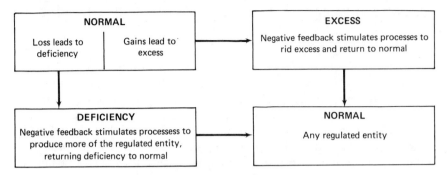

Figure 7–1. Model of homeostasis.

Roy (1980) develops her model of an adaptive system with reference to theories developed in psychology, sociology, and physiology. The person as a patient is viewed as being comprised of parts linked together. Strains may arise both within the linked system or from the external environment. The linked elements of the system include four subsystems: physiologic needs; self-concept; role function; and interdependence. The four subsystems function by adapting: The person adapts according to physiological need; the person adapts self-concept in interaction with others; the role is adapted in response to outside stimulation; and finally, the person adapts according to the subsystem of interdependence. The nurse's role is to act as an external regulator to modify adverse stimuli affecting adaptation.

DeWalt and Haines (1977) were interested in the effect of stressors on the human body and the function of nursing intervention to render the stressors less harmful. They examined the effects of specified local stressors, such as oral breathing, oxygen flow, and intermittent mechanical suction, on healthy oral mucosa. During the first stage, the alarm reaction, there was evidence of increased salivation and paling and drying of the mucosa. During the second stage, the adaptive reaction, decreased salivation and increased dryness of the mucosa was noticed, together with other signs. During the third stage, the exhaustive reaction, a numbness and loss of taste, and a breaking in the continuity of the lip mucosa was noted. Oral hygiene given twice during the fifth and final hours of the experiment seemed to minimize the effects of the stressors.

Downs (1977) studied the effects of stressful conditions on the newborn. Study subjects were women of low socioeconomic status. The data supported the contention that environmental stress was related to neonatal pathology.

SYSTEMS THEORY

A *system* is an organization of parts that are interrelated in such a manner that a change in one part brings about a change in all parts. A system constantly changes as it interacts with the external environment—adaptations and adjustments continuously occur, although these may be subtle and difficult to observe. A system differs from each of its parts and is greater than the sum of its parts. In addition, a number of subsystems form a larger and more complex system. The concept *system* stands for a number of differing ideas. For example, a social system is not the same as a general system. A social system may be a small constellation of roles, such as those in the family (husband–wife–child, or mother–father–brother–sister), or it may be the interrelated systems of an entire society. On the other hand, a general system is a complex adaptive system characterized by an elaboration or evolution of organization that depends on disturbances and variety in the environment to keep it informed.

General systems theory is the end result of a culmination of shifts in the scientific perspective over the last few centuries. First, a system was viewed as one of equilibrium–disequilibrium. The *equilibrium model* depicts a system of simple organization that functions to reach stability and remain steady within a narrow condition of disturbance. Next, a system was viewed as "homeostatic." The *homeostatic model* applies to more complex systems, such as those of the body, which tend to be highly organized in spite of infections or injuries that threaten to reduce the level of organization. The *general system model* is characterized by a complex adaptive system that changes organization in response to changes in the environment. General systems theory is quite complex but centers upon cybernetic processes as crucial in self-correction and change.

The types of systems used by nursing scholars vary from one theorist to another. Johnson (1980) uses a behavioral-system approach, while Neuman proposes a system comprised of an individual interacting holistically with stress and with reaction to stress.

Johnson's Behavioral System

Johnson (1968, 1980) developed her model of behavioral systems for nursing from an interdisciplinary body of theoretical literature and empirical data drawn from psychology, ethology, anthropology, and general systems theory.

The model depicts the patient as a behavioral system, in a manner similar to that of the physician who views the patient as a biologic system (see Figure 7–2). Johnson defines *system* as a "whole which func-

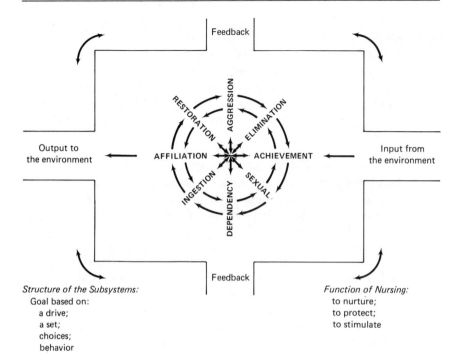

Figure 7–2. Johnson's behavioral system model.

tions as a whole by virtue of the independence of its parts." The "parts" of Johnson's system are seven subsystems of behavior: 1) the attachment or affiliative subsystem; 2) the subsystem of dependence; 3) the ingestive; 4) the eliminative; 5) the sexual; 6) the aggressive; and 7) the achievement. An eighth subsystem, "restoration," is added later by other theorists, using the Johnson behavioral system, but Johnson (1980) rejects this addition.

Each of these subsystems functions to carry out a specialized task for the system as a whole, and each subsystem is structured by a set of behavioral responses organized around a motivational structure. The elements of the motivational structure include "observed behavior"; "drive"; "set"; and "choice." Drive is associated with goal-directed behavior, while the individual's "set" refers to the predisposition to act in a particular way with reference to the goal. The "choice," or "behavioral repertoire," is the set of behavior available to the individual to achieve a particular goal. Johnson suggests that the cross-cultural prevalence of the subsystems indicates that the behavioral response or the releasers for such behavior are genetically programmed. At the same time, she notes that the variability found in human responses indicates the significance of social and cultural factors.

Johnson notes that each of the subsystems must be protected from noxious influences and malfunctions, and each must be stimulated to grow. The function of nursing is to help restore the balance of each subsystem when it is disturbed, and to act to prevent future imbalances.

Johnson summarizes the functions of each of the behavioral subsystems:

1. The attachment or affiliative subsystem functions in both survival and security, and is critical. Likewise, it has empirical consequences for other functions, such as social inclusion, intimacy, and bonding. This subsystem is one of the first to develop and is rooted in the mother-child dyad.
2. The dependency subsystem functions to obtain nurturant responses by manifesting succoring behavior—that which solicits aid, assistance, attention, recognition, and approval. Dependency behavior undergoes a developmental process, progressing from total dependency seen in infants and ill persons, to dependency on self and interdependency on the social group.
3. and 4. The ingestive and eliminative subsystems, intimately associated with the biological system, are controlled by social norms that prescribe the rules for proper eating and elimination.
5. The sexual system functions to procreate and gratify, and is rooted both in biology and in social norms that influence when, where, and with whom sex is allowed. It also influences the gender-role identity.
6. The aggressive subsystem functions to protect and preserve, although collective life limits self-protection to include the protection of the group.
7. The achievement subsystem functions to master or control intellectual, physical, creative, mechanical, and social skills.

Research is needed to study the system and subsystems and to identify, clarify, and explain problems encountered in nursing that are associated with disturbances in the systems. A number of scholars, such as Auger (1975) and Small (1980), use the Johnson model to describe and assess the activity within each subsystem.

Auger uses the case study method to examine and describe the systems of a hospitalized patient. First, she describes the activity in each of the subsystems; then, she discusses the impact of hospitalization upon each subsystem. Finally, she predicts what behavior patterns the patient must learn by the time of discharge.

Small (1980) first completes research on the perceived body image and spatial awareness of visually impaired children, then uses the Johnson model to identify problems in the behavioral subsystems of both the visually impaired and their parents. Small notes that the eye contact deemed to be important in maternal-infant bonding may be missing in cases of visual impairment. The task of the nurse is to encourage the mother to substitute other behavior such as touch and vocalization for the impaired subsystem.

Criticizing Johnson's theory, Stevens (1975, p. 72) notes that attention is upon the subsystems while the nursing processes to be applied are less well formulated. Nor are the relationships among the subsystems of behavior fully explored and described. For example, the relationship between achievement behavior and affiliative behavior are yet to be well explained. In Steven's view, Johnson's theory is one of equilibrium–disequilibrium. The equilibrium sought is that of behavior.

Neuman Health-Care System

Neuman's health-care system draws on systems theory, Gestalt theory, and adaptation theory to present a "total person approach" to the patient problem. The individual is seen as an open system in interaction with the total interface of the environment. The person adjusts to stress and defends against tension producing stimuli that may cause disequilibrium, crises, or stress. Variables that influence the adjustment process include basic physiological condition, sociocultural background, state of development, cognitive skills, age, and sex. The interacting variables determine the amount of resistance an individual can demonstrate to any stressor. The stressors may be intrapersonal (conditioned responses), interpersonal (role expectations), or extrapersonal (financial circumstances).

The model is depicted as a series of concentric rings surrounding a central structure—the basic survival factors common to all human beings (see Figure 7–3). Surrounding the core structure, a series of rings depict the "flexible line of resistance"—internal factors that help defend against a stressor. The next ring, "lines of defense," includes variables such as the individual's coping patterns, life-style, developmental stage, and other factors of resistance. "Flexible lines of defense" surrounding the lines of defense are dynamic factors that alter rapidly and act as protectors. Multiple stressors, or negative factors such as loss of sleep, can reduce defenses and evoke a reaction to stress.

Nursing intervention includes primary prevention to strengthen flexible lines of defense; secondary prevention to treat symptoms, strengthen resistance, and rank need-priorities; and tertiary prevention to maintain adaptation. Craddock and Stanhope (1980) conducted a

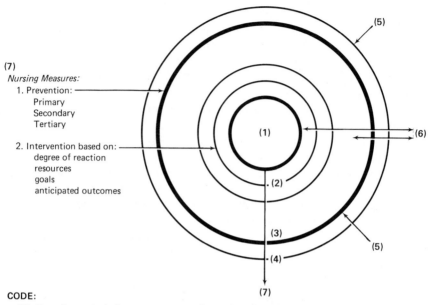

CODE:

(1) *Central core*—basic factors common to all organisms, including temperature range, genetic structures, response patterns, organ strength, weaknessess, ego structure, and knowns or commonalities.

(2) *Lines of resistance*—interval factors that help defend against a stressor.

(3) *Normal lines of defense*—variables such as coping patterns, life-style, stage of development.

(4) *Flexible lines of defense*—a dynamic protective buffer against stressors.

(5) *Stressors identified and classified*—includes loss, pain, change, sensory deprivation.

(6) *Reaction*—individual intervening variables, such as time, resistance.

(7) *Nursing prevention and intervention measures*—primary, secondary, tertiary prevention; intervention based on resources, goals, anticipated outcomes, and degree of reaction.

Figure 7–3. Neuman's Health-Care System.

study to test the usefulness of the Neuman model in nursing practice. The study sample included registered nurses and clients in a private, nonprofit home health-care agency. Each nurse chose clients from their caseloads, which one of the researchers assessed using the Neuman approach. The researcher then interviewed each of the nurses to compare perceptual differences between the nurse providing care and the client receiving care. The results of the study suggested that the Neuman model has the ability to categorize data for assessment and planning.

SOCIAL THEORIES

Social theories, such as theories of social stratification, demography and symbolic interation, are frequently used in nursing research to explain the relationship between poverty and disease, morbidity rates in various social contexts, and the relationship between social roles and social structures. Each of these will be examined briefly.

Social Stratification Theory

Theories of social stratification explain the ranking of individuals and groups in terms of property, power and prestige. The rich have property, power, and access to the best systems of health care, while the poor have none of these. The best single indicator of social class is occupation. Occupational prestige suggests levels of social class (see Table 7–2). Anthropologists such as Warner and sociologists like Myrdal have developed a number of models that identify the basis of stratification in terms of occupation, education, property, lineage, affiliation, reputation, and race. Warner (1949) proposed a six-class system based on his study of New Haven (see Table 7–3).

Myrdal noted that, in comparison with white people, few black people ever make the money or have the property and prestige characteristic of the middle-class. And the number of blacks in the upper class is so low as to be without consequences.

Whether blacks or whites, the poor of the United States tend to be migrant farm laborers, the elderly living on a fixed and inadequate income, ghetto and slum dwellers, and skid row people. Families occupying the bottom of the class system include those handicapped by unemployment, mental illness, alcoholism, illegitimacy and desertion, chronic illness, crime, and ignorance. Harrington (1964) estimated that such poor people comprised between thirty and forty million during the 1960s.

Kitagawa's and Hauser's (1973) report of a recent massive nationwide study of mortality noted that persons in lower classes have higher morbidity and mortality rates for almost every disease or illness. And the gap between the social classes may be increasing. Persons from the lower class usually have a limited education which interferes with their understanding of the health care system. For example, the language of doctors and nurses may be difficult for them to interpret, and they may hesitate to ask for explanations.

Examining the characteristics and perceptions of low-income women, Triplett (1970) noted that the poor not only have more health problems but also receive less care. She drew on theories of social class to design an exploratory study to determine whether or not lower-class women perceive health workers as threatening. Forty white women who lived in an urban area and had at least one preschool child were interviewed. Among the findings, Triplett notes that poor users of preventive health services tended to be heads of their households, to receive welfare assistance, and to have more children than good users.

TABLE 7–2. OCCUPATIONAL PRESTIGE RANKS*

Occupation	Rank	Occupation	Rank
U.S. Supreme Court		Undertaker	44.0
Justice	1.0	Welfare worker for	
Physician	2.0	city	44.0
Scientist	3.5	Policeman	47.0
State governor	5.5	Bookkeeper	49.5
College professor	8.0	Insurance agent	51.5
Chemist	11.0	Carpenter	53.0
Lawyer	11.0	Mail carrier	57.0
Dentist	14.0	Plumber	59.0
Architect	14.0	Automobile	
County judge	14.0	repairman	60.0
Psychologist	17.5	Barber	62.5
Minister	17.5	Corporal in regular	
Mayor of large city	17.5	army	65.5
Priest	21.5	Truck driver	67.0
Banker	24.5	Clerk in store	70.0
Biologist	24.5	Lumberjack	72.5
Instructor in public		Filling station	
schools	27.5	attendant	75.0
Captain in regular		Coal miner	77.5
army	27.5	Night watchman	77.5
Accountant for a		Restaurant waiter	80.5
large business	29.5	Taxi driver	80.5
Building contractor	31.5	Janitor	83.0
Railroad engineer	39.0	Garbage collector	88.0
Electrician	39.0	Shoeshiner	90.0
Trained machinist	41.5		

*Based on Hodge et al. Occupational Prestige in the United States 1925–1964. American Journal of Sociology 70, 286–302 1964.

On the other hand, good users tended to have lower self-esteem, to be more socially isolated, and to admit feelings of loneliness.

Demographic Theory

Demography is the study of population variables, such as age, sex, and race. Population changes reflected in birth rates, death rates, and disease rates are also of primary interest. Many research projects include demographic variables as part of their data collection, and at times, the entire research focuses on demographic characteristics or epidemiological studies.

TABLE 7-3. WARNER'S SIX-CLASS MODEL

	Social Class	Characteristics of People
I	Upper-upper class	old families; old aristocracy; people with money
II	Lower-upper class	aristocracy but not old families; people with money
III	Upper-middle class	nice, respectable people with little money
IV	Lower-middle class	good people but "nobody"; don't have money
V	Upper-lower class	poor whites, poor but honest people
VI	Lower-lower class	poor whites; no account lot; shiftless people

For example, Nakagawa (1972) conducted an epidemiological study of changes in psychiatric symptoms over a 26-year span. She examined trends in the complaints of patients, in the context of changing sociocultural environment and psychiatric treatment. Findings indicate that recent complaints tend to center around drug overuse, somatic problems, and sociocultural problems. On the other hand, the number of persons exhibiting thought-process disorders declined over the years. Nakagawa suggests that such approaches may be useful to search for ways to improve nursing.

Symbolic Interaction: Role Theory

Symbolic interaction focuses on the meanings that roles, symbols, and interaction have for the actors. Symbolic interaction is a dynamic process in which roles change and adjust over time. The theory is often used to study childhood socialization and to examine roles learned in adult life.

The theoretical foundations of symbolic interaction appear in the work of Cooley (1902) and George Herbert Mead (1934). Cooley formulated the concept of the "looking-glass self" to designate the process by which the child develops a self-image by imagining what other people are thinking of the child. Each to each, Cooley notes, is a looking-glass: we see ourselves reflected in the eyes of the others around us. The looking-glass self emerges in three steps: first, we imagine our appearance to the other person; then, we imagine the judgment that the person makes of our appearance; finally, we get a feeling, such as pride or mortification, as we imagine the person's judgment of us. Our self-image is a social image, created symbolically as each puts himself or herself in the place of others and views himself or herself objectively through their eyes. The nurse acts as a looking glass to the children, patients, and clients who see themselves reflected in the nurse's role behavior. And the nurse sees his or her own image reflected in their eyes.

Mead views the "self" as a social phenomenon, but he stresses the process of communication in language, play, and in games. In the use of language, the child comes to see herself or himself as an object: the *I* and the *me* and the *other*. To put himself or herself in the place of the other is to play that role and look back at herself or himself as the other must. Thus, the child or the adult sees herself or himself objectively.

The self emerges first in the child's egocentric play and then in games with others. In team games, the person must not only take the role of significant others, but must have expectations of roles in general. The roles can be rehearsed in imagination before they are played in fact.

A number of nursing perspectives and studies are based on the role of the nurse and patient, and on self-image. For example, Riehl's (1980) model uses the perspective of symbolic interaction to examine the role of the patient vis-a-vis the nurse: to understand the role assumed by the patient, the nurse attempts to put herself in the patient's role, that is, role-taking. Then the nurse attempts to understand how the patient acts in response to attitudes of others and the person's self-image.

CULTURE THEORY

Broadly defined, *culture* is a traditional way of life that has been learned and passed on from one generation to another. Research studies in nursing that use culture as a factor include that of Williams (1972), who studied surgical convalescence among Anglo- and Mexican-American women; Aamodt (1977), who examined the social-cultural dimensions of caring among Papago children; Horn (1977), who studied transcultural nursing among the Muckleshoot people; and Leininger, who made numerous cross-cultural studies. All of these studies explain the relationship between culture and nursing by reference to Leininger's theory.

Leininger (1978) seeks to explain the theoretical perspective of a subfield of nursing that she calls *transcultural nursing*—a set of cross-cultural concepts and hypotheses dealing with behavior, values, and beliefs used by nurses to practice efficaciously (see Figure 7–4). Leininger defines the essence of nursing as caring and proposes a number

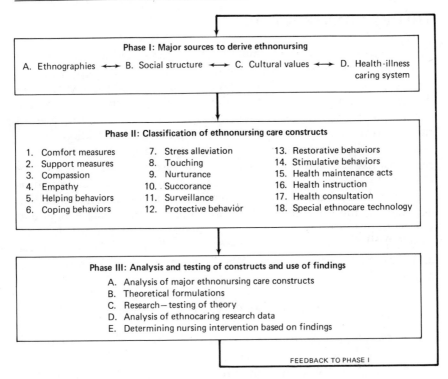

Figure 7–4. Leininger's conceptual and theory-generating model (1978).

of hypotheses useful to the nurse to collect and analyze data. These include the following (abridged):

1. Differences in caring values and behaviors lead to differences in nursing-care expectations of care-seekers.
2. Differences in caring values and norms exist between societies of high and low technology.
3. Nurses with different values who work in other cultures can create conflict and problems.
4. Nurses' dependence on technology can increase interpersonal distance and client dissatisfaction.
5. Differences in folk values and Western nurses' values are reflected in conflict and stress.
6. Culture-specific nursing will elicit more satisfaction from clients then nonculturally oriented services.

THEORY CONSTRUCTION

Researchers test theory by formulating hypotheses deductively from the theory and testing the hypotheses in research. Construction of theory, on the other hand, begins after observation. The researcher uses inductive reasoning to order the observations into categories and concepts, and attempts to relate one concept to the other in a statement—the empirical generalization. From the empirical generalization, the researcher deduces hypotheses for further testing. As the evidence for relationships between concepts grows, the researcher may use creative abilities to propose a general explanation for the interrelationships among the concepts and propositions. Thus, a theory is formulated that summarizes the interrelationships, and predicts the relationships that will be found in future observations. Theory construction involves observation, forming categories, conceptualization, and both inductive and deductive reasoning. Jacox (1981) summarizes the efforts to develop a theory:

1. Specifying, defining, and classifying the concepts used to describe the phenomena of the field.
2. Developing statements or propositions that propose how two or more concepts are related.
3. Specifying how all of the propositions are related to each other in a systematic way.

In the first step, the emphasis is on concepts; in the second step, the emphasis is on the proposition; and, in the third step, the propositions are related to one another.

Dickoff and James suggest that a theory is a mental invention for some purpose—to describe, explain, predict, or prescribe. Theories may be constructed in their view at four different levels:

1. Naming theory (factor-isolating theory) is the lowest level of theory construction but also the most basic. This kind of naming and describing theory is basic because the higher levels depend on its development for their own emergence. Naming theory puts observations into named categories and includes both the name of the phenomenon and its description. Nursing diagnoses are an example of naming theory.
2. Factor-relating theory is the second level of theory. It relates the named concepts to one another. This is also the same level as the construction of empirical generalizations—a statement that proposes the relationship between two concepts.

3. Situation-relating theory is the third level of theory. It explains the interrelationships among concepts or propositions. Once such explanations have been formulated, predictive statements, or hypotheses, may be deduced. The hypothesis may predict causation or correlation.
4. Situation-producing theory is the fourth level of theory. It prescribes the activities necessary to reach defined goals.

Each level of the theory construction presupposes that the lower levels have been developed. Not all theorists would include description and naming as a theory, unless a relationship between the names is shown. However, some theorists, such as Diers, have found the approach useful for proposing research in nursing practice.

SUMMARY

A *theory* is an explanation for the interrelations among facts, concepts, or propositions. The theoretical framework summarizes what is known from past work and predicts what will be found in the future.

A number of theories are used in nursing research, including learning, development, adaptation, systems, social, and cultural theories.

Learning theory includes theories of conditioning, behavior, and social learning. Conditioning, or stimulus–response theory, suggests that learning takes place when a stimulus known to produce a response is presented along with a new stimulus that the researcher wants the subject to learn to associate with the response. Operant conditioning or behaviorism proposes that learning occurs as an individual acts upon the environment to obtain a reward or reduce tension. Social learning theories are closely associated with the stimulus–response–reinforcement theory but place considerable emphasis on the social elements associated with learning.

The Gestalt or cognitive theories of learning propose that learning occurs in association with knowing and thinking on the part of the individual. In this view, the whole picture is more than the sum of its parts.

Development theory seeks to explain changes that take place through time, first on one level and then on another. Piaget's cognitive theory suggests that knowing proceeds through five phases of development, reaching from birth to the fifteenth year of life. Freud's theory of personality development begins at birth and continues throughout life. Erikson's theory incorporates the entire span of human life, as does Havighurst's theory of the tasks of development. Peplau explains that the development of interpersonal relationships between patient and nurse occurs in four phases, during which the nurse assumes reciprocal roles in relation to the patient's roles.

Theories of adaptation, stress, and homeostasis explain the process by which persons adjust internally and externally, in order to function and survive, often in the face of disease and stress. Selye defines *stress* as a state manifested by the General Adaptation Syndrome. The syndrome evolves in three stages: alarm, resistance, and exhaustion. The third stage must be reversed or the individual will die. Adaptation and homeostasis are related in that the organism reacts to gains and excesses or deficiencies by negative feedback that triggers the homeostatic process to correct the imbalance.

Systems theory explains the organization of parts and their interrelationships. A system differs from each of its parts and is greater than the sum of its parts, but a change in one part brings about a change in the whole system. Systems may consist of a simple level of organization, such as the equilibrium model, or it may be as complex as the general systems model. The general systems model is a complex adaptive system that changes organization in response to changes in the environment and the subsequent cybernetic process in the system. Widely used in nursing, Johnson's behavioral system depicts the patient as a system of seven interacting behavioral subsystems. Each subsystem carries out a specialized task for the system as a whole. The nurse nurtures, protects, or stimulates needy systems. Neuman's health-care system also incorporates elements of Gestalt and adaptation theories.

Social theories, such as theories of social class, explain the observations on the basis of forces that are external to the individual. These forces place the individual in a social class, which then determines the style of living and dying, and the chances of becoming sick and getting well. Demographic theories examine populations of persons—the rates at which they are born, get sick, and die. Symbolic interaction theories focus on the meanings that roles, symbols, and interaction have for the actors. Taking the role of the other and looking back upon oneself as an object is a central focus of symbolic interaction.

Broadly defined, *culture* is the traditional way of life that has been learned and shared by groups of people. Differences in nurses' and patients' caring values and behavior are reflected in various ways that may be described and classified.

The process of theory construction begins with observation and inductively arrives at forming concepts, then expresses two or more concepts in a single proposition, and finally explains the relationship among propositions. The explanation for this relationship is called the *theory*. Certain theorists, such as Dickoff and James, suggest that theory construction begins with description and naming of concepts; emerges into a second level, in which the concepts or factors are related to one another; emerges into a third level, in which the interrelationships among concepts or propositions are explained; and finally, emerges into the highest level of theory, in which activities are prescribed to reach certain goals.

STUDY QUESTIONS

1. Examine the theories of learning. Select one of the theories that would be useful to test the use of behavior modification.
2. Identify a nursing problem you would like to study. What theory would assist you?
3. Using Johnson's or Neuman's systems theory, formulate a problem statement or a hypothesis to test in research.
4. Suggest a research project based on the development theory.
5. You have obtained a job in the inner city working with a prenatal clinic. What theory would be helpful to understand the relationships between the poor and their way of life?
6. Suggest a research problem based on theories of adaptation, stress, or homeostasis.
7. You have been asked to help with a new research project to study the health care problems of Cubans who have just arrived in the United States. How could you use Leininger's ethnonursing care concepts to assist you?
8. Discuss the four levels of theory proposed by Dickoff and James. Can you think of observations in nursing that do not have a name? Think of a concept such as anxiety that you have encountered in nursing. What observations are summarized in the name?
9. What theory is the most appealing to you for use in research? Why?

REFERENCES AND SUGGESTED READINGS

Aamodt, A. (1972): The child's view of health and healing. In Batey, M. (ed.), Communicating Nursing Research. Boulder, Colorado: Western Interstate Commission for Higher Education. *The Papago child's view of health and healing.*

Abbey, J. (1980): FANCAP: What is it? In Riehl, J. and Roy, C. (eds.), Conceptual Models for Nursing Practice (2nd ed.). New York: Appleton. *A mnemonic device for teaching, using general system theory and Selye's general adaptation syndrome.*

Auger, J. (1976): Behavioral Systems and Nursing. Englewood Cliffs, N.J.: Prentice Hall. *Chapters two and three include systems theory.*

Bell, J. (1977): Stressful life events and coping methods in mental-illness and -wellness behavior. *Nursing Research 26, 136–141. Selye's stress theory used.*

Bensberg, G. et al (1965): Teaching the profoundly retarded self-help activities by behavior shaping techniques. *American Journal of Mental Deficiency 69, 674–679. Uses learning theory to change behavior.*

Blake, M. (1980): The Peplau developmental model for nursing practice. In Riehl, J. and Roy, C. (eds.), Conceptual Models for Nursing Practice (2nd ed.). New York: Appleton. *Developmental theory.*

Buckley, W. (1967): Sociology and Modern Systems Theory. Englewood Cliffs, New Jersey: Prentice-Hall. *Modern systems theory explained.*

Cannon, W. (1939): Wisdom of the Body (rev. ed.). New York: Norton. *Cannon identifies and names the concept* homeostasis.

Cooley, C. (1902): Human Nature and the Social Order (rev. ed. 1922). New York: Scribner's. *Describes the looking-glass self, a concept of symbolic interaction theory.*

Craddock, R. and Stanhope, M. (1980): The Neuman health-care systems model: recommended adaptation. In Riehl, J. and Roy, C. (eds.), Conceptual Models for Nursing Practice (2nd ed.). New York: Appleton. *Summarizes the theory behind the Neuman model.*

DeWalt, E. and Haines, A. (1977): The effects of specified stressors on healthy oral mucosa. In Downs, F. and Newman, M. (eds.), A Sourcebook of Nursing Research (2nd ed.). Philadelphia: F. A. Davis. *Stress theory used.*

Dickoff, J., and James, P. (1968): A theory of theories—a position paper. In *Nursing Research 17, 197–203. Researching research's role in theory development. In Nursing Research 17, 204–206. Describes the approach of Dickoff and James to study of theory and theory development.*

Diers, D. (1979): Research in Nursing Practice. New York: J. B. Lippincott. *Chapters two and three include theory for nursing research.*

Downs, F. (1977): Maternal stress in primigravidas as a factor in the production of neonatal pathology. In Downs, F. and Newman, M. (eds.), A Sourcebook of Nursing Research (2nd ed.), pp. 129–139. *Uses stress theory.*

Downs, F. and Newman, M. (eds.) (1977): A Sourcebook of Nursing Research (2nd ed.). Philadelphia: F. A. Davis. *Fifteen research reports, many of which state theoretical orientation.*

Erikson, E. (1950): Childhood and Society. New York: Norton. *Neo-Freudian developmental theory.*

Fielo, S. (1975): A Summary of Integrated Nursing Theory (2nd ed.). New York: McGraw-Hill. *Summarizes various theories.*

Festinger, L. (1957): A Theory of Cognitive Dissonance. Stanford, Calif.: Stanford University Press. *Presents Festinger's cognitive dissonance theory.*

Freud, S. (1938): The Basic Writings of Sigmund Freud. New York: Random House. *Psychoanalytic theory.*

Glaser, B. and Strauss, A. (1967): The Discovery of Grounded Theory. Chicago: Aldine. *Used in nursing theory.*

Goslin, D. (1969): Handbook of Socialization Theory and Research. Chicago: Rand McNally. *Sources for developmental theory.*

Grosicki, J. (1968): Effects of operant conditioning on modification of incontinence in neuropsychiatric geriatric patients. *Nursing Research 17, 304. Operant conditioning theory in research and practice.*

Hardy, M. (ed.) (1973): Theoretical Foundations for Nursing. New York: MSS Information Corp. *Eight articles including general systems theory, stress, adaptation.*

Hardy M. and Conway, M. (eds.) (1978): Role Theory: Perspectives for the Health Professions. New York: Appleton. *Role theory used as a unifying theoretical approach in nursing.*

Harrington, M. (1962): The Other America. New York: Macmillan. *Poverty in the United States.*

Havinghurst, R. (1952): Developmental Tasks and Education. New York: Longmans, Green. *Developmental theory.*

Hodge, et al (1964): Occupational prestige in the United States 1925–1964. In *American Journal of Sociology 70*, 286–302.

Holaday, B. (1974): Achievement behavior in chronically ill children. In *Nursing Research 23*, 25–30. (1980): Implementing the Johnson model for nursing practice. In Riehl, J. and Roy, C. (eds.), Conceptual Models for Nursing Practice (2nd ed.) New York: Appleton, pp. 255–263. *Uses Johnson's system model and Piaget's developmental model to assess a case study.*

Horn, B. (1978): Transcultural nursing and child-rearing of the Muckleshoot people. In Leininger, M., Transcultural Nursing. New York: Wiley, pp. 223–238. *Uses transcultural theory.*

Jacox, A. (1974): Theory construction in nursing: an overview. In *Nursing Research 23*, 4–13. *Classic approach to theory construction.*

Johnson, D. (1980): The behavioral system model for nursing. In Riehl, J. and Roy, C. (eds.), Conceptual Models for Nursing Practice. New York: Appleton, pp. 207–216. *Johnson presents the theory behind her systems model.*

Leininger, M. (1979): Transcultural Nursing. New York: Wiley. *A series of articles using transcultural theory.*

Levine, M. (1967): The four conservation principles of nursing. In *Nursing Forum 47*, 45. *Principles of nursing proposed.*

Lowery, B. and DuCette, J. (1976): Disease-related learning and disease control in diabetes as a function of the locus-of-control. *Nursing Research 25*. *Locus-of-control theory.*

Mead, G. (1934): Mind, Self and Society. Chicago: University of Chicago. *The classic dynamic approach to role theory.*

Myrdal, Gunnar et al. (1944): An American Dilemma. New York: Harper and Row. *Social stratification theory with reference to race.*

Nakagawa, H. et al (1972): An epidemiological study of psychiatric symptom pattern change: pilot study findings. In Batey, M. (ed.), Communicating Nursing Research. Boulder: WICHE. *An epidemiological approach to nursing research.*

Neuman, G. (1980): The Betty Neuman health-care system model. In Riehl, J. and Roy, C. (eds.), 2nd ed. New York: Appleton, pp. 119–134. *Systems theory.*

O'Neil, S. (1972): The application and methodological implication of behavior modification in nursing research. In Batey, M. (ed.), Communicating Nursing Research. Boulder: WICHE. *Stimulus-response-reinforcement theory.*

Pavlov, I. (1928): Lectures on Conditioned Reflex (trans. W. H. Gantt). New York: International Publishers. *Classical conditioning theory.*

Peplau, H. (1952): Interpersonal Relations in Nursing. New York: G. P. Putnam's Sons. *Utilizes developmental theory.*

Piaget, J. (1926): The Language and Thought of the Child. New York: Harcourt, Brace, and World. *Theory of development and perception.*

Riehl, J. and Roy, C. (eds.) Conceptual Models for Nursing Practice. (2nd ed.). New York: Appleton. *Three theoretical models presented.*

Robischon, P. (1977): Pica practices and other hand-mouth behavior and children's development level. In Downs, F. and Newman, M. (eds.). A Sourcebook of Nursing Research. Philadelphia: F. A. Davis, pp. 152–170. *Developmental theory.*

Rottkamp, B. (1976): A behavior modification approach to nursing therapeutics in body positioning of spinal-cord-injured patients. *Nursing Research 25,* 181–185. *Behavior modification theory.*

Rotter, J. et al (1962): Internal versus external control of reinforcement: A major variable in behavior theory. In Washburn, N. (ed.). *Decisions, Values and Groups.* New York: Pergamon Press, pp. 473–516. *Locus of control theory.*

Selye, H. (1956): The Stress of Life. New York: McGraw-Hill. *Widely used stress syndrome and theory.*

Skinner, B. (1953): Science and Human Behavior. *Basis for behavior modification procedures, based on operant conditioning theory.*

Small, V. (1980): Nursing visually impaired children with Johnson's model as a conceptual framework. In Riehl, J. and Roy, C. (eds.). Conceptual Models for Nursing Practice (2nd ed.). New York: Appleton, pp. 264–273. *Use of system therory.*

Stillman, M. (1977): Women's health beliefs about breast cancer and breast self-examination. *Nursing Research 26,* 121–127. *Cognitive dissonance theory.*

Stevens, V. (1979): Nursing Theory. Boston: Little, Brown. *A critique of nursing theory.*

Triplett, J. (1977): Characteristics and perceptions of low-income women and use of preventive health services: an exploratory study. In Downs, F. and Newman, M., A Sourcebook of Nursing Research. New York: Appleton, pp. 94–106. *Utilizes social-class theory.*

Wallace, W. (1971): The Logic of Science in Sociology. Chicago: Aldine. *Brief book includes examination of theory.*

Warner, W. et al (1949): Social Class in America. Chicago: Science Research Associates. *Model of social class.*

Windwer, C. (1977): Relationship among prospective parents' locus of control, social desirability and choice of psychoprophylaxis. *Nursing Research 26,* 96–99. *Locus of control theory.*

CHAPTER 8

SAMPLING

Sampling is the process by which the study subjects or objects are chosen from a larger population. Sampling is a crucial part of the research process, since the method of sampling determines whether or not the study sample represents the entire population from which it was drawn. If the sample does represent the entire population, the findings from the sample can be generalized to the population. If the sample does not, the findings apply only to the sample studied.

This chapter is designed to introduce the student to the complex topic of sampling. Upon completion of the chapter, the student should be able to: 1) define basic terms used in sampling; 2) state advantages of sampling; 3) discuss the theory of probability that underlies scientific sampling; 4) distinguish between probability sampling and nonprobability sampling; 5) identify and describe methods of probability sampling and nonprobability sampling; 6) describe steps to select particular samples; and 7) discuss sample size and biases in sampling.

BASIC TERMS IN SAMPLING

Basic terms encountered in sampling include the following: *population, universe, sample, generalization, probability sampling, nonprobability sampling,* and *strata.* Each of these will be briefly examined.

1. *Population is the total group of persons or objects that meets the designated set of criteria established by the researcher.* If the researcher is interested in female patients in the United States, the population consists of all females who are presently patients (or who have ever been patients, if this is what interests the researcher). Thus, the population is all cases that conform to the researcher's established criteria. A list of all cases, objects, or groups of cases or objects in the population is called a *sampling frame.* The total population is also called the *universe* or *target population*—for example, the total number of female patients to whom the results of the research could be generalized. The enormous task of getting a list of all female patients in the population of the United States is obvious. If the list were obtainable from some central computer, the task would only just have begun. The sample drawn from the population would have to be contacted and studied, a formidable undertaking reserved for long-term, well funded projects. Therefore, the *accessible population* is the population of subjects who are available to the researcher—for example, the population of female patients in a hospital at one time; or the female patients attending a weight-loss clinic, a prenatal clinic, or a hypertensive clinic. The list of all such patients would be more easily obtainable and the sample drawn from the list easier to study. At times, all of the accessible population may be studied. However, the findings of a study sample apply only to the accessible population from which the study sample was drawn, and then only if certain sampling techniques—random sampling—insure that each female in the accessible population had an equal chance of being chosen for the sample. Otherwise, the findings apply only to the sample studied, and the researcher is not able to generalize either to the accessible population or any other.

2. *Sample is the subset of cases drawn from the target or accessible population.* A single member of the population or sample is called an *element*, the basic unit from which data are collected. At times, several elements or a set of elements form a *sampling unit*. For example, if the researcher wished to study females attending all of the hypertensive clinics in a city, each clinic would be a sampling unit, and each patient would be an element.

3. *Generalization is the ability to apply the conclusion reached from studying the elements in a sample to the population from which the study sample was drawn.* The researcher concludes that the results of the study sample are the same conclusion that would have been reached if every element in the entire population had been studied. Every researcher wants to be able to generalize the results obtained from the sample, and this may be done if the sample is selected by probability sampling.

4. *Probability sampling is a process in which each element of the population has an equal chance of being chosen for the sample.* Several methods of probability sampling include simple random sampling, stratified random sampling, systematic sampling, and cluster sampling. Each of these is examined below.

5. *Nonprobability sampling is a process for selecting samples without using probability sampling.* Methods used include accidental sampling, quota sampling, and purposive sampling.

6. *Strata are two or more subpopulations.* Strata are comprised of mutually exclusive portions of the population called *stratum*. For example, a researcher studying female patients could divide the population into strata. Each stratum could consist of women of a particular socioeconomic class: upper class, middle class, and lower class. Each stratum would be as homogeneous as possible, with the same education, occupation, and income. A sample could then be drawn from each stratum to examine the influence of social class on female patients.

ADVANTAGES OF SAMPLING

The advantages of sampling include time, money, efficiency, and safety. If a sample of the population will provide reasonably accurate data, it is not necessary to use time and resources to study an entire population. In addition, the study of certain populations could destroy the elements. For example, if the researcher wishes to test the contents of bottles of infusion solution, it is not necessary to open every bottle, which would destroy the usefulness of all. A scientifically chosen sample should give data from which it is possible to generalize. It is not necessary to examine all of the blood in a human body to study its contents—a small sample will do. The gain in accuracy by including a total population is not enough to warrant the additional expense or risks sometimes involved. For example, advantages of sampling are apparent in experiments with drugs or treatments. In order to study the effects of an experimental drug or treatment, it is not feasible to include every patient who has cancer. Unpleasant or unknown side effects should be limited to as few persons as possible. In cases where dangers are suspected, a sample of animal subjects is usually tested. At times, it is not possible to examine or measure all members of a population. For example, studies of autistic children or those with Down's syndrome require long periods of intensive observation. To study a total population would rarely be possible. In such cases, the advantage of a small sample is apparent.

SCIENTIFIC SAMPLING

There are two basic methods of choosing a sample: probability sampling and nonprobability sampling. Based on probability theory, *probability sampling* is a method whereby each element in the population has an equal chance of being chosen for study. Probability sampling reduces the possibility of selecting a biased sample, that is, one in which all of the population are not represented and the researcher is not aware of it. For example, *The Literary Digest* conducted a study to predict the results of the election of 1936, between Roosevelt and Landon. Based on a polling of people whose names were selected from telephone directories or lists of automobile owners, Landon was predicted to win. The sample was biased by being limited to those who had telephones or owned automobiles and neglecting poorer persons who had neither. Based on a biased sample, the prediction of a Landon victory was wrong. In addition, the data summaries based on randomly selected samples may be analyzed, using statistical techniques that can compute sampling error, the measure of how much sample findings differ from population values. An examination of probability sampling and the theory upon which it is based enables the student to understand the process of scientific sampling.

PROBABILITY THEORY

The theory of probability deals with the possibility of events occurring by chance. It establishes the rules for calculating the risks associated with predicting future events. Soon after its inception, probability theory began to be used to solve problems related to the study of populations. The concept of probability may be defined in three ways: 1) a subjective determination of fair odds; 2) relative frequencies expected to occur in a *series of events;* and 3) an equally-likely *set of events* mathematically calculated (Dixon and Massey, 1959, Chapter 20).

1. Subjective probability is a process by which an individual assesses the odds that some hypothesis may be true, based upon what is known. This type of probability is used every day to make practical decisions, for example, whether or not to cross the street against a traffic light. If emergency circumstances warrant it, if it is early in the morning, or if there is no traffic including police on the street, then one may decide he or she has enough knowledge to assess the odds of whether or not he or she will be hit or arrested for crossing the street against a light.

Betting odds are another example of subjective probability; gamblers may estimate that they have enough information on a boxer, football team, or horse to give 2 to 1 odds that a particular one will win. Likewise, scientists may make statements such as, "Based on the present state of knowledge, the odds against life on the planet Venus are 10,000,000 to 1." As scientists learn more about Venus, the odds may rise or fall.

Much of nursing practice depends upon subjectively experienced, anticipated probabilities. For example, the decision to give one type of nursing care may be based upon the nurse's present experience and knowledge of the probability that the patient will experience benefit from this type of nursing care. In general, diagnosis and therapy in the health sciences presently rely heavily upon such subjective internal mental processes, although current medical research is seeking to formalize these probabilities in order to make more accurate diagnoses by using computers. As yet, however, people have not been able to supply the computer with as much information to use systematically as the experienced clinician has available in memory to use less systematically. Health care still has strong subjective elements.

2. Mathematical probability, the second conception of probability into which both the "equally likely set of events" and "relative frequency" fall, is a mathematical one. The probability of relative frequency expresses the notion that the frequency of the occurrence of a given event is relative to the nonoccurrence of that event, in any series of events that could produce either occurrence or nonoccurrence. For example, a nickel tossed into the air has an equal chance of turning up heads relative to the chance of not turning up heads, that is, of turning up tails. The probability equals the number of ways the coin can fall divided by the total number of possible outcomes. The relative frequency is simply a proportion: if an event is sure to happen, it has a probability equal to 1; if an event cannot happen it has a probability equal to 0. Thus, the probability of any event must be a number between 0 and 1. In the case of tossing the nickel, probability may be expressed by the following formula:

$$\text{Probability} = \frac{\text{the number of ways the coin can fall}}{\text{the total number of possible outcomes}}$$

$$\text{Probability of heads} = \frac{1 \text{ (heads } or \text{ tails)}}{2 \text{ (heads } plus \text{ tails)}}$$

$$\text{Probability } P = 50\% \text{ (or .5, or } \frac{1}{2}, \text{ or } 50/100)$$

Therefore, if a coin is tossed into the air 100 times, heads would probably turn up 50 times. This definition of probability, called the *frequency definition*, is based on the classical theory of probability. The basic definition of classical probability is very simple: the probability, symbolized as p, of a coin tossed in the air coming up heads is 1 in 2, or $\frac{1}{2}$, or

50/100, or .5—four different ways of writing the same thing, that is, the frequency definition of probability.

3. Equally-likely probability, a second mathematical approach, is related to a set of events (rather than a series, as above) that are likely or possible to occur. For example, if we select one person from a well mixed group of 50 persons, we may consider any of the 50 equally likely to be chosen; or, if we draw a card from a well shuffled deck of 52, we would expect to have an equal chance of selecting any particular one of the 52 cards; or, if we draw a name written on a slip of paper from a box containing 100 identical well mixed slips (except for the names), we expect that any one of the slips is equally likely to be chosen. A comparable situation may occur when a sample of individuals has been scientifically drawn from a population for a public-opinion poll or when a group of patients has been scientifically chosen to estimate the characteristics of a population.

Probability enters into the very issues of what is knowledge and evidence. It is basic to the process of setting up and carrying out experimental questions and measurement procedures, and it is the foundation of the mathematical techniques used for both evaluating research and formulating what the results mean.

PROBABILITY SAMPLING

Probability sampling includes the following four methods of data collection: 1) simple random sampling; 2) systematic sampling; 3) stratified sampling, and 4) cluster sampling. The essential characteristic of all of these methods is that the researcher can specify for each element of the population the probability that it will be included in the sample. However, the most carefully selected sample will contain some degree of sampling error (random variation from the truly accurate sample), but, if probability sampling is used, it is possible to estimate the amount of sampling error. In addition, the researcher who uses probability sampling can specify the size of the sample needed to have a degree of certainty that sample findings do not differ by more than a specified amount from those of the total population. Each method of random sampling will now be examined.

1. Simple random sampling is the basic probability design that gives each element in the population an equal chance of being chosen. The first step in random sampling is to define the population: to specify all the cases that conform to some designated characteristic. Theoretically, this could be all of the people who reside in the United States. The survey or accessible population is that from which the survey sample is actually selected as a practical matter: for example, all nurses who work in a certain state or selected states. In order not to mislead those who read the research report, it is essential that the researcher record precisely what the population was and how the sample was selected.

Once the population is defined, a number is assigned to each unit or element in the population. A simple random sample is then chosen, by using a table of random numbers, which may be found in any statistics textbook. The researcher enters the table of random numbers at some random starting point, for example, making a blind stab. Once the starting point is identified, the researcher goes up, down, or diagonally in a systematic manner, noting the numbers and selecting those that correspond from the total population, until the previously selected sample size has been obtained (see Table 8–1).

2. *Systematic Sampling is the process by which every nth element is drawn from a list of the entire survey population.* For example, a survey population that lists 10,000 units may be used to select a systematic sample of 1,000

TABLE 8–1. A SAMPLE TABLE OF RANDOM NUMBERS

25	19	64	82	84	28	31
23	02	41	46	04	97	19
55	85	66	96	28	82	80
68	45	19	69	59	03	68
69	31	46	29	85	65	16
37	31	61	28	98	24	65
66	42	19	24	94	02	72
33	65	78	12	35	79	16
76	32	06	19	35	04	75
43	33	42	02	59	40	64

To select a random sample of 20 cases from a target population of 90 cases, take the following steps:
1. Assign a number to each case, from 01 to 90; or use the last two digits of the Social Security number or patient number; or arbitrarily assign a number.
2. On the table of random numbers, arbitrarily pick a two-digit column.
3. With closed eyes, select a random start in that column.
4. Beginning with the starting number, continue to sequentially select every 2-digit number in that column and in the next, if necessary, until 20 cases have been selected.
5. In the event a random number not included in the sequence 01 to 90 occurs (i.e., 96), skip that number and proceed to the next one listed.

by selecting every tenth unit on the list. The researcher enters the list at a random point (by making a blind stab, or selecting a number from one to ten by simple random sampling) and selects that unit plus every tenth element that follows.

If certain precautions are taken to insure that the list arrangement does not introduce a bias, systematic sampling is considered superior to simple random sampling (see Babbie, 1975, p. 155). A study during World War II (Babbie, 1975) used unit rosters to select a systematic sample: every tenth soldier was selected. However, the rosters reflected the table of organization in each military unit: in each squad of ten soldiers, sergeants first, then corporals, then privates. When the researchers chose every tenth person on the roster, they ended up with a sample that contained only sergeants. However, had they entered the list at another point, no sergeants would have been represented. The list introduced a systematic bias. Therefore, the researcher should carefully examine the nature of a list before using it.

3. Stratified random sampling is possible when the composition of the total population is known, with respect to some significant characteristic. Stratification involves grouping the units of a population into homogeneous strata prior to sampling, and then using simple, systematic, or cluster (see below) sampling to select the study sample. For example, a study of nurses can begin by dividing the population into nurses with an R.N. degree, those with a B.S.N. degree, those with an L.P.N. degree, and so on. Each stratum is homogeneous and insures that appropriate numbers of each element will be drawn in a random sampling of each stratum. While there will be heterogeneity in the sample as a whole, each homogeneous subset or stratum will be better represented, thereby insuring a sample with smaller sampling errors. The general principle is that, if stratification will result in homogeneous strata, then it is desirable to stratify. Stratification may take place before a random sample is drawn from the population or afterwards.

4. Cluster sampling is the process in which the population is first divided into existing categories, or clusters, and then the elements or units to be included in the study samples are selected by random sampling from each cluster. When the research is dealing with a large, spatially scattered population, this approach is helpful. In such cases, obtaining a list of every element in the population may be expensive, if not impossible. For example, a study of the population of nursing students in the United States would require a list of every student nurse in every nursing school, in order to draw a random sample. A cluster sampling method would first require that nursing schools be placed in clusters, for example, all schools in each state or geographical region. A sample of the *nursing schools* could then be drawn by random sampling, either simple, systematic, or then be drawn by random sampling, either simple, systematic, or stratified. Then, a list of the *student population* of the randomly selected nursing schools could be requested, from which a sample of the students themselves may be randomly drawn. It is clear that a ten percent sample of the schools that represented the total population of schools is a more manageable and realistic number with which to work.

Likewise, cluster sampling is helpful in getting permission to conduct research. For example, administering an interview in schools, hospitals, or factories would require disrupting activities in general, in order to utilize a random sample of the entire population. If the population were divided into clusters (all surgical wards, all medical wards, etc.) from which the study subjects were then drawn, disruption, work, and expense would be minimum.

NONPROBABILITY SAMPLING

The major advantages of nonprobability sampling are convenience, economy, and time, although these must be balanced against the risks involved in not using probability sampling. The major forms of nonprobability samples include (1) accidental sampling, (2) quota sampling, and (3) purposive sampling.

1. Accidental sampling is a process in which samples are fortuitously chosen, for example, the first five hundred people in a shopping center, on a college campus, or on the street. There is no known way of ascertaining the biases introduced in such samples; therefore, the findings may be misleading, since there is no control whatsoever.

2. Quota Sampling is a means by which samples reflect certain characteristics of the population being studied, without the use of random selection. For example, a study of attitudes toward abortion in New Orleans, used quota sampling to reflect as nearly as possible the composition of the New Orleans population. Since the population of New Orleans is 70 percent Catholic and 30 percent Protestant, the sample reflected these proportions. Since New Orleans is 40 percent black and 50 percent white, the sample likewise reflected these percentages. Finally, since 5 percent of New Orleans' residents live in area A (the rich), 25 percent live in area B (the middle class), 50 percent live in area C (the working class), and 20 percent live in the slums (the lower class), similar percentages were drawn from these areas.

Other identifying characteristics could also have been used, such as education or occupation. The more carefully the quota sample is drawn, the more confidence one has that it reflects the characteristics of the total population. Therefore, the study of attitudes toward abortion in New Orleans is more representative of the population as a whole. Demographic characteristics of an area are generally available from census material or the health department. Quota sampling does entail certain risks. Unless trained, interviewers tend to interview their friends in excessive proportion and tend to concentrate on areas where there are large numbers of potential respondents, such as college campuses and business districts, which are then over-represented. Where home visits are required, interviewers may concentrate on particular times of the day when only certain people are at home, or on particular housing types, for example, avoiding housing of the very poor and the very rich.

3. *Purposive sampling is the process of picking cases that are judged to be typical of the population, restricting observations to subgroups.* For example, in the light of results of past elections, the researcher may choose a state or county as a barometer of an election outcome. Sampling errors and biases cannot be computed, and such sampling should not be used when the possible errors are serious or if probability sampling is at all practical.

SAMPLE SIZE

The size of the sample depends upon the size and nature of the population and the type of question asked. However, larger samples are better than smaller ones, regardless of the size of the target population. The more variable the characteristic being measured, the larger the population should be. If one were measuring different kinds of schizophrenia in the general population, one would need a very large sample to arrive at a stable estimate of how schizophrenia is distributed in the population. However, if the target population consisted of those persons in mental institutions, one would need a much smaller population, since a mental institution is a self-selected population that presumably includes a number of schizophrenics. The size of the sample may be smaller if the population is known to be homogeneous: in this case, the sample may be expected to represent the population.

Probability theory and random sampling are the basis of all statistical analysis and of research inference in general. Without the use of random sampling, the ability to generalize from a sample is greatly weakened.

BIAS IN SAMPLING

Bias may be defined as a systematic difference between a population, or *true value*, and the corresponding value taken from that population. Bias can occur for the following reasons: (1) the entire population is not included (for example, the Literary Digest telephone survey excluded persons without telephones); (2) faulty measurement, that is, the specific item to be measured is not measured (for example, nursing attitudes rather than nursing behavior is measured); (3) nonresponse, that is, self-selection of those who do not answer on the basis of some factor, such as health; (4) faulty design or schedule; (5) faulty interviewing and poor questions on the survey, which lead to incorrect information from the response; and (6) faulty tabulation and interpretation of analysis. Bias may be reduced by carefully identifying the target population; by using valid and reliable measures, including scales, questionnaires, and interview schedules and trained interviewers; and by using meticulous care in tabulating and analyzing data. Bias is further discussed in Chapter 12.

SUMMARY

Sampling is the process by which study subjects or objects are chosen from a larger population. A critical element of the research process, sampling determines the extent to which research findings from the study sample can be generalized to the larger population from which it was drawn.

Basic terms used in the study of sampling include *population*, or *universe, sample, generalization, probability sampling, nonprobability sampling*, and *strata. Population*, or *universe*, is the total category of persons or objects that meets the criteria established by the researcher. The *accessible population* is the category that is available to the researcher for study. A *sample* is a subset of cases drawn from a population. An *element* is one unit of the sample from which data are collected. A *sampling unit* is comprised of several elements. *Generalization* is the ability to apply the conclusions reached from the study of a sample to the population from which the sample was drawn. *Probability sampling* is a process in which each element of the population has an equal chance of being chosen for the study sample, while *nonprobability sampling* does not use probability methods. *Strata* refers to two or more subpopulations comprised of individual, mutually exclusive layers called *stratum*.

The advantages of sampling include time, money, efficiency, and safety. When the study of a small sample will provide reasonably accurate data, it is not practical to study a population. At times, such as in testing drugs, it is unwise to study more subjects than necessary. Studies that require long and intensive observation and interpretation require a limited number of subjects. In such cases, the study of populations is rarely feasible.

There are two methods of choosing a sample—probability sampling and nonprobability sampling. Probability sampling reduces the possibility of *bias*, that is, selecting a sample, without the researcher's knowledge, in which all of the population are not represented. Probability sampling also allows the researcher to compute *sampling error*, a measure of the extent to which sample findings differ from the true value of the population.

Probability theory from which probability sampling is drawn deals with the possibility of events occurring by chance. Probability may be subjective, that is, a determination of fair odds based on individual experience, or it may be mathematically calculated as the relative frequencies expected to occur in a series of events or in an equally-likely set of events.

Probability sampling includes simple random sampling, systematic sampling, stratified sampling, and cluster sampling. Simple random sampling involves obtaining a list of the total population and selecting a sample by any method that gives each unit in the population an equal chance of being chosen. A common way is to assign numbers to each element in the sample, then to select numbers to be in the sample by using a table of random numbers. A systematic sampling begins with a list and selects every nth element. However, precautions must be taken to insure that the list does not introduce a bias. Stratified random sampling involves grouping the elements of a population into homogeneous strata prior to sampling, then using any method of probability sampling to select the correct percentage of subjects from each stratum. Cluster sampling is used to consolidate large groupings from which samples are selected by a method of probability sampling.

Nonprobability sampling involves selecting a sample without using a method of probability sampling. Major forms of nonprobability sampling include accidental sampling, or choosing the sample by convenience; quota sampling, or choosing the sample to represent the same percentage of characteristics found in the population; and purposive sampling, or selecting typical cases for the study sample.

The size of the sample depends upon a number of factors, such as the size and nature of the population and the kind of question the researcher wishes to answer. In general, larger samples are better than small samples. The more heterogeneous the population, the larger the sample should be, while the more homogeneous the population the smaller the sample may be.

Bias is defined as the systematic difference between the true value of the population and the corresponding value taken as a sample from that population. Bias can be caused by not including the entire population in the sampling process or by faulty measurement of the sample. Bias may be reduced by carefully defining the population and by using random sampling to select a study sample.

STUDY QUESTIONS

1. Identify a target population from which you wish to draw a sample for research. Define how to identify units of the population.
2. Use the units above to draw the following: a) a simple random sample; b) a systematic random sample.
3. What is the theory of probability? What does it have to do with sampling?
4. Give three definitions of probability. How do they differ? How are they the same?
5. How would you use quota sampling to study abortion in your town?
6. If you wished to study blood pressure among blacks of your town, how would you get a sample that was representative?

REFERENCES AND SUGGESTED READINGS

Babbie, E. (1973): The Practice of Social Research. Belmont, Calif.: Wacsworth. *Chapters 6 and 7 include the logic of sampling and examples of sample designs.*

Brink, P. and Wood, M. (1978): Basic Steps in Planning Nursing Research. North Scituate, Mass.: Duxbury Press, (pp. 93–100).

Dixon, W. and Massey, F. (1957): Introduction to Statistical Analysis. New York: McGraw-Hill. *See Chapter 4, Universe and Sample.*

Fox, D. (1976): Fundamentals of Research in Nursing (3rd ed.). New York: Appleton, pp. 158–177. *Chapter 8 includes excerpts from nursing.*

Johnson, A. (1977): Social Statistics without Tears. New York: McGraw-Hill. *See Chapter 9, Taking Samples.*

Knapp, R. (1978): Basic Statistics for Nurses. New York: Wiley, Chapter 4.

Lin, N. (1976): Foundations of Social Research. New York: McGraw-Hill, Chapter 9.

Messick, D. (1968): Mathematical Thinking in Behavioral Sciences. San Francisco: W. H. Freeman, Part 1.

Phillips, B. (1966): Social Research. New York: Macmillan, Chapter 15. *Sampling, etc.*

Phillips, J. and Thompson, R. (1967): Statistics for Nurses. New York: Macmillan, Part II.

Selltiz, C., Wrightsman, L., and Cook, S. (1976): Research Methods in Social Relations (3rd ed.). New York: Holt, Rinehart, and Winston, Appendix A— An Introduction to Sampling.

Walizer, M. and Wienir, P. (1978): Research Methods and Analysis. New York: Harper & Row, Chapter 15.

PART 4

Research Designs

CHAPTER 9
Research Designs

RESEARCH DESIGNS

Research design refers to the way the researcher plans and structures the research process. The design provides guideposts to keep the research headed in the right direction. There is no such thing as one correct design—designs vary from one study to another. Each researcher chooses the design that is most useful for the research purpose, whether to observe in order to know, to know in order to predict, or to predict in order to control and prescribe.

If the purpose of the research is to observe, describe, explore, and assemble new knowledge, a descriptive or exploratory design is used. If the purpose is to predict a causal relationship between variables or to establish correlation, an experimental or correlational study design is used. The survey design is used to obtain information from the self-reports of people in the natural setting in order to provide either quantitative descriptions or to discover relationships. The documentary or historical design is used to describe or compare data collected in the past. Secondary analysis, the use of available research data, is used to obtain new information from data that has already been scientifically collected for another study. A methodological research design is used to describe, develop, test, or evaluate research instrumentation (see Table 9–1).

Upon completion of this chapter, the student should be able to: 1) identify and describe various research designs used in nursing research; 2) define concepts, such as *control, randomization,* and *manipulation,* used

TABLE 9–1. TYPES OF DESIGNS, EXAMPLES, AND PURPOSES

Type of Design	Examples	Purpose
Descriptive Exploratory	1. Case Study 2. Comparative Study 3. Classificatory Study 4. Concept-formulation	To assemble new information; to describe in order to know; to analyze characteristics.
Experimental	1. True or Classic 2. Solomon Four-Group (true experiment) 3. Two After-Groups Control (true experiment)	To know in order to predict change; to explain.
Quasi-experimental	1. Four Cell (without randomization) 2. Time Series (single group) 3. Multiple Time Series (control-type group added) 4. Equivalent Time-Samples, etc. (see Campbell and Stanley, 1963, for this and others)	To know in order to predict, explain.
Pre-experimental (absence of, or nonequivalent, control group results in decreased value as an *experiment*)	1. "One-Shot" Case Study 2. One Group Before/After No control group. 3. Static Group Comparison Control group is not equivalent to experimental group.	To describe, to suggest limited predictions or explanations.
Survey	1. Questionnaire 2. Interview	To describe or explain.

TABLE 9–1. TYPES OF DESIGNS, EXAMPLES, AND PURPOSES
(Continued)

Type of Design	Examples	Purpose
Documentary-Historical	1. Public Records (census material) 2. Private Records 3. Mass Media	To describe, explain, or interpret.
Other (examples of many other designs are available)	1. Methodological 2. Ex-Post-Facto 3. Correlational	To develop or evaluate methods To describe, predict. To explain variation.

by researchers in various designs; 3) state the purpose of each research design; and 4) discuss the advantages and disadvantages of each research design.

DESCRIPTIVE-EXPLORATORY DESIGNS

With the descriptive-exploratory design, the researcher plans to assemble new information about a phenomenon. The researcher describes, compares, classifies, and conceptualizes new knowledge from what may have been unorganized or unrelated facts or data. Exploratory descriptive designs differ from descriptive designs in that exploratory designs may be more focused in order to formulate problems for more precise investigations later, or to describe new information that may subsequently be used to develop hypotheses. On the other hand, the descriptive design accurately describes characteristics of an individual, a situation, or a group; or examines the frequency with which an event occurs or is associated with another event (Selltiz et al, 1976, p. 90). Types of designs with the purpose of describing or exploring new information include: 1) the case study, 2) the comparative study, 3) the classification study; and 4) the concept-formulation study.

1. The case study is a basic type of descriptive design used in nursing to examine a single unit, such as an individual, group, community, culture, situation, problem, or process. In general, case studies are widely used by practicing professions such as law, anthropology, social work, psychiatry, and medicine. Nurses use the case study design in research to conduct intensive and lengthy investigations. For example, Martinson (1979) studied sixty-six families, case-by-case, over a period of six years, to investigate the feasibility and desirability of home care for the dying child. Others have used the case study design to study health in a cross-cultural perspective (Leininger, 1978). Resio and Verhonick (1973) used the case study design to analyze the characteristics of patients who had developed decubitus ulcers. Data included 375 variables collected from 96 patients. This type of design is similar to the pre-experimental design (explained below) but emphasizes description rather than change.

There are several advantages of the descriptive case study design: First, the case study is often a source of stimulating insights. At times, the researcher is able to create a *Gestalt*—a whole—from diverse bits of information. The exhaustive approach of the case study brings the individual or group to life as human beings rather than study objects. Second, particular diagnoses may be studied, not only to point up the patterns of illness but also to cast light on what is "normal," "wellness," or "health." Third, the case study is useful to describe processes of development—women becoming nursing mothers, infants becoming children, patients going through stages of an illness. Fourth, the design is helpful to study adjustment—the experience of adjusting to handicaps or diseases is illuminated for patient and nurse. And fifth, the design has the advantage of being flexible; the researcher may structure the design in terms of the time and material available.

The greatest disadvantage of the case study is the question of representativeness. There is no way of knowing whether the study is representative of a larger population. And for all intents and purposes, replication is impossible.

2. *The comparative study is a description or exploration of more than one unit or case.* The researcher examines two or more individuals, groups, communities, cultures, situations, or processes, in order to discover how they are alike and how they differ. For example, customs of health care may be compared cross-culturally; or the concept of *restlessness* may be compared in several different patients, such as the dying, the coronary, a patient who has hyperinsulinism, or one who is simply bored (see Norris, 1975, p. 107). Comparisons may be made on one dimension, such as the frequency of high blood pressure in blacks and whites; or an index may be developed to enable the researcher to compare several dimensions. For example, an index of social class that includes education, occupation, and income allows the researcher to compare lower-class blacks with middle-class blacks, or with lower-class and middle-class whites.

3. *Classification studies put observations into categories and name the categories.* Classification may precede or follow observation. The researcher seeks to describe behavior, signs and symptoms, attitudes, demographic variables such as age, sex, race, or any other characteristic of interest. Then the researcher puts those that are alike in the same category and names the category. For example, Strauss et al (1974, p. 560) drew on one and a half years of field work to classify pain into categories such as "on-going pain," "inflicted pain," "expected pain trajectories," and "unexpected pain trajectories." Brill and Kilts (1980, p. 154) classified nursing diagnoses as "immediate," based on verified descriptions of present behavior; "foreseeable," based on description of previous health responses; and "possible," or potential diagnoses based on similar descriptions.

Classification research is useful in a number of ways (Simon, 1978, p. 47). Classification aids summarization: after putting data into categories, the researcher can count the frequency. For example, summaries may be made of the number of patients with on-going pain or inflicted pain. Classification also aids comparison: it reveals the similarities and differences among categories. Classification leads to clarification: the researcher gains a better understanding of the phenomena being classified. Finally, classification leads to explanation: the researcher can establish the relationships among categories, which, taken together, describe and explain the total situation or process.

4. *Concept-formulation studies organize the researcher's observations and experiences into a meaningful and coherent whole, expressed by a word or concept.* Concepts stand for the mental images the researcher forms from observations or facts. *Conceptualization* is the process of ordering the observations, or data, by means of appropriate concepts. This is a difficult task. The concept is not a simple and directly observable item but a complex combination of interrelated observations. Observations of persons crying, weeping, sobbing, and lamenting may be ordered into one concept—*grieving*. Concept formulating is somewhat like an operational definition in reverse: the researcher observes, measures, and describes complex behavior and then invents a word to stand for it. The names are the concepts. Concept formulation is accomplished by inductive reasoning—beginning with observations and organizing them by logical thought into concepts. The researcher who is able to name the concepts and state a relationship between the concepts has formulated an empirical generalization and taken a significant step toward the formulation of a theory. Theory is the ultimate aim of all science.

Advantages and Disadvantages of Descriptive Designs

An advantage of descriptive and exploratory designs is the broad range of data and richness of detail that the researcher assembles. By observing and comparing, the researcher is able to gain a holistic view. As human conduct is observed and compared, hidden motives of behavior, or the latent rather than manifest patterns, may become apparent. The patterns and processes as a whole may be comprehended. From the wealth of description, classification and concept formulation are possible. The researcher may be able to move from observation and description, classification and conceptualization, to empirical generalization— stating a relationship between two concepts. At this point, the researcher has taken a significant step toward the development of a theory that explains what was observed and predicts what will be observed in later research.

A disadvantage of descriptive research is the inability to generalize the findings from the study of one community or one case to a broader population. Because the procedure is not standardized, descriptive studies cannot be replicated or evaluated. Even the same researcher may not be able to repeat precisely what was done before. Descriptive studies may not always be accurate; errors may creep into the study, and the observer's viewpoint may be biased in various ways. That is, the observer may have a tendency to observe in a manner that consistently differs from what a true accurate observation is. For example, a woman may consistently fail to observe male behavior, while a man may consistently observe men, rather than children or women. Yet, the objective of descriptive or exploratory research is not to generalize but to describe what is, to test ideas that may later be tested more rigorously. Comparative description, the classification of data into categories, and the formulation of concepts from descriptive data may be useful in a more general sense, especially if these are used to show relationships that may be tested and may lead to forming conceptual or theoretical frameworks.

EXPERIMENTAL DESIGNS

Experimental designs and variations fall into three major categories: the "true," or classical experimental design, the "quasi-experimental" design, and the "pre-experimental design." These differ in the amount of control the researcher uses. The true design maintains maximum, rigorous control by using the processes of *randomization* and *manipulation,* while the quasi-experimental and pre-experimental designs lack elements of control. An examination of what is meant by concepts such as *control, randomization,* and *manipulation* is useful to understand the experimental designs.

Control, Randomization, Manipulation

Control has several meanings in research. Broadly speaking, it is the researcher's ability to regulate and check all possible elements of the research. Major means of control include randomization and manipulation. *Randomization* is the process that first insures every unit in the target population an equal chance of being chosen for the study sample, and then insures that each unit in the study sample has an equal chance of being assigned to either the experimental or the control group (see Chapter 8). *Manipulation* refers to the process by which the researcher manages the independent variable in order to study its effect on the dependent variable.

To make sure that the design insures the collection of verifiable data (i.e., has validity), the researcher must also control extraneous variables that may influence the findings. *Extraneous variables* are those factors, present in large numbers in the environment, that are not interesting to the researcher but may act upon the dependent variable and confuse the effect of the independent variable. Eight classes of extraneous variables may especially interfere with research on human subjects: history, maturation, testing, instrumentation, statistical regression, selection, mortality, and interaction among these (see Chapter 12). To help control these variables, the researcher uses both experimental and control groups whose units are first randomly selected from the target population, and then (R) randomly assigned to either the experimental or the control group. The classic or true experiment clearly illustrates this control (see Figure 9–1). Two time periods (*before* and *after*) refer to the groups before the independent variable X is introduced into the experimental group but withheld from the control.

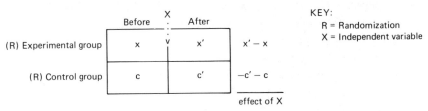

Figure 9–1. The true experimental design.

The characteristic steps to take in the true experiment design are:

1. Delineate the population or universe to be studied (i.e., the set of subjects or objects that share a common observable characteristic).

2. Select a sample from the population by random sampling.
3. By random assignment, subdivide the sample into two subsamples.
4. Specify one subsample the experimental group and the other the control group.
5. Before introducing the independent variable, observe and record all important characteristics of the two groups.
6. Introduce the independent variable into the experimental group but withhold it from the control group.
7. After introducing the independent variable, observe the dependent variable in both the experimental and the control groups.
8. Compare the changes that occur in the experimental group with those that may have occurred in the control group.
9. Record the difference.
10. Compare these values with statistically computed values that judge the significance of the difference, and indicate whether or not the observed differences could have occurred by chance.

The degree to which the findings are significantly greater than would be expected to occur by chance alone indicates the degree to which it is probable that a causal connection has been established.

At times, the researcher may supplement randomization with other processes, such as the use of homogeneous populations.

The Solomon Four-Group True Experimental Design

The Solomon four-group experimental design includes the four-cell classic experimental design above, plus two additional after groups, an experimental after-group and a control after-group (see Figure 9–2). The

	Before	X	After	KEY:
(R) Experimental group	x	v	x'	R = Randomization
(R) Control group	c		c'	X = Independent variable
(R) Experimental group	—	X ... v	x''	
(R) Control group	—		c''	

Figure 9–2. The Solomon four-group true experimental design.

two after-groups assist to control whatever effects of testing or measurement the before-groups may have experienced. For example, if the researcher wished to measure the effect of teaching a diabetic patient about diet, the researcher may give a test before the teaching, introduce teaching as the independent variable X, and then give the same test after the teaching to measure the effect the teaching has had. But the researcher cannot be sure that the first test in the before period did not influence the effect and cloud the action of the independent variable, the teaching, The use of two groups, neither of which were tested in the before period, helps control the effect of the testing. This design enables greater comparison. If all comparisons are in agreement, the ability to generalize increases. However, more work is involved.

Two After-Groups Control Design

The two after-groups control design is comprised of two randomly selected groups, neither of which is pretested or premeasured in the before period of time. The independent variable is introduced into the experimental group and withheld from the control group. These two groups are identical to the last two groups of the Solomon four-group design. The process of randomization is sufficient in itself to assure a lack of bias (Campbell and Stanley, 1966, p. 25). In situations where pretesting or premeasuring is not feasible, this design is appropriate (see Figure 9–3).

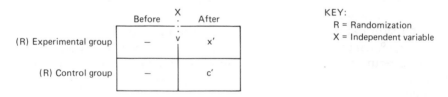

Figure 9–3. The after-groups control design.

Examples from Nursing Research

Numerous examples of experimental designs from the clinical area are reported in the nursing research literature. However, the researcher often cannot use random sampling, since the study subjects must be taken as they arrive in the clinic or hospital rather than being drawn from a target population by random sampling. In such cases, randomization takes the form of random assignment: the existing sample of patients is randomly sudivided into the experimental group and the control group. The resulting groups should be equivalent: the design should insure the collection of verifiable data (i.e., it has internal validity), but the loss of random sampling weakens the ability to generalize to a target population (i.e., it does not have external validity). In such cases, a basic strategy is to run a series of small sample experiments, whose cumulative results enable the researcher to generalize with more confidence (Woolridge et al, 1968). This suggests the need to replicate studies, an invitation to nurses and students whose cumulative replications will add to the ability to generalize from the original study.

Various hosptial settings, such as the operating room, premature nursery, and recovery room, contain a fairly well controlled environment and have been used by researchers such as Hasselmeyer, and Dumas and Leonard. Hasselmeyer (1961) conducted an experiment in the premature nursery to determine the effect of continually supporting the backs of premature infants with a diaper roll. She randomly assigned 59 infants to either the experimental group or the control group, introducing the diaper roll into the experimental group only. All other conditions were kept constant, including the amount of feeding, clothing, and handling. Each of the 59 infants was observed for definite periods of time by trained observers, using a scale developed to measure the dependent variable, the behavior of the infants.

Dumas and Leonard (1963) studied the effect of nursing on the incidence of postoperative vomiting. Patients on the operating schedule were randomly assigned into an experimental group, who received interaction with an experimental nurse, and a control group, who did not receive the experimental interaction. Vomiting in the recovery room was used as the dependent variable to indicate stress.

Other experimental studies in nursing include Cleland's (1977) investigation of the prevention of bacteriuria in hospitalized female patients with indwelling catheters; and Brown and Grunfeld's (1980) examination of infants' taste preferences for sweetened or unsweetened foods.

QUASI-EXPERIMENTAL DESIGNS

A quasi-experimental design is one in which full experimental control—usually randomization—is not possible. The use of quasi-experimental designs requires that the researcher be aware of the points on which the results are questionable. If neither random sampling nor random assignment is used, it is not possible to generalize from the findings. And judging whether the independent variable (experimental manipulation) resulted in observed differences between the experimental group and the control group requires more careful evaluation. Three examples of the quasi-experimental design follow:

The Four-Cell Design Without the Use of Randomization

The study subjects in this design are not randomly selected or randomly assigned. Instead, the groups are naturally assembled collectives, such as in classrooms or clinics. The researcher chooses the study subjects to be as similar as availability permits. To judge the similarity of the two groups, a pretest or premeasurement is made in the "before" time period. The more similar the scores on the pretest, the more effective this control becomes (see Figure 9–4). The independent variable is introduced into the experimental group only, after which both the experimental and control groups are tested or measured in the "after" period. Even though the researcher is not able to use random selection or assignment of study subjects, the use of a control group helps the researcher determine whether or not the independent variable actually made a difference in the experiment.

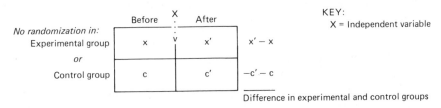

Figure 9–4. Four-cell design without randomization.

McGillicuddy (1977) used a somewhat similar design. She studied two groups of hospitalized children: one group had the mother rooming-in with the child and the other group did not. Each group had pre-hospitalization and post-hospitalization tests to measure changes in the child's behavior.

Huckabay (1978) used two samples of students to study the effect of an innovative teaching program. One group of students was taught with an innovative teaching program while the other group was taught with lecture and discussion methods. Both groups were tested before and after the teaching programs to determine any differences in the students' learning behavior.

The Time Series Experimental Design

The time series experimental design, a single group experiment, is comprised of a series of observations in the "before" time period to establish a baseline. The experimental (independent) variable is then introduced, followed by another series of observations to examine the effect of the independent variable (see Figure 9–5). For example, Hanson (1973) stud-

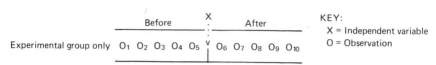

Figure 9–5. The time-series experiment.

ied the effects of administering cold and warm tube feedings on the temperature and heart rate of five volunteer subjects. The variables, temperature and heart rates, were established during the feedings and compared with those recorded when the feedings reached the stomach.

DeWalt and Haines (1977) used a similar design. The researchers studied the effect of stressors (oral breathing, continuous flow of oxygen, and intermittent mechanical suctioning) on the healthy oral mucosa of a volunteer. Observations of the subject took place in a laboratory setting, at fifteen-minute intervals over a five-hour period, to determine both the effects of the stressors on healthy oral mucosa and the effectiveness of nursing intervention to minimize the effects of the stressors.

The Multiple Time Series Design

Considered an excellent quasi-experimental design (Campbell and Stanley, 1966, p. 55), the multiple time series design is similar to the one-group time series experimental design, except that a control group is added. The independent variable is introduced into a series of observations on the experimental group but withheld from the series of observations made on the control group. The use of the control group, and the manipulation of the independent variable in the experimental group, increases the certainty with which the researcher can generalize findings.

PRE-EXPERIMENTAL DESIGNS

Pre-experimental designs is the name given to three designs that are considered weak experimental designs (Campbell and Stanley, 1963, pp. 6–13). The weakest of the three is the single group, or single case study, that is studied only once, following a treatment or an agent presumed to cause change (see Figure 9–6). Because the study design has a total absence of control, it is considered to be of little value as an experiment. At least one comparison is needed before scientific evidence is possible. However, many variations of this design exist, including the *ex-post-facto* design in which the researcher attempts to explain a phenomenon that has already occurred.

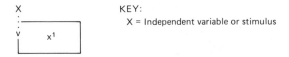

Figure 9–6. One-group studied once after stimulus.

Before and After Experimental Group: One Group Design

The second pre-experimental design is one in which the top two cells of the experimental design are used without a control group. That is, only one group is observed before and after the independent variable is introduced (see Figure 9–7). Loss of the control groups decreases the usefulness of the study but may be necessary in cases where it is not possible or feasible to have control groups. For example, Fieve et al (1971) used the design to measure the effects of lithium in treating manic psychosis. Six psychotic patients diagnosed as manic were tested by using the Psychiatric Evaluation form. The patients were then put on a regimen of lithium and later tested again. The before scores served as a control group. The differences in the before and after scores were considered a measure of the effectiveness of lithium.

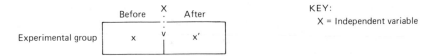

Figure 9–7. The experimental group only, before and after.

The Static Group Comparison Design

With this pre-experimental design, a group that has experienced the independent variable is compared with one that has not (see Figure 9–8). Lindeman and Van Aernam (1977, p. 49) used this design to study the effects of structured and unstructured preoperative teaching on the postoperative behavior of study subjects. The experimental group was comprised of subjects admitted during a specified time period, while the control group consisted of subjects admitted during a different time period. The experimental group received the independent variable, structured preoperative teaching, while the control group did not. The weakness in such a design is that the groups may not have been equivalent.

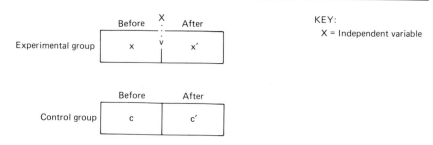

Figure 9–8. Static group comparison design.

Advantages and Disadvantages of the Experimental Designs

The advantages of the experimental design follow from three of its major characteristics—control, randomization, and manipulation. When the variables are narrow, well defined and controlled, it may be possible to establish a causal relationship, the process in which the independent variable or stimulus invariably precedes the effect. This is most clearly seen in the classical experimental design. Used when better designs are not feasible, quasi-experimental designs introduce a design that is similar to the classical experimental design, although randomization is often lacking. Experimentation is important in the task of theory testing and adds to the accumulating body of knowledge.

However, there are many disadvantages to be found in the use of the experimental approach. First, neither may work well with the study of human subjects, a complex and complicated process. There are few if any valid criterion measures, or measures of the dependent variable, available to indicate the effects of independent variables upon human subjects. In addition, the experimental setting may not accommodate the variables, some of which are too broad for the laboratory or for any artificial setting. Moreover, the independent variable may take years to manifest itself. The correlation between smoking and cancer is an example of the long time span necessary in some cases. Likewise, cooperation may be difficult when the researcher wishes to use the experimental method on human subjects who have full knowledge of the nature of the experiment. Finally, the widespread use of random assignment alone, rather than in conjunction with random sampling, interferes with the researcher's ability to generalize from the sample to a broader population, without a large number of studies to bolster the claim.

THE SURVEY

Survey research is a mode of inquiry that relies heavily upon the validity of verbal reports. A well known example of a survey is the United States Census. It combines a distinct method of data collection (interviews and questionnaires) with a special form of data analysis by statistical means. Surveys tend to study the effect of social forces in the field which are not under the researcher's control. In this case, the major controls are statistical rather than experimental, the critical factors being the use of random sampling to select a representative sample from the target population, and the statistical analysis and interpretation of data.

Modern survey research is not old, dating back to the 1930s, when Gallup and Roper brought the mode of inquiry and the form of statistical analysis together. It requires that standardized information be collected from or about subjects selected from a larger population by random sampling. The size of the sample is often quite large, although some studies have used less than 100 cases. The units of analysis range from individuals to groups, communities, or organizations. Common methods of data collection include the interview, mailed questionnaire, telephone interviews, and the survey that retrieves data from existing records or archival material.

Aims of the Survey Design

The survey may be either descriptive or explanatory. The aim of the descriptive survey is to look for data about the distribution and frequency of some datum in a population or subgroup. For example, the descriptive survey may seek to learn how respondents answer a question on abortion, in order to compare the responses of different groups, such as the married and single, males and females, or Catholics and Protestants. Or the descriptive survey may seek to determine how one or more characteristics are distributed in a population; for example, who has diabetes, high blood-pressure, malnutrition, and where do they live in a particular community?

On the other hand, explanatory surveys seek to discover why the distribution takes the form it does. Why does malnutrition occur among the poor, teenagers, or the elderly? Why does it occur in one sector of the community more often than it does in another?

Time Factors in the Survey

The survey may be *static*, that is, a *cross-section* of the population is examined at one point in time; or the survey may be *longitudinal*, including elements of change over a period of time. Longitudinal studies may be either *retrospective,* beginning at one point in time and tracing a phenomenon backward; or they may be *prospective,* beginning in the present and following a group or phenomenon forward over a period of time.

Longitudinal studies of change also include trend studies, cohort studies, panel studies, and follow-up studies. A trend study repeatedly asks the same question of equivalent samples of different individuals, while a panel study interviews the same subjects at two or more points in time. A cohort study examines a category of persons born during a particular time period. For example, a cohort of women born in 1940 may be studied in 1990 to determine the number of children ever born to them. At fifty years of age, the women are presumably past the child-bearing period and may be considered as having completed families. Follow-up studies seek to determine any change or development in individuals or groups who have been previously studied.

In all of these cases, two or more groups may be used, one exposed to an independent variable and one not. The absence of random assignment of the sample to either experimental or control groups distinguishes this form from the classic experimental design. The location of the research also differs, surveys being conducted more often in the field than in the laboratory.

Advantages and Disadvantages of the Survey Design

A major advantage of the survey is that data are gathered from a more natural setting. The variables are examined as they are found in the existing social milieu. A large amount of data can also be gathered at a fairly reasonable price. Surveys using the questionnaire are likely to cover a wide geographical area, reach many people, insure respondents' anonymity, and require less skill to administer. With careful pretesting of the instruments used, and with the use of random sampling techniques, the survey has a considerable degree of representativeness. No other method can reach as large a population as rapidly and be as accurate.

A major weakness of the survey design is that it only collects self-reports. This means that recall may be selective or that the respondent may not be willing to express attitudes or beliefs on sensitive topics. Standardization of the questionnaire also means that the least common denominator is represented. In addition, the response rate may be low, thereby introducing a bias. Finally, unless the researcher uses the interview, which is more expensive, the researcher is not able to observe the study subjects directly and loses the "feel" of the situation.

Examples from Nursing Research

The survey is widely used in nursing research to collect data by questionnaire or interview. At times, it may be combined with other research methods, or it may be used alone. Hurwitz and Eadie (1977) used both the survey and dream analysis to study the psychologic impact on nursing students of participating in abortion procedures. Using a series of questionnaires, together with dream reports written at the same time, data was collected over a four-week period, during which the students were assigned to various clinical experiences. In the first week, the clinical experience took place in abortion units, the questionnaire included a question on the students' feelings about abortion, and four basic questions were asked on the students' dreams, which were included each week. The following weeks did not include abortion experiences but did have other surgical experiences. Questionnaire data were analyzed by using the chi-square statistic, while dream data were analyzed by content analysis.

Stillman (1977) used a questionnaire to investigate the nature of women's health beliefs about breast cancer and breast self-examination, and the extent of breast self-examination. A convenience sample of 122 members of a women's organization filled out a questionnaire developed by the researcher and comprised of five sections. The data were analyzed by the use of descriptive statistics.

Ford (1973) studied the cultural criteria and determinants for the acceptance of modern medicine among reservation Indians of South Dakota. The researcher used several research designs, including unstructured interviews that focused on beliefs, attitudes, and interpersonal relations. The sample included "Yuwipi and herbal medicine men and women and their clients, peyote leaders and their clients, and persons using modern medicine" (Ford, 1973, p. 45). Analysis of data was descriptive, and used case study presentations.

THE DOCUMENTARY-HISTORICAL RESEARCH DESIGN

The historical research design is structured to collect and interpret data by examining material that already exists. The steps in the design are: 1) identify the major sources of material relevant to the research problem or hypothesis; 2) ascertain the location of the materials and documents, and determine its accessibility; 3) obtain permission to use the materials; 4) examine the data thoroughly; 5) establish categories of the data; 6) review current interpretation of the data; and 7) examine the data for new perspectives and explanations.

The major sources of data are public records and documents, private records, and the mass media. These may include *primary sources,* first-hand descriptions of observation, or *secondary sources,* publications that refer to or analyze primary sources.

Public Documents

Public documents include official governmental reports, such as statistical data (census data, birth rates, death rates, morbidity rates, etc.); police records (suicides, violence, drug use, child abuse); production data (agricultural production, industrial output, etc.); and health data (immunizations, life expectancy, etc.). Such data affords an economical approach to research and may be found in many libraries. Courthouse documents, such as court cases, wills, deeds, and taxation data, are also often useful.

Records of hospitals and health departments are official confidential documents that require special permission for study. Nurses who have open access to patients' records during clinical practice should obtain permission to use the same records for research studies.

Private Documents

Private documents include diaries, notes, letters, journals, and autobiographies that give a glimpse of the private worlds of the authors. The problems associated with using private documents are considerable, including questions of validity. Moreover, personal documents are often inaccessible, although the researcher may use records from her or his own family and friends that would not be available to other scientists.

The Mass Media

Books, magazines, movies, plays, and innumerable other popular sources may be worthwhile records for the researcher who seeks to examine what is being communicated about nursing, sickness, health, living, and dying. For example, television shows use the dramatic potential of the hospital to portray nurses, doctors, and patients in particular roles. Such depictions may have an impact on the public's view of nurses and nursing. This impact may be subsequently reflected in support for or against health agencies or personnel.

Folk beliefs concerning health and disease may likewise be examined by analyzing advertisements to cure ills or prevent disability. Magazines, newspapers, billboards, and television commercials help sell millions of dollars of drugs, palliatives, and cures, Little work has been done in this area, although a method of data collection related to records (content analysis) is well known.

To assess the validity of archival sources, the researcher may apply both external and internal criticism. *External criticism* is concerned with the document itself: Are the letters purported to be from patients in mental institutions actually written by the patients themselves? Is the diary of the child in the rehabilitation center a fake? *Internal criticism* is concerned with the content of the document: Was the primary witness able to tell the truth? Is the primary witness accurately reporting in the document when compared with other sources?

The comparatively low cost of acquiring such data makes historical analysis and record review attractive. However, there are the risks of error implicit in archival and historical sources, such as errors arising from selective deposit, selective survival, and selective editing of the data. The competency of the person who collected and recorded the data may determine the usefulness of the materal. Official sources tend to be more reliable than nonofficial records, but the researcher must carefully evaluate all documents. In using historical materials, the researcher must also distinguish between primary sources and secondary sources. Primary sources include first-hand descriptions of observations, such as minutes of a meeting, interview schedules or questionnaires used in a survey, research reports, hospital records, diaries, films, newspaper eye-witness accounts, or ethnographies and case studies. Secondary sources include books, articles, speeches, or publications that refer to, describe, compare, or analyze primary sources. Each of these has its use in historical designs, but it must be clear which the researcher is using.

Examples of Documentary Research Methods in Nursing Research

Using records from two state hospitals in Washington State, Nakagawa (1972) presents an historical epidemiological investigation that extends over a 26-year span. The sample was chosen by systematic selection: every fifteenth name on the roster of 9,257 names of patients who were admitted to the hospital for the first time. A detailed system to code the data at the time of record review was developed and used together with content analysis, a method of data collection (see Chapter 11). In order to examine the items and categories for change over time, the researcher compiled the 617 cases into groups. The trends over the 26-year span were shown by changes in proportions of an item or category among the intervals.

Advantages and Disadvantages of the Documentary Design

The major advantage of historical research designs is that data collection may be less expensive, because the observations are already collected and documented. However, the researcher must assemble, classify, and analyze the documents. Private and public documents not only may cover a long period of time, they may have been collected for purposes other than the research and may, therefore, be unbiased. However, the disadvantages of the historical design are considerable: The data may have gaps—they may be incomplete in the very areas crucial to the research problem. Records may also be lost, damaged, or otherwise inaccessible. The recorder may have been unwilling or unable to observe and record accurately. Bias may have intruded into the data-collecting process, or records may not be accurate. Yet, if critically examined, the documentary-historical approach provides nursing with a source of knowledge helpful to understand the nursing process.

METHODOLOGICAL DESIGNS

Methodological designs are plans for the development of tools used in research, such as scales, tests, or measuring instruments. The steps in the methodological design differ from the phases and steps generally used in research in that the methodological design involves invention and evaluation rather than sampling and data collecting. Downs and Fitzpatrick (1976) sought to develop an instrument to measure the quality of nursing care. They investigated the reliability and validity of a tool that assessed body position and motor activity. Such research is of vital importance, since it gives the researcher a confident means of collecting data.

EX-POST-FACTO AND CORRELATION DESIGNS

The ex-post-facto study is one that occurs "after the fact." The researcher attempts to explain a phenomenon that has already occurred. Something has happened in the life of an individual or a group of individuals that the researcher wishes to explain or describe. For example, birth defects can only be studied after the fact. The birth of the so-called thalidomide babies was presumed to be a result of the use of the drug thalidomide during pregnancy. The researcher could not manipulate the independent variable, the drug thalidomide, for ethical reasons. However, once the appearance of the birth defect was documented, researchers could look for preceding factors that may have been the presumed cause, or may be correlated with the effect.

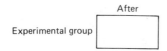

Figure 9–9. Ex-post-facto design.

The ex-post-facto study design is similar to the pre-experimental design described earlier. Goode and Hatt (1952, p. 85) suggest its similarity to the single-cell design (see Figure 9–9). The basic logic of the experiment and the ex-post-facto design is the same: the researcher wishes to establish the relationship between the independent variable and the dependent variable (Kerlinger, 1973, p. 379). The difference between the experiment and the ex-post-facto design is that control is lost in the ex-post-facto design. The independent variable cannot be manipulated, and the subjects cannot be randomly selected from the target population or randomly assigned to the experimental group or control group. Accompanying these differences is an associated problem: proper interpretation of data. Therefore, interpretation of ex-post-facto findings should be tentative, even when hypotheses are carefully selected and tested.

The value of ex-post-facto studies lies in the fact that many important research problems cannot be studied by experimentation. Ethical research prohibits the researcher from introducing a variable that may harm the study subjects. Certain variables cannot be manipulated, such as environmental, economic, and social factors, or personal characteristics of individuals, including sex, age, or diagnosis. The ex-post-facto study investigates cases in which these variables have been manipulated by life events: the environment has become polluted, jobs have been lost, or sex changes have been attempted. A second value of the ex-post-facto study is the relative "naturalness" of the design. Study subjects are not studied in a laboratory, but at home, at work, or in a situation where they have been placed by life.

Correlation and Causation

Correlation is the pattern of variation in two phenomena. Correlation, sometimes called concomitant variation or association, is a process which examines how a change in the amount of one variable is accompanied by a comparable change in the amount of another variable.

A causal relationship is also an association, but one that is strong enough to have predictive powers. To infer that one variable is the cause of another, the researcher must have three types of evidence: 1) the cause X and the effect Y must vary together in the way predicted by a specific hypothesis; 2) Y must not precede X in time; and 3) other factors did not determine Y (Selltiz et al, 1976, p. 489). As Mill (1930) puts it: when two or more cases of a given phenomenon have one and only one condition in common, then that condition is regarded as the cause of the phenomenon. When the researcher is unable to judge with certainty that the effect was directly caused by the stimulus, then the change is said to be associated or correlated with the stimulus rather than caused by the stimulus. Some researchers are wary of causality. Kerlinger (1973, p. 393) warns that the study of cause and causation is an endless maze. Particularly in the study of human subjects, causal relationships should be regarded as difficult to establish.

Correlational designs are similar to ex-post-facto studies in that neither expects to determine causality. However, correlational designs differ from ex-post-facto designs in that correlational designs may examine past events but may likewise include other time frameworks.

Time Frameworks
Correlational designs may include either prospective studies or cross-sectional studies. A well known prospective study, the Framingham Heart Study, followed 5,209 persons for over two decades. Gibbs et al (1974) utilized a record review of 15 months and interviews during a three month period to study reproductive health care patterns among the poor of San Antonio.

Amborn (1976) conducted a brief cross-sectional correlational study to examine the clinical signs associated with the amount of suctioned tracheobronchial secretions. Data was collected from 35 study subjects over a one-hour period.

Elder (1976) used a predictive correlational study to explain variables that may influence a dependent variable. A large number of variables (education, religion, sexual experience, age, etc.) were used to predict the willingness that nursing students demonstrated to participate in the provision of contraceptives.

Advantages and Disadvantages of Ex-Post-Facto and Correlational Designs
Both designs have the advantage of examining the results of factors that could not be studied because of ethical restraints. In the ex-post-facto design, life has introduced the presumed independent variable. The researcher examines the effect, searching among the processes of the past to identify a possible agent whose presence is correlated with the effect. The disadvantage of the ex-post-facto design is the loss of control—both manipulation and randomization.

Correlational designs are useful to examine the extent to which changes in one factor vary with changes in one or more other factors. The disadvantage of the correlational design is the researcher's tendency to attribute causality to descriptive relationships. However, carefully designed with good hypotheses, correlational studies provide information that may be used to predict.

SUMMARY

The research design is the plan and structure of the research, whether it is a descriptive-exploratory design, an experiment, a survey, a documentary-historical design, or a methodological design. Each of these differs in the method of data collection, the degree of control, the unit under study, the site of the research, and the purpose. However, all of the designs are useful in nursing research.

The descriptive-exploratory design proposes to observe, describe, explore, and assemble new knowledge. Four types of descriptive designs are the case study, the comparative study, the classificatory study, and the study that seeks to conceptualize from descriptive data. The case study is a basic type of descriptive design that examines a single unit in depth. The case study is often a source of stimulating insights and is useful to study change and adjustment. The greatest disadvantage of the case study is the researcher's inability to generalize from only one case. The comparative study allows the researcher to describe how the units under study are alike and how they differ. Comparison may be made on one dimension, or an index of several dimensions may be useful. Classification studies put observations into categories and name the categories—classification follows description and is derived from it. Classification aids summarization and comparison and clarifies description. It also is a step that leads to explanation, when the researcher is able to establish relationships among the categories. Concept-formulation studies seek to organize description into a coherent whole that is expressed by a word or concept. Conceptualization is the process of ordering observations, by means of appropriate concepts. Formulating concepts from descriptive data is difficult, but provides the basis for an empirical generalization that states the relationship between two or more concepts. The advantages of descriptive designs are the advantages conferred by the studies above. Beginning with observation, the researcher inductively reasons to describe and denote patterns of descriptive data. Yet, the primary objective of descriptive or exploratory research is not to generalize but to provide the data base for ideas that may be tested later more rigorously.

With the experimental design, the researcher has maximum control over the independent variable and over the selection and assignment of subjects to different experimental conditions. A major means of control is randomization—the process that first insures every unit in the target population an equal chance of being chosen for the study sample, and then insures each unit in the study sample an equal chance of being assigned to either the experimental or the control group. A second means of control is manipulation—the process by which the researcher treats or manages the independent variable, in order to study its effect upon the dependent variable. The researcher must also control extraneous variables, those factors present in large numbers in the environment that are not interesting to the researcher but may act upon the dependent variable and confuse the effect of the independent variable. Three types of true experimental designs include: 1) the classic experimental design, comprised of a randomly chosen and assigned experimental group and a control group that is measured before and after the independent variable is introduced into the experimental group; 2) the Solomon four-group, which adds two after-groups to the classic experimental design (an additional after-experimental group and an additional after-control group); and 3) two after-groups, an experimental and a control group. All groups of the true experimental design are randomly chosen from a target population and assigned to either the experimental or control group. All groups enable the researcher to manipulate the independent variable, in order to study its effect.

With quasi-experimental designs, full experimental control, usually randomization, is not possible. If neither random sampling nor assignment is used, the researcher cannot generalize from the findings of the sample to the population. And the researcher must carefully judge whether the independent variable resulted in observed differences between the experimental and control groups. There are many quasi-experimental designs, including a four-cell experimental group similar experimental designs, including a four-cell experimental group similar to the true classical experiment, except for the lack of randomization. Other designs include the time series experimental design, in which one group is observed several times before and after the introduction of the independent variable; and the multiple time series design, which is similar to the time series design, except that a control group is added.

Pre-experimental designs include: 1) the single group design, which is studied only once following a treatment or an agent presumed to cause change; 2) one group studied before and after a stimulus is introduced; and 3) the static group design, in which a group that has experienced the independent variable is compared with one that has not. Although none is strong, the weakest of these three is the single group design.

The advantages of the experimental design follow from the level at which the researcher is able to control through randomization and manipulation. The most effective designs are the true designs; the most ineffective are the pre-experimental designs. Quasi-experimental designs usually lack randomization but are recommended if it is not possible to carry out the true experiment. The disadvantages of the experimental design are the difficulty of experimenting on human subjects and the limitations of the laboratory setting. Time is also a factor that handicaps the experimental study of human subjects—the independent variable may take years to manifest itself.

The survey is a mode of inquiry that relies heavily upon verbal self-reports. The national census is an example of survey research design. The method of data collection by questionnaire and interview is combined with a special form of data analysis by statistical means. Random sampling is used to select a representative sample from the target population (or, in the case of the national census, the total population is surveyed). Units of study range from individuals to national populations. The survey may be either descriptive or explanatory. The descriptive survey collects data about the characteristics or frequency of specified units and processes. The explanatory survey seeks to discover the relationship between variables. A survey may examine a population at one point in time—the cross-section; or it may study change over a period of time—the longitudinal study. The longitudinal study may be retrospective, beginning at one point in time and tracing a phenomenon backward; or it may be prospective, following a group or phenomenon forward over a period of time. The trend study repeatedly asks the same question of equivalent samples of the population, while the panel study interviews the same subjects at two or more points in time. The cohort study examines a group of persons who were born at the same time and thus experienced similar events, while the follow-up study examines change or development of those who have been previously studied.

A major advantage of the survey is that data are gathered from a natural setting. In addition, large amounts of data may be collected from a broad geographical area. The major weakness of the survey design is the reliance on respondents' self-reports, which may be selective or incorrect. In the case of the questionnaire, lack of response is also a disadvantage, because the returns may not be sufficient to represent the population.

With the documentary-historical design, the researcher examines records and documents already in existence. Major sources of data include official and unofficial documents, statistics, audio-visual media, and general historical data. To assess the validity of archival sources, the researcher uses external criticism concerned with the document itself, and internal criticism concerned with the writer's ability and willingness to tell the truth or report accurately. The researcher must distinguish between primary sources, or first hand descriptions of observations, and secondary sources, such as books, articles, speeches, or publications that use primary sources. The major advantage of documentary or historical research designs is that the data have already been collected. But therein lies its weakness: the data may have gaps, or be incomplete, lost, damaged, or inaccessible, or the recorder may not have been willing or able to observe and record accurately, without bias.

A methodological design is a plan for the development of tools or measures, such as scales and tests. This design emphasizes development and evaluation, rather than sampling and data collection.

Ex-post-facto designs examine the data after life or nature has introduced the independent variable. The researcher does not have direct control, either because the effect has already been manifested or because it is not possible to manipulate the independent variable. Instead, the researcher investigates the effects of the independent variable after they have occurred. Ex-post-facto study designs are useful because of the ethical constraints on manipulation when human subjects are used. The researcher cannot introduce or manipulate the independent variable, but in cases where it has been introduced, the researcher can try to study its presumed effect.

Correlational studies examine how variables change in terms of one another. Correlational designs may be prospective, beginning at one point in time and following study subjects forward; or they may be cross-sectional, studying the changes in the amount of one variable in relation to changes in another, in a concurrent time framework. Correlational studies are useful to provide information about the extent of changes between associated variables.

STUDY QUESTIONS

1. What is a research design?
2. Name six designs, and suggest nursing research for each.
3. What are the two kinds of experimental designs? What distinguishes each kind?
4. Draw a model of the classical experimental design and of the quasi-experimental design. Compare each with the other, referring to what is present and absent.
5. What are the major means of control in research?
6. What are the steps to take in carrying out an experimental design?

7. How does the Solomon four-group experimental design differ from the classic experimental and from the after-group-only control design?

8. What are some settings in the hospital that nurses have used to conduct research with the experimental design? What problems can arise in using such a design?

9. What is a pre-experimental design? Why do Campbell and Stanley consider this kind of design ineffective as an experiment? Why is it used?

10. What are the advantages and disadvantages of the experimental design?

11. What is a survey? What different time factors may be used in a survey?

12. What are the major advantages and disadvantages of the survey design?

13. How can survey designs be combined with other research designs?

14. What is an historical-documentary research design?

15. What are good sources of documents? What are the advantages and disadvantages of each source?

16. Compare a descriptive case study with a methodological research design.

17. Compare causation, correlation, and ex-post-facto designs. What are the advantages of the correlational and the ex-post-facto design?

REFERENCES AND SUGGESTED READINGS

Amborn, S. (1976) Clinical signs associated with the amount of tracheobronchial secretions. *Nursing Research 25,* 121–126. *An exploratory correlation design.*

Austin, A. (1957): History of Nursing Source Book. New York: G. P. Putnam's Sons. *Excerpts from authors' writings on nursing from historical perspective.* (1958): The historical method in nursing. *Nursing Research 7,* 4–10. *Means used in the historical design.*

Branch, H. (1979): Women in pain. In Kjervik, D. and Martinson, I. (eds), Women in Stress: A Nursing Perspective. New York: Appleton, pp. 237–255. *Includes use of the case study.*

Brown, M. and Grunfel, C. (1980): Taste preferences of infants for sweetened or unsweetened food. In *Research in Nursing and Health 3,* 11–17. *Experimental design using random assignment.*

Campbell, D. and Stanley, J. (1966): Experimental and Quasi-experimental Designs for Research. Chicago: Rand McNally. *Includes experimental, quasi-experimental, and pre-experimental designs, and factors jeopardizing validity.*

Christy, T. (1975): The methodology of historical research. In *Nursing Research 24,* 189–192. *The use of historical design.*

Cleland, V. (1977): Investigations in the clinical setting. In Verhonick, P. (ed.), Nursing Research II. Boston: Little, Brown, pp. 33–76. *Experimental design in the clinical setting.*

Cornell, S. (1974): Development of an instrument for measurement of the quality of nursing care. *Nursing Research 23,* 108–117. *Methodological design to develop a research tool.*

DeWalt, E. and Haines, A. (1977): The effects of specified stressors on healthy oral muçosa. In Downs, F. and Newman, M., A Sourcebook of Nursing Research. Philadelphia: F. A. Davis, pp. 24–32. *Experimental research.*

Downs, F. and Fitzpatrick, J. (1976): Preliminary investigation of the reliability and validity of a tool for the assessment of body position and motor activity. *Nursing Research 25,* 404–408. *Methodological design.*

Downs, F. and New, M. (eds.) (1977): A Sourcebook of Nursing Research. Philadelphia: F. A. Davis. *Fifteen articles on research identify research design.*

Dumas, R. and Leonard, R. (1963): The effect of nursing and the incidence of post-operative vomiting; a clinical experiment. *Nursing Research 12,* 12–15. *Experimental study.*

Elder, R. (1976): Orientation of senior nursing students toward access to contraception. *Nursing Research 25,* 338–345. *Correlational study.*

Fieve, R. et al (1971): A critical trial of methysergate and lithium in mania. In Kuper, D. (ed.), Lithium and Psychiatry Journal Articles. Medical Examination Pub. *An experimental study.*

Ford, V. (1973): Medicine among the Teton Dakota, Rosebud Indian Reservation, South Dakota. In Batey, M. (ed.), Communicating Nursing Research. Boulder, Colo.: WICHE. *Research using the survey and other designs.*

Goode, W. and Hall, P. (1952): Methods in Social Research. New York: McGraw-Hill, Chapter 7.

Gibbs, et al (1974): Patterns of reproductive health care among the poor of San Antonio, Texas. *American Journal of Public Health 64,* 37–40. *Longitudinal study.*

Hasselmeyer, E. (1961): Behavior Patterns of Premature Infants. Washington, D.C.: Govt. Printing Office. *Experimental design.*

Hanson, R. (1973): Effects of administering cold and warmed tube feedings. In Batey, M. (ed.), Communicating Nursing Research. Boulder, Colo.: WICHE. *Time series experimental design.*

Holaday, B. (1980): Implementing the Johnson model for nursing practice. In Riehl, J. and Roy, C. (eds.), Conceptual models for Nursing Practice. New York: Appleton, pp. 255–263. *Case design used.*

Huckaby, L. (1978): Cognitive and affective consequences of formative evaluation in graduate nursing students. *Nursing Research 27,* 190–194. *Quasi-experimental design.*

Hurwitz, F. and Eadie, F. (1977): Psychologic impact on nursing students of participation in abortion. *Nursing Research 26,* 112–120. *Questionnaire and dream collection.*

Josten, L. (1979): Child abuse. In Jervik, D. and Martinson, I., Women in Stress: A Nursing Perspective. New York: Appleton, pp. 218–236. *Case reports.*

Kerlinger, F. (1973): Foundations of Behavioral Research (2nd ed.). New York: Holt, Rinehart, and Winston, Part 6, Designs of Research, pp. 300–423.

Kjervik, D., and Martinson, I. (eds.) (1979): Women in Stress: A Nursing Perspective. New York: Appleton. *Twenty articles survey various stressful situations.*

Lo Rocco, S. and Polit, D. (1980): Women's knowledge about the menopause. In *Nursing Research 29,* 10–13. *Survey of 500 women in greater Boston.*

Leininger, M. (1978): Transcultural Nursing. New York: Wiley. *Twenty-six articles, a number of case studies.*

Lindeman, C. and Van Aernam, B. (1977): Nursing intervention with the presurgical patient—the effects of structured and unstructured preoperative teaching. In Downs, F. and Newman, M. (eds), A Sourcebook of Nursing Research (2nd ed.). Philadelphia: F. A. Davis, pp. 45–63. *Pre-test/post-test static group design.*

McGillicuddy, M. (1977): A study of the relationship between mothers' rooming-in during their children's hospitalization and changes in selected areas of children's behavior. In Downs, F. and Newman, M. (eds.), A Sourcebook of Nursing Research (2nd ed.). Philadelphia: F. A. Davis, 64–77. *Use of interviews, questionnaires, comparative groups.*

Miller, D. (1970): Handbook of Research Design and Social Measurement (2nd ed.). New York: David McKay. *Part I includes guide to research designs.*

Mill, J. (1930): A System of Logic (8th ed.). New York: Longmans.

Nakagawa, H. et al (1972): An epidemiological study of psychiatric symptom pattern change: pilot study findings. In Batey, M. (ed.), Communicating Nursing Research. Boulder, Colo.: WICHE. *An historical epidemiological approach.*

Norris, C. (1975): Restlessness: a nursing phenomenon in search of meaning. *Nursing Outlook 23,* 103–107. *Illustration of description of nursing phenomena in the clinical area.*

Notter, L. (1972): The case for historical research in nursing. *Nursing Research 21,* 483. *Historical design.*

Resio, D. and Verhonick, P. (1973): On the measurement and analysis of clinical data nursing. *Nursing Research 22,* 388–393. *Case study analysis of characteristics of decubitus ulcer data.*

Selltiz, C. et al (1976): Research Methods in Social Relations (3rd ed.). New York: Holt, Rinehart, and Winston. Chapters 4 and 5.

Stillman, M. (1977): Women's health beliefs about breast cancer and breast self-examination. *Nursing Research 26,* 121–127. *Survey design by questionnaire.*

Stouffer, S. (1950): Some observations on study design. *American Journal of Sociology 55,* 356–359. *Models for experimental designs.*

Verhonick, P. (ed.) (1975): Nursing Research I. Boston: Little, Brown. *Six articles.* (1977): Nursing Research II. Boston: Little, Brown. *Seven articles.*

Wooldridge, P. et al (1968): Behavioral Science, Social Practice and the Nursing Profession. Cleveland: The Press of Case Western Reserve University. *Discusses the use of small samples with high internal validity to claim external validity.*

PART 5

Collecting the Data

CHAPTER 10

RESEARCH METHODS

Research method refers to the way the researcher collects data, whether by observation, questioning, or measuring. The method of data collection is related both to the problem being studied and to the research design. The researcher uses methods of observation and measurement to collect data in the experimental design; questioning and measurement in the survey design; and all three methods in the historical design.

Observation, questioning, and measurement are basic but not mutually exclusive methods of data collecting. They are often used in various combinations. For the purpose of examination, however, the three methods will be separated. This chapter will concentrate on observation, while the following two chapters will analyze methods of asking questions and measuring.

Upon completion of this chapter, the student should be able to: 1) state the factors that must be kept in mind to plan an observational study; 2) describe the observer's role in participant and non-participant observation; 3) explain what the observer watches; 4) describe classification as a means of observation; 5) define *operational definition* as a method of observation; 6) discuss instrumentation and its role in observation; 7) describe the role of scaling in observation; and 8) discuss the strengths and weaknesses of the observational method of data collecting.

OBSERVATION

Observation—the ability to see, examine, and record information—is the basis of all modern science. The role of the observer, and what the observer watches, require careful attention in research. Methods and means by which the researcher observes include sampling, classification, operational definition, instrumentation, scaling, and measuring. Sampling has been examined earlier (Chapter 8). Classification, operational definition, and instrumentation will be examined in this chapter, with some reference to scaling and measuring. Scaling and measuring will be examined in more depth later (Chapter 12).

SCIENTIFIC OBSERVATION

While all human beings continuously observe throughout their lives, observation becomes scientific only when it fulfills certain conditions: 1) the observation is undertaken with specific objectives in mind; 2) it is systematically planned and recorded; 3) all observations are checked and controlled; and 4) the observations are related to scientific concepts and theories. Scientific observation is best exemplified by the true experimental design (see Chapter 9). However, the researcher may not always be able to fulfill all of the conditions for scientific observation. Aamodt (1972) points out that explanations for health and healing at the sociocultural level are neither well understood nor described. In such cases, observation is perforce highly exploratory. Relying upon one observer, such research is at times as much an art as a science. Yet, such studies pave the way for studies that *can* meet the criteria for scientific observation. For example, the researcher who studies the autistic child, the catatonic schizophrenic, or people of different cultures may well rely solely on the observation of behavior over a considerable period of time to describe what is meant by *autism, schizophrenia,* or a particular *culture.*

In any observational study, a number of factors must be kept in mind. Kassenbaum (1970) suggests that the role of the observer involves considerable preparation. First, the researcher must be aware of the *selective attention* he or she habitually displays as an observer; the researcher must also consider the selective attention he or she wishes to display. For example, nurses may selectively observe patients on the basis of sex and age: men may be observed differently from women, and children differently from adults. The bias in the observations must be recognized and corrected. Second, the researcher must specify what he or she is reporting, whether overt behavior alone, or inference from the behavior to the intentions of the subject. Third, the researcher must select, sharpen, and make explicit both what he or she plans to observer, and what the researcher actually observes. Fourth, the researcher should think carefully about the experiences, reliving in his or her mind the observations made before, during, and after the researcher records them. Finally, the researcher should be sensitive to the impact of his or her presence upon those observed and should record these impressions often, in a systematic and careful manner.

A number of roles are available to the observer. The researcher may become an accepted member of the group being studied to participate in the processes being observed. Or, the researcher may stay aloof from participation and observe only. Once the researcher selects the role, he or she must identify *what* to observe and measure and *how* the observations will be made, that is, the means of observing, measuring, and recording the data. Each of these processes is now examined.

The Role of the Observer: Participant or Nonparticipant Observation

The role of the observer may be one of full participation or of nonparticipation. In participant observation, the researcher finds a role that is acceptable to the subjects under study and assumes it full time, in order to interact with the subjects and observe behavior in its "natural" state. The objective of participant observation is to obtain a depth of experience that is not available by watching alone. In nonparticipant observation, the researcher remains aloof from interaction. In this case, the objective is to exchange depth of subjective experience for a more objective approach to data. Part-time participation may involve a combination of participant and nonparticipant observation.

Participant observation has been used by nurses such as Chapman, Horn, and Kendall to collect ethnographic data or clinical observations. For example, Chapman (1977, p. 17) conducted an experiment in the clinical area to study the effects of different nursing approaches upon the postoperative responses of male herniorrhaphy patients. She was able to use a number of previous studies reported in the literature to plan her study, check and control the experimental variables, and relate the observations to scientific concepts and theories. She assumed the role of participant observer by presenting herself to the patient as a member of the nursing staff. At the same time, she used a mechanical aid to enhance her observations—she wore a small tape recorder with a microphone to record nurse–patient interaction for later classification by independent judges. Chapman solved the ethical problem faced by researchers in such situations by obtaining the informed consent of all subjects prior to their admission to the study. Horn (1978) spent three years as a participant observer in weekly well-child clinics on the Muckleshoot Indian reservation to observe and describe social and cultural factors influencing child-rearing practices and health care. Similarly, Kendall (1978) conducted an ethnographic study in a small Muslim village in central Iran to study maternal and child nursing.

Instead of a participant observation study, Marshall (1972) used nonparticipant observation to study the reactions of patients to sounds in the intensive coronary care units. Marshall did not wish to become involved in patient care, and, at the same time, she wished to protect the patients from additional stress. She used an instrument already in place (cardiac monitor) and added a tape recorder in an unobtrusive position to document the effect of sounds in the unit upon the patients' cardiac responses.

Both participant and nonparticipant observation may vary in terms of the degree of structure used. If it is not clear what data will be found or which measurements or scales are useful, unstructured observation is necessary. However, unstructured observation is realistic only if the investigator has the time to spend observing and interacting with the study subjects, or devising and testing measures and scales. On the other hand, structured observations are used if the researcher knows what will be observed and has a system of classification, instrumentation, operational definitions, and scales with which to work. If more than one observer is at work, structure is essential. In such cases, the researcher must develop standardized methods of observation and must train observers to use each method, in order to insure uniform observations.

Participant and nonparticipant observation are used to study all types of observable behavior. Observation is also used to examine records, or written observations of the past. In such cases, the observer's role is primarily judgmental and analytical. The researcher makes a judgment of whether the writer has made a valid observation, and uses techniques such as content analysis to analyze the material in terms of the concepts and theories being used. However, each research method must specify *what* will be observed and *how* it will be observed.

What the Observer Watches

What the observer watches depends upon the research design, the instruments available, and the theory that underlies the study. The experimental design is structured and controlled—it clearly specifies what will be observed and how. On the other hand, the survey depends upon indirect observation. The researcher questions the subjects about matters the researcher cannot observe. The historical design depends upon the study of documented observations of the past. The methodological design, the ex-post-facto design, and the correlational design combine methods of observing, questioning, measuring, and evaluating.

What the observer watches is influenced by the instruments available. Electronic devices to monitor internal conditions enable the researcher to observe what he or she ordinarily could not. Audio-tapes and video-tapes capture processes that the researcher can examine later in detail. Such devices may be set to monitor observations at random times during the day and night—a feat not convenient or possible for the usual observer. Factors such as silence, duration of interaction, and fidelity of content may simultaneously be captured, a nearly impossible undertaking for one observer or even several observers.

What the observer watches is structured by the theory or assumptions with which the observer begins. For example, observations of behavior modification may differ from observations of health practices in folk culture, and they may differ according to the unit of study and the site of the study. Observations of a family studied in its home will differ from observations of a family studied in the hospital setting. The observer may choose to watch individual behavior or processes, such as dying or sleeping.

What the observer watches is also related to the amount of control and manipulation the observer can exert. Observations in a highly controlled experiment differ from observations in uncontrolled, opportunistic, "natural" environments. The observer who is manipulating an independent variable and watching closely the effect on the dependent variable is involved in a highly structured observation. On the other hand, the researcher who is collecting descriptive data has the advantage of watching a broader set of factors but must deal with a myriad of uncontrolled behaviors.

Uncontrolled observation in which the researcher does not intervene tends to fall into five categories of "simple observations" (Webb et al, 1966, p. 115). These simple observations include: 1) exterior physical signs, 2) expressive movement, 3) physical location, 4) language behavior, and 5) time duration. These categories were devised primarily for unobtrusive measures in social sciences, but they are also helpful to the researcher in health science and may be adapted for use. Each of these categories will be examined, with examples from nursing studies where these are available.

1. Exterior physical signs express current or past behavior and often may be observed unobtrusively. These physical signs include voluntary changes of the body, such as beards, haircuts, tatoos, and clothing. Beards, length of hair, and haircuts are easily discernible signs related to life-style, affluence, state of mind, or occupation. For example, neglect of the hair may suggest certain emotional factors at work. Webb et al suggest that tatoos may be associated with delinquency, since more delinquents than nondelinquents are tatooed. On the other hand, tatoos may be a sign of military service and conformity to group pressure. Clothing is a particularly significant exterior sign that may reflect social status and image or the meaning of the situation to the patient. For example, Kane (1958) examined the meaning of clothing that out-patients wore to interviews. He followed this study with an examination of clothing worn by an out-patient (1959), and later examined the meaning of the form of clothing (1962). Klein *et al* (1972) examined the use of clothing—uniforms or street clothes—worn by members of the psychiatric staff, while Petrovich et al (1968) compared the use of uniforms and street clothes worn by psychiatric nurses. The white uniform of the nurse or physician may be associated with restraints or painful treatments, causing patients—especially children—to react with fear to anyone in a white uniform.

Exterior physical signs that have long been observed by nurses include: clinical signs of disease and physical disorder, such as the rash associated with measles; the color changes, edema, or dyspnea associated with heart disease; and vital signs, such as temperature, pulse, blood pressure, and respiration, which are used to infer or estimate internal physiology.

2. *Expressive movements communicate inner emotions that are ordinarily not observable. Kinesics,* the study of communication by observing body motion, is a fairly new field in nursing research, although kinesthetic needs have been examined by Hasselmeyer (1964), Barnard (1973), and others. Kinesics includes the unobtrusive study of facial expression, gestures, and body position that express emotions. Wolff (1948) observed the gestures of mental patients at meals and work and found evidence of a relationship between mental condition and the way patients moved their hands. Other body movements that have been examined include touch, dance, and the expressive responses to music. McCorkle (1974) investigated the effects of touch on seriously ill patients, while Burnside (1973) examined the effects of touch on the care of the aged. Ammon (1969) studied the effects of music on children in respiratory distress, while Gunning and Holmes (1973) and Puttock (1972) investigated the use of dance therapy with psychotic children.

3. *Physical position or physical location refers to the clustering, dispersion, or position assumed by persons of different ages, sexes, and psychological states, such as fear or stress.* For example, certain persons assume the fetal position under stress. Webb et al (1966, p. 124) report that fearful persons tend to cluster closely to one another, while Leipold (1963) reports an increase in the spacing distance between individuals experiencing stress. The degree of space preferred at various times of the day, together with the degree of sociability manifested, was observed by Rodgers (1977), who reported that the amount of personal space preferred was greater in the morning than in the afternoon.

4. *Language behavior, or conversation, includes both the content and the persons who communicate with one another.* Baziak and Dentan (1965) report that nurses and physicians often use medical words that are incomprehensible to their patients. Mahl's (1956) study of stuttering and slips of the tongue in the clinical setting reveals how the disturbances of speech and the silences are clues to inner meanings. Webb et al suggest that conversation samples may be collected unobtrusively by noting who talks with whom, for how long, and about what. However, eaves-dropping may raise ethical questions, although observations of public conversations may not. Communication with patients and familes may be accompanied by silences, smiles, frowns, or humor that convey more to the patient than the content of the conversation. Robinson (1970, p. 117) noted the importance of such communication, but this has been little explored.

5. *The observation of time, the duration, fluctuation, and time-movement studies, have received considerable attention in nursing.* For example, Alderson (1974) studied the effect that increases in body temperature have on the perception of time. Felton (1970, p. 1973) examined the effects of biological rhythms on nurses' efficiency, work shifts, and sleep patterns. Time-movement studies to establish staffing standards in nursing are numerous.

MEANS AND METHODS OF OBSERVATION

The means and methods by which observations are made in research include: 1) classification, 2) operational definition, 3) instrumentation, 4) scaling, and 5) measurement. All of these processes are related (see Figure 10–1). *Classification,* the assignment of persons, places, or things to named categories, is an integral part of organizing observations. A scale may be an instrument that measures observations. Measurements that are incorporated into operational definitions, instruments, and scales may come before data is collected or after. In spite of the intimate interrelationships among the means and methods of observation, each of these processes may be separated from one another for analytical purposes.

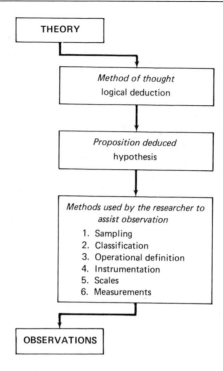

Figure 10–1. Relationships among theory, methods of observation, and observation.

Classification

Classification is the systematic assignment of subjects, objects, or ideas to named categories. The names suggest the basic units that will be observed. Basic units may be either specific motor behaviors, such as touching, or concepts such as anxiety, that must be defined by operational definition, in order to be observable and measurable.

The names assigned to the categories should follow as closely as possible those defined in the literature. Once categories have been established according to theory, reclassifying or re-naming them suggests a change in the theoretical approach. For example, changing the name of a mental illness from *dementia praecox* to *schizophrenia* suggests a change in the theory that explains such an illness.

Classification may be a goal in itself, or it may be a means to order what will be observed. For example, nursing research that seeks to establish categories such as "patient needs" or "nursing diagnosis" uses classification as a goal. Such classification identifies what needs to be observed and measured in nursing and, as such, is basic to the discipline. However, classification is more commonly used as a step in the research process that occurs before observation and helps the researcher organize what will be observed; or, it is a step that occurs after observation and helps the researcher order similar observations that were made. Research that begins with theory, assumptions, or ideas from which hypotheses are deduced or objectives are developed, uses classification before observation to specify exactly what the researcher predicts will be observed. Classification done after observation is inductive: the researcher develops categories from what was observed and assigns names or develops concepts that describe the similar data assigned to each category.

Classification begins with the formulation of the research proposal or working hypothesis that identifies what the observables will be. For example, the following hypothesis identifies four categories into which observations will fall:

Infants born to mothers who smoke will have a lower birth weight than infants born to mothers who do not smoke.

The four categories of data to be observed are mothers who smoke; mothers who do not smoke; birth weights of infants born to mothers who smoke; and birth weights of infants born to mothers who do not smoke. Yet, this fourfold classification is too broad for most research projects. For example, mothers who do and do not smoke include many different categories of mothers: those with the first child, those with many children, young mothers, older mothers, single mothers, married mothers, black mothers, and white mothers. Each of these categories contain variables that may influence birthweight as much as the independent variable, smoking. Therefore, the researcher must identify particular categories for study that control as many extraneous variables as possible. For example, selecting mothers with their first child will control the factor of multi-parity. In order to be mutually exclusive and exhaustive, all categories must be carefully defined. In order to be observable and measurable, all variables must be defined by operational definition.

Mutually exclusive categories are those with data that unequivocally fall into one and only one category. In the example above, mothers either smoke or do not smoke: mothers who fall into one category are excluded from the other. *Exhaustive categories* are those that include all possible cases of the variable to be observed. "Marital status" must include all possible types: never married; presently married and living together; presently married and separated; formerly married and widowed; formerly married and divorced. Such categories must be established before data are collected, not only to identify what will be observed, but to include such categories on interview schedules or check lists for observing, interviewing, or reviewing records.

After collecting data, the researcher may discover that an unexpected category of marital status exists: a mother whose marriage has been annulled. To assure that the categories are exhaustive, a new category must be established after data are collected to include this case.

To establish observable and measurable categories, precise definitions of the variables to be observed are mandatory before observation. Two types of definitions are common: the verbal or nominal definition, which defines concepts in words; and the operational definition, which defines variables in terms of observation and measurement. Formulating the operational definition is crucial prior to observing data.

The Operational Definition

The *operational definition* is a set of directions or procedures that designate precisely how to observe, measure, and record the phenomenon to be observed. In order for one researcher to be able to collect data in the same manner as another, the operational definition is essential. Few if any operational definitions are accepted by all scientists. No operational definition corresponds exactly to every researcher's view of what should be observed and measured. An operational definition is useful for a number of reasons: 1) it specifies exactly what a particular researcher plans to observe; 2) it communicates precisely how the variable to be observed will be measured and how the measurement will be recorded; and 3) it facilitates the possibility of detecting measurement errors and leads to a better interpretation of the observation. For example, Lindeman and Van Aernam (1977) developed a number of operational definitions, such as "subjects" and "stir-up-routine," to study nursing intervention with the presurgical patient.

Subject was defined by six criteria: 1) fifteen years and older; 2) admitted under nonemergency conditions; 3) scheduled for surgery other than eye, ear, nose, and throat; 4) scheduled for general anesthetic; 5) able to cooperate for tests of ventilatory function; and 6) not on intermittent positive pressure breathing therapy. *Stir-up routine* was defined as the conscientious application of three precepts at definite intervals during the postoperative period: 1) the patient must inflate his lungs adequately; 2) the patient must cough; and 3) the patient must move or be turned.

Touch was defined by McCorkle (1981, p. 115), using the following operational definition: "Gentle physical contact made by the investigator's hand at the patient's wrist during the entire interaction with an increase in pressure at the beginning of each one of the three specific questions asked by the investigator." McCorkle defined the seriously ill patient as: "A hospitalized patient admitted to a specified area for seriously ill patients, such as intensive care and coronary care units, or a patient designated seriously ill by his physician and diagnosis. The patient's condition had to be one in which there was a chance of recovery during the present hospitalization, but not necessarily a cure of his illness."

Using the operational definitions above, researchers may duplicate the "subject" studied by Lindeman and Van Aernam, and the "seriously ill patient" studied by McCorkle. The "stir-up-routine" could be replicated, as well as "touch."

Operational definitions are used to measure visible and invisible variables. For example, a rash may be visible to all observers, but no two may describe the rash in exactly the same way without an operational definition. On the other hand, anxiety may not be visible. To make anxiety observable and measureable, a set of directions that specify how to observe, measure, and record the phenomenon is necessary. The complexity of the concept and the lack of agreement in defining it is exemplified by the fact that at least 120 specific procedures to measure anxiety were extant in 1961 (Cattell and Scheier). Since that time, other procedures have been added.

The operational definition defines the phenomenon to be observed in a narrow manner in order to increase objectivity in observation and precision in measurement. However, as operational definitions become more and more specific, it is clear that data are lost, and the complexity of a concept such as *anxiety* is reduced to a simple level. This is a part of the price to pay in order that the study may be replicated and the phenomenon observed and measured.

For example, for two researchers to investigate the variable in the hypothesis stated above,* *smoking* and *mother* should be given an operational definition. Without an operational definition, questions immediately arise, such as what to do with the mother who was a heavy smoker but quit before she became pregnant. Such queries are answered by the operational definition, which removes ambiguity by giving the procedures for defining *mother*. For example, the following set of directions define what is meant by *mother* for the purpose of one study: 1)

---

*The hypothesis states: infants born to mothers who smoke will have a lower birth weight than infants born to mothers who do not smoke.

she is a primipara; 2) she is between the ages of 19 and 34; 3) she is currently married and living with her spouse; 4) she is not suffering from designated chronic diseases (diabetes, nephritis, etc.); 5) she was delivered of a living child in the public hospitals of Central City; 6) she was drawn by random sampling from the target population of primiparas in Central City during a designated time period; 7) she gave informed consent to be interviewed.

Smoking mother may be more simply defined as: 1) a mother who meets the definition of *mother* above; 2) who reports she smoked for five or more months during pregnancy; and 3) who reports she smoked on the average of five cigarettes per day.

Although data are lost by the operational definition, precision in observation and measurement are gained. Once the researcher establishes the categories of observables, the researcher must next locate or devise the instruments for the observation.

Instrumentation

In research, *instrumentation* refers to the construction and use of instruments in the observation, measurement, and analysis of data. Instruments are devices, tools, implements, questionnaire items and response categories, interview schedules, papers, or documents that facilitate observation and measurement. Instruments include both "hardware"— computers, thermometers, tape recorders, cameras, transducers to indicate various responses, timers, counters, and radio transmitters—and "software"—paper and pencil instruments, such as scoring charts, interview schedules, questionnaires, assessment guides, and scaling devices (see Table 10–1).

The primary instruments of observation are the human sensory organs. However, these allow for the observation of only a small part of the phenomena in the environment. Instruments and the know-how to use these enable the researcher to extend the senses' accuracy and range. The most sophisticated instruments have been invented in the realm of time, motion, and weight, although the instruments used to observe human behavior, health, and sickness are becoming more developed. A number of these instruments may be used with little technical knowledge, while others require experts both to use the instruments and to interpret the data. For example, the use of an instrument to measure temperature or blood pressure may easily be learned, while the use of x-rays and computers is much more difficult. However, a review of the records that interpret data already collected by sophisti-

TABLE 10–1. INSTRUMENTS TO ASSIST OBSERVATION*

Instrument	Function
Accelerometer	A transducer; measures rate of change in a moving object.
Algesimeter	Measures pain threshold
Audio analgesia	An audio signal for analgesia.
Biofeedback devices	Displays signals of a person to that person.
Calorimeter	Measures heat loss.
Cardiotachometer	Measures heart rate.
Dhronometer	Measures periods of time.
Decibel meter	Measures sound levels.
Dolometer	Measures subjective pain levels.
Dynamometer	Measures force.
Electrocardiograph	Measures electrical potentials of heart muscle.
Electrogoniometer	Measures angular positions of body limbs.
Electroencephalograph	Measures electrical activity of brain.
Electronystagmograph	Measures gastric motility.
Electromyograph	Measures electrical activity of muscles.
Electronystagmograph	Measures eye movements induced by electrical stimulation.
Ergodynamograph	Records work associated with muscular activity.
Esthesiometer	Measures touch sensibility.
Galvanic skin resistance device	Measures DC resistance of skin.
Kinesthesiometer	Measures ability to perceive own body position.
Mobat	Measures blood alcohol concentration viz. expired breath.
Opthalmograph	Measures movements of eye during reading.
Plethysmograph	Measures changes in blood volume.
Pneumograph	Records respiratory movements.
Stabilograph	Measures human motor response instability.
Transducer	Transfers energy between two or more systems.

*Rugh and Schwitzgebel (1977).

cated instruments and analyzed by experts enables the researcher to gather such data second-hand.

Direct observation and assessment relies primarily on the well trained observer, who watches, listens, palpates, smells, uses instruments that extend these senses, and records each observation precisely. The researcher may use one of the many instruments described in the literature or devise his or her own instrument.

"Hardware" includes easy-to-use devices such as the flashlight, tuning fork, tongue blade, thermometer, sphygmomanometer, stethoscope, and weight and height scales. Instruments that require more expertise are the tonometer (to show changes in intraocular pressure), Snellen chart and Rosenbaum pocket vision screener (to examine visual acuity), ophthalmoscope, otoscope (to examine the ear), nasal speculum, and vaginal speculum (see Table 10–2 for other instruments). If the client gives informed consent, hardware instruments such as tape recorders, movie cameras, and videotapes are invaluable to document observations. Such instruments collect data in the natural setting, hospital, clinic, or laboratory to be analyzed in detail at a later date. Other instruments include timing devices, such as wrist watches or stop watches, infrared photography, two-way mirrors, electric eyes, and various instruments that measure moisture, pressure, activity, or count mechanical movement.

"Soft-ware" includes paper and pencil instruments, such as clinical assessment instruments that give a step-by-step procedure; instruments such as the Apgar score to determine need for resuscitation of the newborn; interview schedules; questionnaire forms; and numerous tests and schedules to assess and/or measure concepts such as *fear, depression,* and *anxiety.*

Instruments to observe and assess the physiological and psychological states include devices noted above and also those of considerable biomedical complexity. For example, instruments are available to convert a physiological event into an electrical signal that may be recorded, transmitted, or displayed. The transducer, a device that transfers or converts energy from one form to another, is used with an amplifier, an instrument that amplifies or modifies the transducer's electrical signal, and either an oscillograph, which writes down information, or an oscilloscope, which records information photographically. The electrocardiogram and the electroencephalogram require special training both to collect and analyze data, but the researcher may use these instruments in a second-hand manner by examining experts' reports.

The sphygmomanometer and the stethoscope are familiar instruments used in physiological studies. Less familiar instruments are the pneumotachometer, which measures airflow; the spirometer, which measures pulmonary volume; the myograph, which measures muscular contraction; and the tromometer, which measures involuntary tremors of the muscles in the fingers. To measure the strength of muscles, a dynamometer is used. To measure reaction time, a chronoscope is used, as well as various watches and stop watches that measure length of time, pressure, and movement.

Numerous other laboratory instruments such as the microscope enable the researcher to assess the health status of the subject. In addition, the patient's chart or record is an instrument itself for observing laboratory findings and physicians's examination.

Scaling

Scaling is a process of determining magnitude or quantity (see Chapter 12). Before observations, the researcher develops or locates a scale to help collect the data. A scale transforms an hypothesis into something that is observable.

Four general types of scales are: 1) the nominal, 2) the ordinal, 3) the interval, and 4) the ratio. The nominal scale names and measures whether subjects' characteristics are the same or different: sex (male *or* females); pregnant (yes *or* no); level of education (high school, college, graduate school). The researcher names the categories of observations to be made, and the nominal scale "measures" the frequency of the observation. The researcher can count the number of men and women, blacks and whites, and pregnant and nonpregnant females. However, the nominal scale is limited to such discrete and noncontinuous categories. Categories can neither be ranked nor measured in any other way.

Frequently used to plan for observations of attitudes, the ordinal scale allows the researcher to rank observations. For example, the quality of nursing care may be measured by an ordinal scale that asks the patient to rank the care received as good, better, or best.

The interval scale enables the researcher to measure quantitative observations that have no zero point: the temperature of a patient may be measured by a Fahrenheit or a centigrade thermometer that is divided into equal units, but without a zero point.

The ratio scale enables the researcher to plan to measure observations that do have a zero point, although this value may never be produced. For example, length, weight, and height may be measured by a ratio scale with equal intervals and a zero point.

Bias in Observation

Bias in observation—the tendency to observe subjects or processes in a manner that differs consistently from true observation—may be introduced in a number of ways. The *Hawthorne effect* refers to the change in subjects' responses because subjects know they are participating in a study, rather than because of factors the researcher wished to study. Bias may also be introduced because observers may see the data differently: a short nurse may get a different blood pressure reading than a

TABLE 10–2. SELECTED OBSERVATIONS AND INSTRUMENTS

Observation	Instruments
Achievement	Kahl's Achievement Orientation Scale (1968)
Activity	Activity Inventory, Brodie (1977)
Aggression	Geen and Stonner (1971)
Angles of the limbs	Goniometer
Anal sphincter pressure	Kohlenberg (1973)
Anxiety	Anxiety Scale Questionnaire, Cattell and Scheier (1968); Timed Behavioral Checklist, Paul (1966)
Aptitude and ability	Eckland (1965)
Assertiveness	Rathus Assertiveness Schedule (1973)
Attitudes toward	Guttman Scales; Likert Scales; Semantic differential Scales; see Miller (1970) for others
Physical fitness and exercise	Richardson (1960)
Mental illness	Cohen and Struening (1959)
Mentally retarded people	Bartlett, Quay, and Wrightsman (1960)
Blindness	Cowen, Underberg, and Verrillo (1958)
Disabled people	Yuker, Block, and Campbell (1960)
Menstruation	McHugh and Wasser (1959)
Mental hospitals	Souelem (1955)
Authoritarianism	F-Scale, Adorno et al (1950)
Bacterial counts	Microscope
Blood alcohol concentration	MOBAT—commercial device to estimate via breath
Blood volume	Plethsymograph; commercial instrument
Blood pressure	Sphygmomanometer (mercury, anaeroid, electronic)
Community attitude	Community Attitude Scale (see Miller, 1970, pp. 272–277)
Community solidarity	Community Solidarity Index, Fessler (1952)
Development	Bayley Scale of Infant Development; Denver Developmental Screening Test. Frankenburg and Dodds (1967)
Depression	Depression Adjective Check List, Lubin (1965)
Distance	Social Distance, Boggardus Social Distance Scale
Electrical activity of organs	
Brain	Electroencephalograph
Heart	Electrocardiograph
Muscles	Electromyograph

TABLE 10–2. SELECTED OBSERVATIONS AND INSTRUMENTS
(Continued)

Observation	Instruments
Equilibrium	Movement of platform, Shipley and Harley (1971)
Eye-foot coordination	Mirror-visual instrument, Mikaelian (1972)
Fear	Fear Scale, Geer (1964)
Force	Dynamometer, commercial instrument
Galvanic skin response	Galvanic Skin Resistance Device, commercial instrument
Gross motor movement	Self-winding watch, Schulmann and Reisman (1979)
Gastric motility	Electrogastrograph, commercial instrument
Head movement of infant	Pressure change in air pillow, Vietze et al (1974)
Hearing	Audiometer, commercial instrument
Heat loss	Calorimeter, commercial instrument
Heart rate	Cardiotachometer, commercial instrument
Length	Various measurement scales; mecometer for infants
Life changes	Life Change Inventory, Costantini et al (1974)
Locus of control	Rotter et al (1972)
Micturation	Moisture Detection Device
Motion	Kinomometer, Kinesimeter
Morale	Minnesota Survey of Opinion (see Miller, 1970)
Occupational categories	NORC (1972)
Oral hygiene	Chemical agents, Evans et al (1968)
Pain	Algesimeter, threshold; Dolometer, subjective pain.
Respiration	Air flow, Pneumotachometer; volume, spirometer; Pneumograph
Social desirability	Scale of Social Desirability, Crowe and Marlowe (1960)
Social participation	Chapin's Social Participation Scale (see Miller, 1970)
Salivation	Measurement method, Brown (1970)
Sleep	Rapid eye movements
Social interaction	Inventory, Methuen and Schlotfeldt (1962)
Social status	Hatt and North Occupational Ratings

tall nurse. To reduce bias in observation, Simon (1978, p. 278) suggests that: 1) observers be carefully trained; 2) the area of discretion within which bias may operate be reduced by carefully specifying the observer's task; 3) detailed instructions be given; 4) immediate and detailed reporting be required; 5) mechanical devices such as tape recorders and cameras be used when possible for checking observations; and 6) several researchers observe, record, and compare observations.

SUMMARY

Research methods are the means by which data are collected. Common research methods used in nursing include observation, questioning, measurement, and a combination of these. Observation is the basis of all modern science and is used in experimental, descriptive, and historical research designs. The role of the researcher who uses observation as a primary means of collecting data may be one of participant or nonparticipant observer. Such roles may be used in various settings, including the clinic and the community. Both types of roles vary in terms of the degree of structure used and the selection of what will be observed. Highly structured observation is essential in experiments, while uncontrolled observation is used in cases of nonintervention, or simple observation. Five categories of simple observation useful in nursing research are: exterior physical signs (clothing, body markings, clinical signs), expressive movements (gestures, touching, expressions), physical positioning (clustering or dispersing), language behavior (conversation), and time observations (perception of time, time-movement).

The methods by which observations are made and summarized include classification, operational definition, instrumentation, and scaling. In addition, measurement may accompany or follow observation (see Chapter 12). *Classification* is the systematic assignment of subjects to named categories that are mutually exclusive and exhaustive. The *operational definition* is a set of directions or procedures that designate precisely how to observe, measure, and record observed phenomena. *Instrumentation* is the construction and use of tools to observe, measure, and analyze data. Numerous instruments have been devised to observe and assess people's health status. *Scaling* is a process of determining magnitude or quantity. Qualitative scales, such as the nominal and ordinal scales, determine the category of the variable to which study subjects belong. The ordinal scale not only determines the category but ranks the categories in terms of a graded order such as poor, good, better, or best. An *interval scale* is a quantitative scale, with equal intervals but no absolute zero point. Temperature measured in centigrade is an example of the interval scale. The *ratio scale* is a quantitative scale that does possess an absolute zero point, although zero may not be produced. Examples of the ratio scale include length, weight, and height.

Bias in observation—the tendency to observe subjects in a manner that differs consistently from true observation—may be introduced by the study subject or by the observer. The *Hawthorne effect* refers to the change in subjects' responses because subjects know they are participating in a study, rather than because of factors the researcher wished to study. Bias may be introduced by the observer who sees data differently.

STUDY QUESTIONS

1. What is the connection between research methods and research designs?
2. Describe how you have used the three methods of research to collect data in nursing. Is the same process used to collect data in nursing practice and nursing research?
3. What methods help the nurse observe in research?
4. If you are to observe scientifically, what conditions must you meet?
5. You are planning a research project that involves the observation of autistic children. What do you think your role as observer should be?
6. You have a grant to study the effects of visitors on patients in the intensive coronary care unit. What method could you use to protect the patients from stress and keep you from being involved in patient care?
7. In deciding what you can observe in a study of schizophrenic patients who come to a community clinic, what are some factors to consider?
8. What exterior physical signs can you observe in a prenatal clinic that may alert you to special problems of health care that need research?
9. You are the nurse in a home for the elderly who are able to care for themselves to a considerable extent. How would research on expressive movements enable you to encourage the patients to exercise more effectively?
10. Describe a research project on communication between student nurses and clinical supervisors that involves silences, smiles, frowns, or laughter.

11. Diagram the relationship between theory, methods, and observation.
12. In planning an observational research project, what are some methods that will help you observe?
13. You wish to study the effect of different methods of teaching diabetic patients to give insulin to themselves. What categories will help you observe the data and record it effectively?
14. Make an operational definition of *diabetic patient* that describes those you will teach in question 13 above.
15. Referring to Tables 10–1 and 10–2, identify any instruments with which you are familiar.
16. If you plan to use classification in research, what scale would be helpful?
17. What does the ordinal scale measure that the nominal scale cannot?

REFERENCES AND SUGGESTED READINGS

Aamodt, A. (1972): The child's view of health and healing. In Batey, M. (ed.), Communicating Nursing Research. Boulder, Colorado: Western Interstate Commission for Higher Education, pp. 38–56. Response to critique. In Batey, M. (ed.), Communicating Nursing Research. Boulder, Colorado: Western Interstate Commission for Higher Education, pp. 57–58. *A participant observation study: Aamodt lived for 13 months with a family and served as a volunteer teacher-aide in mission school, in order to observe children of the Papago in many settings.*

Alderson, M. (1974): Effect of increased body temperature on the perception of time. *Nursing Research 23,* 43–49. *The patient's perception of time associated with rise in temperature.*

Ammon, K. (1969): The effects of music on children in respiratory distress. In *ANA Clinical Sessions.* New York: Appleton. *A study of the effects of music on children with respiratory distress.*

Barnard, K. (1973): The effect of stimulation on the sleep behavior of the premature infant. In Batey, M. (ed.), Communicating Nursing Research. Boulder, Colorado: Western Interstate Commission for Higher Education, pp. 12–33. *Behavioral observations of the sleep state of infants, during the 32nd to the 35th week of gestation, to collect data on sleep-wake patterns.*

Batey, M. (1973): Communicating Nursing Research. Boulder, Colorado: Western Interstate Commission for Higher Education. *Fifteen studies in nursing research, many with critiques and responses to critiques. Includes participant-observation and nonparticipant observation studies in the field and in the hospital.*

Baziak, A. and Denton, R. (1965): The language of the hospital and its effect on the patient. In Skipper, J. and Leonard, R., Social Interaction and Patient Care. Philadelphia: J. B Lippincott. *The medical jargon used by nurses and physicians is incomprehensible to laymen.*

Burnside, J. (1973): Caring for the aged: touching is talking. *American Journal of Nursing. Therapeutic communication through touching is discussed.*

Carlson, C. (ed.) (1970): Behavioral Concepts and Nursing Intervention. Philadelphia: J. B. Lippincott. *Contains article by Robinson on humor.*

Cattell, R. and Scheier, I. (1961): Neuroticism and Anxiety. New York: Ronald. *Includes discussion of measures of anxiety.*

Chapman, J. (1977): Effects of different nursing approaches upon selected postoperative herniorrhaphy patients. In Downs, F. and Newman, M. (eds.) A Sourcebook of Nursing Research. Philadelphia: F. A. Davis, pp. 15–23. *Use of participant observation in clinical area experiment.*

Ciminero, A., Calhoun, K., and Adams, H. (eds.) (1977): Handbook of Behavioral Assessment. New York: Wiley. *Seventeen articles that review behavioral assessment comprehensively.*

Felton, G. (1970): Effect of time cycle changes on blood pressure and temperature in young women. *Nursing Research 19*, 48–58. *Biological rhythms, efficiency, and sleep patterns of nurses.* (1973): Rhythmic correlates of shift work. In Batey, M., Communicating Nursing Research. Boulder, Colorado: Western Interstate Commission for Higher Education. *Interval sampling of body temperature and urine every three hours to determine effect of biological rhythms.*

Grant, E. (1971): Facial expression and gesture. In *Journal of Psychosomatic Research 15*, 391. *Contains a check list of one hundred units of muscle change associated with facial expression.*

Gunning, S. and Holmes, T. (1973): Dance therapy with psychotic children. *Archives of General Psychiatry 28. Communicating through dance.*

Habenstein, R. (ed.) Pathways to Data. Chicago: Aldine. *Thirteen articles report research in hospitals, hometowns, etc.*

Hasselmeyer, E. (1961): Behavior Patterns of Premature Infants. Washington, D.C.: Government Printing Office. *Examines kinesthetic needs in the premature.*

Horn, B. (1978): Transcultural nursing and child-rearing of the Muckleshoot people. In Leininger (ed.), *Transcultural Nursing.* New York: Wiley, pp. 223–38. *Participant observations study of the culture of the Muckleshoot Indians of Washington State.*

Holsti, O., Loomba, J. and North, R. (1968): Content analysis. In Lindzey, G. and Aronson, E. (eds.), The Handbook of Social Psychology (2nd ed., Vol. 2). Reading, Mass.: Addison-Wesley. *An authoritative article on content analysis.*

Kassenbaum, G. (1970): Strategies for the sociological study of criminal correctional systems. In Habenstein, R. (ed.), *Pathways to Data.* Chicago: Aldine, pp. 122–138. *Outlines strategies for nonparticipant observer research, using participant observers as sources of data.*

Kane, F. (1959): Clothing worn by out-patients to interviews. *Psychiatric Communications. Nonparticipant observation of the clothing worn by out-patients.* (1959): Clothing worn by an out-patient: a case study. *Psychiatric Communications. Case-study method of unobstrusive observation.*

Kendall, K. (1978): Maternal and child nursing in an Iranian village. In Leininger, M. (ed.), Transcultural Nursing. New York: Wiley, pp. 399–416 *Participant observation in nursing research.*

Klein, R. et al (1972): Psychiatric staff: uniforms or street clothes? *Archives of General Psychiatry 26* (Jan.). *Street clothes worn by health personnel may be better than uniforms.*

Leininger, M. (1978): Transcultural Nursing. New York: Wiley. *Twenty-six articles, many of which report research that uses participant observation methods.*

Leipold, W. (1963): Psychological distance in a dyadic interview as a function of introversion-extraversion, anxiety, social desirability, and stress. Unpublished doctoral dissertation, Univ. of North Dakota. *Uses unobtrusive measures to note seats taken in interviews by introverted and anxious students.*

Lindeman and Van Aernam, (1977). Nursing intervention with the pre-surgical patient—the effects of structured and unstructured pre-operative teaching. In Downs, F. and Newman, M. (eds.) *A Sourcebook of Nursing Research.* Philadelphia: F. A. Davis. *Use of sound on slide instruments.*

Mahl, G. (1956): Disturbances and silences in the patient's speech in psychotherapy. *Journal of Abnormal and Social Psychology 53,* 1–15. *Data collected in psychotherapy sessions by observation.*

Marshall, L. (1972): Patient reaction to sound in an intensive coronary care unit. In Batey, M. (ed.), Communicating Nursing Research, Boulder, Colorado: WICHE, pp. 81–97. *Nonparticipant observation, using electrocardiographic oscilloscopes and tape recorders to study effects of ward sounds on heart rate.*

McCorkle, R. (1974): Effects of touch on seriously ill patients. In *Nursing Research 23. Effect of touching observed.*

Petrovich, D. et al (1968): Nursing apparel and psychiatric patients: a comparison of uniforms and street clothes. *Journal of Psychiatric Nursing 6. Street clothes worn by health personnel compared with uniforms.*

Puttock, D. (1972): Dance therapy. In *Nursing Times 68. Nonverbal communication by means of dance.*

Robinson, V. (1970): Humor in nursing. In Carlson, C. (ed.), Behavioral Concepts and Nursing Intervention. Philadelphia: J. B. Lippincott. *Unobtrusive measure.*

Rodgers, J. (1977): Relationship between sociability and personal space preference at two different times of day. In Downs, F. and Newman, M., A Sourcebook of Nursing Research (2nd ed.). Philadelphia, F. A. Davis, pp. 171–177. *Study of personal space, sociability, and time of day.*

Rugh, J. and Schwitzgebel, R. (1977): Instrumentation for behavioral assessment. In Ciminero et al (eds.), Handbook of Behavioral Assessment. New York: Wiley, pp. 79–113. *Good source of useful instruments for research.*

Skipper, J. and Leonard, R. (eds.) (1965): Social Interaction and Patient Care. Philadelphia: J. B. Lippincott, *Collection of articles dealing with patient care.*

Webb, E. et al (1966): Unobtrusive Measures. Rand McNally. *Chapter Five deals with simple observation.*

Wolff, C. (1948): A Psychology of Gesture. London: Methuen. *Hand gestures studied to examine correlation between emotional make-up and gesture.*

REFERENCES FOR SELECTED INSTRUMENTS

Adorno, T., Frenkel-Brunswik, E., Levinson, D., and Sanford, N. (1950): The Authoritarian Personality. New York: Harper. *Includes the F-Scale, which measures authoritarianism—a syndrome of organized beliefs and symptoms.*

Akutagawa, D. (1965): A Study in Construct Validity of the Psychoanalytic Concept of Latent Anxiety and a Test of Projection Distance Hypothesis.

Unpublished doctoral dissertation, Univ. of Pittsburgh. *Fear Survey Schedule—fifty items, self-rating schedule.*

Boggardus, E. (1959): Social Distance. Yellow Springs, Ohio: Antioch Press. *The social distance scale measures the grades and degrees of intimacy between social groups.*

Bonjean, et al (1967): Sociological Measurement: An Inventory of Scales and Indices. San Francisco: Chandler. *Variety of scales and indices.*

Buros, O. (ed.) (1978): The Eighth Mental Measurement Yearbook. Hyland Park, N.J.: Gryphon Press. *Helps locate information on standardized tests.*

Cahell, J. and Warburton, F. (1967): Objective Personality and Motivation Tests. Chicago: University of Chicago Press. *Paper and pencil instruments.*

Chapin, F. (1970): Social participation scale. In Miller, D., Handbook of Research Design and Social Measurement (2nd ed.). New York: David McKay. *General scale of participation in professional, civic, and social organizations.*

Chesney, M. and Tasto, D. (1975): The development of the menstrual symptom questionnaire. *Behavior Research and Therapy 13, 237–244. Fifty-one items distinguish between verbal symptoms of spasmodic and congestive dysmenorrhea.*

Chun, K., Cobb, S., and French, J. (1975): Measures of Psychological Assessment, Ann Arbor: Survey Research Center. *Psychological measure.*

Eckland, B. (1965): Academic ability, higher education and occupational mobility. American Council on Education. *Measures of intelligence and achievement.*

Evans et al (1968): A new measure of effects of persuasive communications: a chemical indicator of tooth brushing behavior. In *Psychological Reports 23, 731–736. Measures effectiveness of communication.*

Fessler, D. (1952): The development of a scale for measuring community solidarity. In *Rural Sociology 17, 144–152. Useful to determine relationships between community progress and solidarity.*

Geer, J. (1965): The development of a scale to measure fear. *Behavior Research and Therapy 3, 45–53. Fear scale.*

Gesell, A. et al (1956): Youth: the Years from Ten to Sixteen. New York: Harper and Row. *Developmental approach.*

Hollingshead, A. and Redlich, F. (1958): Social Class and Mental Illness. New York: Wiley, pp. 39–391. *A two-factor index of social position is included.*

Kohlenberg, R. (1973): Operant conditioning of human anal sphincter pressure. In *Journal of Applied Behavior Analysis 6, 201–208. Conditioning as an instrument.*

Lubin, B. (1965): Adjective checklists for measurement of depression. *Archives of General Psychiatry 12, 57–62. DACL—the Depression Adjective Checklist—one of the few scales considered sensitive to behavioral treatment programs. Subject rates self.*

Mikaelian, H. (1972): A technique for measuring eye-foot coordination without visual guidance. *Behavior Research Methods and Instrumentation 4, 17–18. A mirror-visual system to measure eye-foot coordination.*

Miller, D. (1970): Handbook of Research Design and Social Measurement. New York: David McKay. *Part II: Guides to Methods and Techniques of Collecting Data in Library, Field, and Laboratory.*

Moreno, J. (1972): Psychodrama. Beacon, New York: Beacon House. *Sociometric technique.*

Osgood, C. et al (1957): The Measurement of Meaning. Urbana: University of Illinois Press. *The semantic differential technique to measure the affect feeling meaning of cognition.*

Rathus, S. (1973): A 30-item schedule for assessing assertive behavior. *Behavior Therapy 4,* 398–406. *The Rathus Assertiveness Schedule. Subjects rate themselves.*

Reeder, L. et al (1976): Handbook of Scales and Indices of Health Behavior. Pacific Palisades, Ca.: Goodyear. *Handbook useful to identify indices of health behavior.*

Richardson, F. and Tasto, D. (1976): Development and factor analysis of a social anxiety inventory. *Behavior Therapy 7,* 453–462. *Social Anxiety Inventory.*

Schulmann, J. and Reisman, J. (1959): An objective measurement hyperactivity. *American Journal of Mental Deficiency 64,* 455–456. *Instrument to measure hyperactivity.*

Shipley, R. and Harley, R. (1971): A device for estimating stability of stance in human subjects. *Psychophysiology 7,* 287–292. *A linear-differential transformer senses movement of a platform to measure equilibrium and stability.*

Vietze et al (1974): A portable system for studying head movement in infants in relation to contingent and noncontingent sensory stimulation. *Behavior Research Methods and Instrumentation 6,* 338–340. *Pressure changes in air pillow triggers switches.*

Walk, R. (1956): Self-ratings of fear in a fear-invoking situation. *Journal of Abnormal and Social Psychology 52,* 171–178. *"Fear thermometer" assesses momentary anxiety level in response to a feared stimulus.*

Wallace, W. (1971): The Logic of Science in Sociology. Chicago: Aldine, Chapter 4. *Hypotheses, instrumentation, scaling.*

Zuckerman, M. (1960): The development of an affective adjective checklist for the measurement of anxiety. *Journal of Consulting and Clinical Psychology 24,* 457–462. *State of anxiety measured.*

CHAPTER 11

ASKING QUESTIONS: QUESTIONNAIRE AND INTERVIEW METHODS

When it is not possible or desirable to observe directly, questionnaires and interviews are the primary means of collecting data. Both methods are effective for obtaining information about attitudes, opinions, perceptions, beliefs, feelings, motivations, private behavior, past behavior, and anticipated behavior. In addition, both are useful for collecting demographic data that characterize a population, such as age, sex, occupation, marital status, and health status. Both rely heavily on verbal reports, either oral or written. However, they differ in that the questionnaire obtains information from a respondent who answers a list of fixed questions with little or no assistance from the researcher, while the interview always involves interaction, either face-to-face or by telephone.

Upon completion of this chapter, the student should be able to: 1) state how to construct a questionnaire and an interview schedule; 2) describe elements of the questionnaire, including the covering letter, instructions, questions, response categories and precoding, inducements to respond, and the informed consent form; 3) differentiate among the structured, semistructured, and unstructured interview; 4) describe the focused interview and the clinical interview; 5) identify and define several projective techniques; 6) discuss other data collection methods, such as the critical incident, content analysis, and Q methodology; and 7) contrast and compare the interview and questionnaire methods, listing advantages and disadvantages.

THE QUESTIONNAIRE

The construction of a questionnaire requires thought, planning, and testing. The researcher must convince and motivate an unseen respondent and give the respondent clear, written instructions, in order that the respondent may understand and respond properly to the questions. The researcher must formulate clear, unambiguous questions, arrange them in the proper order, and organize the questionnaire, in order to make taking data from it as easy and as accurate as possible. We shall examine how to construct a questionnaire, with attention to each of these factors.

Construction of the Questionnaire

The questionnaire is comprised of the following elements: 1) covering letter, 2) instructions to respondents, 3) questions, 4) response categories and precoding, 5) demographic data, and 6) inducements to respond. Each of these elements will be examined.

The Covering Letter. The covering letter begins with the identification of the sponsoring institution and the researcher. The sponsorship of the project refers to the person or agency who endorses or supports the study. The name of a highly respected person or agency is a guarantee to the respondents that the project is worthwhile, that the data will not be misused, and that confidentiality will be maintained. Colleges and universities consistently rate high, their sponsorship usually producing excellent cooperation. The name of a person who is important to the study subjects is likewise helpful. Thus, a covering letter on which the name of the sponsoring institution appears, or which is signed by a well known person, is valuable in gaining cooperation, introducing the questionnaire, and introducing the researcher to the respondents. In general terms, the letter must explain why the research is being done, how the respondents were selected for the study, and why their answers are important. The letter should clearly state whether or not the respondents will be expected to participate further in the study, and should guarantee anonymity and confidentiality to the respondents. A statement that information collected will be used for statistical purposes only, and that all data will remain completely confidential, will reassure the respondent that privacy will be guarded. An informed consent form may follow the letter and precede the questionnaire, or it may follow the questionnaire. In either case arrangements must be made to protect the respondent, so the respondent will return the signed consent form to the researcher with confidence.

Instructions to the Respondents. Instructions should appear throughout the questionnaire to guide the respondent to make appropriate responses. If only one response is proper, the instructions should clearly state this. Where more than one response is possible, this should likewise be indicated. It is particularly important to give directions each time the response pattern changes in any way. Since no explanation or interpretation beyond the written word is possible, clear and simple directions are mandatory. Instructions should be carefully tested by having persons who are not in the sample answer the questionnaire and indicate where the instructions are unclear or ambiguous. Where understanding is doubtful, sample questions and responses may be included in the instructions.

The Questions. The questions are the heart of the questionnaire. The researcher depends upon the questions to collect information about the research problem. Therefore, the questions should be carefully examined and tested for the following: a) appropriateness, b) content, c) wording, and d) order.

1. Two kinds of questions are appropriate in a questionnaire: the standardized or structured question, and the open-ended question. The *standardized* question, also called the *fixed-alternative, closed-ended,* or *highly structured* question, consists of several alternative responses from which the respondent must choose the one most appropriate and accurate:

	YES	NO
There are plenty of opportunities on my job to use my nursing education.	☐	☐
I like the type of patients I work with in the community.	☐	☐
The doctors and nurses in the agency work as a team.	☐	☐

The fixed-alternative closed-ended questions above may be answered quickly and are easy to analyze. However, there are disadvantages, such as the omission of possible alternatives to a simple *yes* or *no* answer, superficial examination of complex problems, and forced responses. In cases where the range of alternative responses is unknown, or the issues are sensitive or need exploration, an open-ended question may be more informative:

> How much opportunity do you have on your present job to use your nursing education? _____

While the analysis of open-ended questions takes time and skill, the researcher gains a wealth of information on sensitive topics that cannot be explored with simple yes or no answers. In addition, material heretofore not investigated can be explored. In fact, both kinds of questions may be used.

2. *The content of the questions arises from the research problem and proposal.* Each facet of the problem must have questions to collect data. The researcher must decide the following: What data must be collected? How many questions is it practical to ask? How many questions should be devoted to collect data from each area? Given a specific number of questions, what must the content of each question be?

It is helpful to develop a question guide that includes the content that must be covered; content that may be helpful but is not essential; the estimated number of questions needed to cover the content; the total number of questions it is practical to ask. A choice may then be made either to increase the length of the questionnaire in order to ask all necessary questions, or to reduce the number of questions.

Determining what should be the content of questions is not easy. A review of the literature to identify key concepts is often helpful. For example, Neumann proposed to study job satisfaction among nursing service personnel. She began her study with a review of the literature to determine the concepts and definitions used in previous studies. Next, she conceptualized *job satisfaction* as a multidimensional set of attitudes or feelings, determined partly by individual characteristics and partly by environmental factors that the worker perceives (Neumann, 1973, p. 166). Finally, she devised a questionnaire of seventy statements, designed to measure job satisfaction.

3. *The wording of the questions and the alternative responses is a crucial and difficult process.* The researcher should develop a check-list that includes all positive and negative characteristics of questions and should examine each question in the light of these attributes. Positive characteristics include clarity, brevity, simplicity, and applicability to the study sample. Negative characteristics include "double-barreled" questions, double negative questions, embarrassing or sensitive questions, jargon-filled questions, complex questions, leading questions, questions that bias, and questions that are inappropriate to the study sample (see Table 11–1 for a check-list).

"Double-barreled" questions ask two questions in one. They often contain words such as *either, therefore, and, both,* and *or.* Examples of such questions include the following: "Are nurses overworked, or do you think they are just inefficient?" "Nursing supervisors have more information about patients than student nurses do; Therefore, do you think students should question procedures established by nursing supervisors?" "When did you stop keeping up with nursing research?"

TABLE 11–1. CHECK-LIST FOR POSITIVE AND NEGATIVE CHARACTERISTICS OF QUESTIONNAIRE QUESTIONS

Positive Characteristics

1. Clarity: Can the question be interpreted in more than one way?
2. Brevity: Can the question be shortened and still retain its meaning?
3. Simplicity: Is the vocabulary at a simple level (such as that of a newspaper) which is appropriate to the study sample?
4. Applicability: can the repondents in the study sample be reasonably expected to answer accurately?

Negative Characteristics

1. Double-barreled questions: Does the question ask two questions in one? Does it first make a statement with which the respondent may not agree, and then ask a question on the basis of that statement? Does the question have a hidden premise?
2. Double-negative questions: Does the question include words such as *don't* or *not?*
3. Leading questions: Is the question asked in such a way that the respondent knows a particular response is desired?
4. Sensitive questions: Is the question asked in such a way that the respondent may become embarrassed, angry, or emotionally upset?
5. Jargon-filled questions: Does the question use professional, technical, or slang terms with which the respondents are not familiar?
6. Complex questions: Does the question use long phrases and complex sentences?
7. Questions that bias: Does the question contain information that would encourage the respondent to view one answer as more likely "right"? Does the question contain emotionally loaded words, such as *motherly, patriotic,* or *Communist?*
8. Inappropriate questions: Does the question assume prior knowledge inappropriate to the sample?

"Double negative" questions use two negatives to indicate a positive statement. For example, the respondents may be asked to state if they agree or disagree with the following double negative question: "I don't think it is not a wise policy to have nursing students in the operating room." It is not immediately clear if a *yes* response means that the respondents feel students should or should not be in the operating room.

"Embarrassing" or "sensitive" questions are any that are so blunt that they offend the respondent. Asking "Did you have premarital intercourse?" or "Did you ever have venereal disease?" may be important to the research proposal, but may be so embarrassing that the respondent will not answer.

"Jargon-filled" questions use language unfamiliar to the respondent, either technical or slang. Questions about *urination* are preferable to those about *micturition,* while asking "How many marijuana cigarettes do you estimate you smoke per week?" is preferable to asking "How many times do you get stoned in one week?"

"Complex questions" must be read more than one time to understand their meaning. For example, the following question asks, "When nursing data are sought on matters such as wages in different specialities, such as maternal-child health, do you think a tabular form drawn up on the questionnaire itself, with all required items clearly stated, leaving blank spaces for proper entries, is preferable to a series of questions utilized to elicit the data?" Such questions must be simplified or discarded.

"Questions that bias" are phrased so that the respondent is encouraged to answer in one way rather than another. For example, using popular or unpopular persons or groups influence answers: "Do you agree with the A.N.A. president that . . ."; or "Do you think your country is wrong to. . ."; or "The communists believe that . . . do you agree?"

"Inappropriate questions" use language that respondents are not able to understand, require information that study subjects will not likely have, request attitudes that few respondents have thought about, or call for a feat of memory that is unlikely for the average person. "How many patients have you cared for since you became a nurse?" is an inappropriate question, because an accurate response is not likely.

The way questions are asked may influence the respondent to answer in a more comfortable and honest manner. The following suggestions may be helpful:

a. Substitute euphemisms for value-loaded language. Ask, "How do you discipline your child?" rather than "How do you punish your child?"

b. Indicate that other people have what might ordinarily be considered socially undesirable attitudes. For example, ask a question about suicide in the following manner: "Many people have thought about suicide at one time or another. Have you ever thought about suicide?" rather than bluntly asking "Have you ever thought about suicide?"

c. If it is desired that the respondent express criticism, give the respondent an opportunity to voice praise where praise is due. For example, you may ask, "What was the most helpful nursing care you received?" before you ask "What would you suggest to improve nursing care on Ward X?"

d. Rather than ask about a person or event the respondent may not be familiar with, structure the question so that the respondent will be able to admit lack of knowledge gracefully. Ask first, "Have you ever had the opportunity to read about Madame Curie?"; then ask, "Do you think Madame Curie is representative of women's capacity to be scientists?"

e. Achieve some balance of social desirability. Don't ask, "How often do you have intercourse a day?"; rather ask, "Some couples engage in intercourse several times a day, while others have intercourse several times a year. How often do you have intercourse?"

f. Structure a question in such a way that any undesirable characteristic is assumed: "How many sexual partners did you have before marriage?" is more apt to get a response than "Did you engage in premarital intercourse before marriage?"

4. *In general, the ordering of questions should precede from general to specific, regardless of whether the question is open or closed.* The procedure is sometimes called the *funnel technique,* beginning with broader questions and narrowing down to precise, specific ones. The entire sequence of questions should follow some logical order, with no abrupt transitions. For example, the time sequence should move from questions about the past, to the present, and then to the future. The order in which questions are asked can influence what answers are given to subsequent questions. Ordering can also affect whether or not the respondent will answer the questionnaire: sensitive questions that are placed first may cut off response, while interesting but neutral questions that appear first may stimulate cooperation. Demographic data are sometimes placed in the beginning of the questionnaire but should generally be placed at the end to avoid a dull beginning.

"Contingency questions" should be answered only by some respondents; therefore, they must be accompanied by clear instructions to avoid frustrating and confusing the respondent. Two methods for ordering contingency questions are:

1. Have you ever nursed a dying child?
   ☐ Yes
   ☐ No
   If yes, how many times have you nursed a dying child?
   ☐ Once
   ☐ 2 to 5 times
   ☐ over 5 times
2. Have you ever nursed a dying child?
   ☐ Yes. Please answer questions 6–10.
   ☐ No. Please skip questions 6–10. Go directly to question 11
   on page 3.

The Response Categories and Precoding. Once the questions have been
formulated, the researcher must provide the respondent with a good
set of answers. Since the respondent must be able to communicate answers without error, the range and wording of answers must be considered with the same careful attention that the questions were devised,
or the questionnaire is in vain.

The response categories must be mutually exclusive and exhaustive:
the respondent must be able to choose one and only one alternative,
but the alternative must be appropriate for each respondent. For example, the question that asks for religious affiliation should include the
following categories:

☐ Protestant
☐ Catholic
☐ Jewish
☐ Other (please specify: _____)

Several different types of responses to fixed-alternative questions
are: Likert-scale responses, rank-order responses, check-list responses,
and other scale responses (see Chapter 9).

1. *Likert-Scale Responses*
   Instructions: Beside each of the statements listed below, please
   indicate whether you strongly agree (SA), agree (A), disagree
   (D), strongly disagree (SD), or do not know (DK).

	SA 1	A 2	D 3	SD 4	DK 5
Supervisors should have a master's degree.	☐	☐	☐	☐	☐

2. *Rank-Order Responses*
   Instructions: Please rank-order the following activities, in terms of what you prefer to do in nursing. Write *1* before the activity you prefer most; *2* before the activity you next prefer, and so on. Please rank-order all listed activities.

   _____ Bedside care

   _____ Administration of a ward

   _____ Giving medications

   _____ Teaching patients

   _____ Supervising students

   _____ Writing reports

3. *Check-List Responses*
   Instructions: Please check the data you use to orient the disoriented patient.

	ALWAYS	FREQUENTLY	SELDOM	NEVER
Nicknames	☐	☐	☐	☐
Have patients sign name	☐	☐	☐	☐
Have calendar available	☐	☐	☐	☐
Radio	☐	☐	☐	☐
Holiday decorations	☐	☐	☐	☐
Identifying meal times	☐	☐	☐	☐

Precoding is the use of numerical codes on the questionnaire responses, so that responses may either be read by machine or counted easily by hand. For example, the codes 1 for female and 2 for male may appear beside the response category:

Please indicate your sex:

_____ 1. Female

_____ 2. Male

Precoding may also be used to specify the positions of each response item on the machine-readable form (computer cards):

> Please write the year and month of your birth:
>
> _____ year   Columns 17–18
> _____ month

Precoding at the response category saves time and effort when processing the responses for data analysis.

Demographic Data. Sometimes questionnaires begin with demographic questions, although many researchers prefer to end the questionnaire with these questions because they tend to be routine and somewhat dull. Demographic data include facts about age, marital status, occupation, educational level, sex, race, number of persons in the household, or other helpful information. For many such questions, standardized wording such as that used in the United States Census is helpful. Demographic data are often useful as a criterion measure (dependent variable) to identify the effect of independent variables, such as treatment or behavior, on different races, ages, or sexes of the respondents.

Inducements to Respond. Researchers have tried a number of approaches to encourage participation in the study. These include enclosing a small pencil with which to write, a coin, or the promise that results will be sent to respondents who request them. However, the most effective seems to be an appeal to the respondents' altruistic nature, by indicating the good that the study may accomplish. For example, letting the respondent know that he or she can help scientists better understand the phenomenon under study may be a considerable inducement to reply. The questionnaire's physical appearance is also important in eliciting a good return. The questionnaire should be attractive, with reasonable length, appropriate size, and inviting color and line-spacing.

Colors should be pretested for effectiveness, but in general, lighter colors, especially yellow and pink, have been found to elicit the highest percentages of returns. A questionnaire of several pages or a planned sequence of questionnaires may benefit by alternating light colors. However, regardless of color, it is important to show more paper than printing. A page of closely typed lines and questions may immediately discourage the respondent.

The size of the questionnaire may vary. A double postcard, with the questionnaire portion to be torn off and returned, has been successful in market surveys. Standard letter-size questionnaires ($8\frac{1}{2} \times$ ⁓⁓) are widely used, since one-page forms encourage the respondent to answer immediately. However, it is important to provide adequate space for comments. A few well answered questions are preferable to many undecipherable answers. In cases where the questionnaire must be long, successfully motivating the respondent may be more important than either the kind of form or the length.

Hand delivery of questionnaires may be an important way to stimulate response. The researcher can deliver the form, explain the project, and elicit cooperation. The researcher may then collect the completed form or have the form mailed back in a self-addressed and stamped envelope. A variation of this technique is to first mail the questionnaire and covering letter and then visit the respondent to pick up the completed form, checking for completeness.

If the questionnaire is mailed, a follow-up mailing may be an effective method to stimulate returns that are not forthcoming. The follow-up mailing should occur two to three weeks after the initial mailing. Usually, the original mailing and two follow-up mailings result in a return from most people who care to respond at all. The overall response is one guide to assess how representative the sample return is. Statistics used to analyze research data often assume that all members of the sample return their forms. This is seldom true. Some social scientists regard a fifty percent return as adequate, sixty percent as good, and seventy percent as very good (Babbie, 1975). Others expect lower returns, from ten to twenty percent (Parten, 1950).

Various Questionnaire Techniques

1. The Delphi technique is a method of data collection that uses questionnaires that are mailed to a panel of experts in successive waves, with feedback from previous questionnaires included with successive questionnaires. Lindeman's (1975) use of this technique is probably the best known example in nursing. Lindeman selected her panel of experts from persons identified by professional nursing organizations and funding agencies. To determine the five areas in which nursing research was needed, four rounds of questionnaires were mailed to 433 panel experts. Of the 433 experts, 341 responded to all four rounds of questionnaires. The first round asked the experts to identify five areas in which nursing research was needed. Of the 2000 responses, 150 were selected as the most frequently mentioned. These were used in the second round, and respondents were asked to indicate three factors: whether nursing should lead research in this area; the value of the item for nursing as a profession; and the impact of the item on patient welfare. The third round of questionnaires included both the range of response and the average response from the previous questionnaire, and experts were asked to comment on these. The fourth round of questionnaires contained both summaries of the third round and comments obtained.

The findings of the study indicated that the highest priorities in the area of patient care were patient education, the alleviation of pain, and the development of indicators to measure the quality of nursing care. The highest priorities in the area of the nursing profession were research into the nursing process, the research process itself, and the development of instruments to measure the quality of nursing care.

2. Sociometric data are concerned with interpersonal and interorganizational relationships and may be collected with questionnaires. In this case, the questions asked may be "Who are your best friends?"; "Who are the persons that you respect most in the group?"; "Who are the persons you would prefer to work with among your colleagues?" The respondents return a list of names indicating their social choices. The researcher then analyzes this data to find the chosen linkages among persons of the group. Analysis of sociometric data includes constructing graphs, such as the sociogram. A *sociogram* consists of dots that represent the persons, statuses, or offices involved. The lines connecting the dots represent the nominating and the nominated persons. The depicted relationships may be either *symmetric* (reciprocal, or mutual choices), or *asymmetric* (nonreciprocal choices). The graphic approach is limited to the number of dots and lines that can be visually depicted.

Sociometric techniques have not been widely used in nursing. Beard and Scott (1975), studying the efficacy of group therapy by nurses for hospitalized patients, is one of the few studies that used this method.

Examples from Nursing Research
The questionnaire is widely used in nursing research. For example, Moore-Nunnally and Aguiar (1974), developed two questionnaires— one to determine patients' attitudes toward the prenatal care they were receiving, the other to determine patients' knowledge levels and attitudes toward their labor and delivery experience. The prenatal questionnaire consisted of 52 items: eight questions on demographic data, 38 questions on attitudes and care the patients did or did not receive, 5 open-ended questions, and 1 question that rated overall opinion on a one-to-eleven scale. The labor and delivery room questionnaire consisted of four parts: part A collected data not available on the patient's chart; part B elicited attitudes toward prenatal classes, labor, and delivery, in five open-ended questions; part C elicited further attitudes, in a series of 25 attitude statements; and part D collected data about pregnancy, labor, and delivery, in nine multiple-choice questions.

In a study of the psychological preparation of surgical patients, Schmitt and Wooldridge (1973) used a questionnaire to measure attitudinal variables at the time of patients' discharge. Both the experimental and the control group were asked to recall how well they had slept and the level of anxiety they felt the evening before and the morning of surgery. Questions were designed to determine what the patients remembered about the surgery, including the operating room and the recovery room. In part, the questionnaire was expected to elicit whether or not the experimental group, who had extra preparation for surgery, would report less anxiety, better sleeping patterns, and would be better able to recall experiences about the surgery.

THE INTERVIEW

The *interview* is a method of data collection in which an interviewer asks questions of the respondent, either face-to-face or by telephone. The interview is comprised of three components: the interviewer, the interview schedule or guide, and the respondent. Each of these represents a wide range of variables. For example, the interview schedule may be highly structured, requiring the most formal type of interaction between interviewer and respondent. On the other hand, the schedule may be only a guide that the interviewer either has memorized or holds in hand, while encouraging the respondent to talk freely. In both cases, however, the interview schedule must be carefully formulated and the interviewer must be rigorously trained. First, we shall examine the interview schedule and the training of the interviewer. Following this, we shall investigate interviews that use various approaches.

The *interview schedule or guide* is a written form constructed with the same attention to instructions and questions that is used for the questionnaire. However, three differences are immediately apparent in the case of the interview: 1) the questions and responses are both spoken; 2) the face-to-face interaction commonly used may decrease the feeling of anonymity; and 3) the interviewer is able to observe as well as question. Each of these has important consequences in the interview.

Instructions on the interview schedule are of two kinds: instructions to the interviewer, which are not to be read, and instructions to the respondent, which must be read. In certain cases, instructions to the interviewer may contain a statement about how to proceed. An interview could be destroyed if the interviewer read *his* or *her* instructions aloud (Babbie, 1975, p. 120): "If the respondent is nearly illiterate, then . . . ." On the other hand, when a formal interview is used, instructions to the respondent must be delivered from a *verbatim* script from the beginning of the interview to the end. The questions must be clearly understood when spoken, and the interviewer must be able to record the responses quickly and accurately. To increase feelings of confidentiality and anonymity in cases of sensitive questions, a separate brief questionnaire may be filled out by the respondent to indicate responses such as income or sexual behavior. These may be placed in an envelope and attached to the interview schedule. A second technique is to hand the respondent a small card containing several categories and have the respondent answer the question by indicating the appropriate category. For example, a question about income may include the following categories from which the respondent selects one:

- Category (A) income under $5,000
- Category (B) income between $5,000 and $ 9,999
- Category (C) income between $10,000 and $14,999
- Category (D) income between $15,000 and $19,999
- Category (E) income between $20,000 and $24,999
- Category (F) income over $25,000

The interviewer's observations increase the depth of the data collected. For example, the interviewer can note the quality of the dwelling, the condition of the yard and furnishings, the appearance of the respondent, the reaction of the respondent to various questions, and demographic data such as sex and race.

The training of interviewers includes how to follow question wording, how to record responses, how to probe for responses when this is appropriate, and how to present one's self in the interview situation. As noted earlier, the interviewer must follow the exact wording and phrasing in a formal interview, without a single change. In the case of open-ended questions, the responses should be written precisely as they are spoken—bad grammar and all. Where gestures and tones are significant to reveal meaning, these may be added in the margin of the interview schedule. Probes may be required to elicit responses to open-ended questions, but these may take the form of silence, or simply asking, "Anything else?" (Babbie, 1975, p. 272). Probes should be neutral: all interviewers should use the same probes, when these are necessary in a formal interview. Where more than one interviewer is used, interview training to deal with these and other questions should be done in a group. The researcher should begin with a description of the study, include general procedures, and then examine the interview schedule in detail, question by question. Demonstration interviews and return demonstrations by the interviewers who are being trained are also helpful. The pilot study helps test the efficiency of the training, and a discussion following pilot interviews can deal with troublesome issues. While actually collecting data, the researcher must work closely with the interviewers, supervising the process from beginning to end. In cases where student groups are working together on an interview project, meetings should be held frequently to compare notes and discuss problems.

In contrast with the standardized and structured questionnaire, the interview schedule may take a variety of forms. The interview may use a highly structured schedule such as those in the formal interview described above. Or, the interview may be partially structured, or totally unstructured. Each of these will be examined.

Standardized and Structured Interview Schedules

This form of the interview includes a schedule of questions that are asked in the same order, with the same wording, and according to identical procedures used by every interviewer. The goal of the interviewer is to be a neutral medium through which questions are asked and responses recorded. If the interviewer affects the responses in any way, a bias is interjected that could be mistakenly interpreted as a characteristic of the respondent rather than an influence of the interviewer. Therefore, questions must be asked in a standard way, with as little interaction with the respondent as possible.

Partially Structured Interviews

In situations where the researcher wishes to conduct a more intensive and general study on a smaller sample, partially structured interviews are useful. In these cases, the interview is more fluid and allows the interviewer latitude to move in interesting and productive directions. Two partially structured interview techniques are the "focused interview" and the "clinical interview."

Focused Interview. This kind of interview is partially structured by a schedule of questions and topics that the interviewer wishes to cover. However, the interviewer is free to deviate from the schedule, so long as the material is covered by the conclusion of the interview. Focused interviews are useful to ascertain how the respondent defines certain situations, such as being in the hospital, in terms of variables such as age, sex, culture, social class, or diagnosis. The responses may be used for many purposes: to test hypotheses previously defined, to formulate new hypotheses from unanticipated responses, or to gather data on specified research problems.

Clinical Interview. A clinical interview combines observations with questioning. Nurses use the clinical interview to gather data on the status of patients or clients, to identify nursing needs, to diagnose, and to plan nursing care and intervention. The clinical interview is widely used in individual casework, in psychiatric clinics, and in field work with participant or nonparticipant observation.

The clinical interview may focus upon a specific situation, such as the development of an illness, the place of an individual within the family, or the relationship of an individual with the family and the community at large. The clinical interview combines observation and questioning with inductive reasoning to establish concepts and categories and to generate theory.

The clinical method begins with the observation of data, and then uses the inductive approach to summarize and categorize the data. The relationship between the concepts or categories may be established by an empirical generalization. Hypotheses may then be generated from the empirical generalization for testing. The clinical method may also include experiments, although the usual approach is to wait for processes to unfold rather than make processes occur as the experiment usually does.

The clinical method has its disadvantages. The case history of an entire life is complex and beyond the researcher's ability to comprehend in its entirety. In addition, the researcher may introduce a bias in observation or questioning, or the client may fail to recall what happened in the past with complete accuracy. As a whole, clinical research may be more effective for formulating hypotheses than for extensive testing.

The Unstructured Interview

The unstructured interview may include elements of both the focused and the clinical interview, but these are integrated into a general approach that encourages the respondent to broach topics and explore them as long as the respondent wishes. An unstructured interview may begin by simply asking the respondent to talk about whatever he or she has in mind, or to "tell what things were like" when he or she was younger. While time-consuming, lengthy, and difficult, this approach helps the interviewer get inside the respondent's private world to discover factors that influence daily life, to investigate ways in which the external world is integrated with the respondent's internal world, or to uncover evidence of abnormal processes at work in the respondent's mind or personality. To assist in this process, the interviewer often uses projective techniques.

Projective techniques are designed to collect data in response to nonstructured or ambiguous stimuli that elicits behavior often unconscious on the part of the respondent. Projective techniques are often used in totally unstructured interviews, in which the respondent is encouraged to control the interview by expressing feelings, fantasies, fears, and doubts freely, without disapproval or even advice from the interviewer. In such cases, the function of the interviewer is simply to create an atmosphere of trust and to encourage the respondent to talk, by using simple phrases such as "tell me more" or "that is interesting." The researcher who plans to use projective techniques that require trained persons to analyze the data should recruit these people early in the research project.

Projective tests commonly used in unstructured interviews include the following: the Rorschach Test, the Thematic Apperception Test, word-association, sentence completion, doll play, figure drawing, psychodrama and sociodrama, and many others. Each of these will be briefly examined.

1. The Rorschach Test consists of ten cards, each of which contains an inkblot— an unstructured, ambiguous stimulus. The subject is asked, "What might this be?" and then tells what he or she sees in the inkblot, thereby giving it structure and revealing what is in his or her own unconscious. In order to interpret findings, the test requires training; therefore, it is useful only in extensive research. It has been used effectively in cross-cultural studies, such as that in which DuBois collected Rorschach material on the people of Alor. This material was independently analyzed by the psychiatrist Kardiner, who reached the same conclusion as DuBois and others about the Alorese basic personality structure (DuBois, 1944).

2. The Thematic Apperception Test consists of a series of pictures of various situations, persons, or processes. The subject is asked to tell a story about what he or she sees in the picture, thus revealing what is in the subject's own mind. Nineteen of the twenty cards contain black and white pictures; the last card is blank, allowing the subject to imagine a picture and describe it. The responses are scored according to the variable the researcher is exploring. Some variables measured are achievement motivation, attitude toward minority groups, attitude toward authority, and need for affiliation.

3. Word association tests, a variation of free association, attempt to draw from the respondent's mind all of the data that the respondent has stored in the process of daily life. The subject is verbally presented with a list of words, one by one, to which he or she responds with the first word that comes to mind. The interviewer notes both the rate of response and the content, to analyze these for areas of emotional disturbance. In order to elicit internal conflicts or attitudes, the word list combines both neutral words and words with emotional implications, such as love or hate.

4. The sentence completion test is similar to the word association test in that the respondent is supplied with a stimulus—a set of incomplete sentences—and asked to respond by completing the sentences in any manner desired. The researcher later puts the responses into categories, or rates them according to a previously set design.

5. Doll-play is a technique often used with children. The child is given a doll or dolls, and the researcher observes what the child does with the dolls. At times, the researcher may tell the child the name of each doll, whether father, mother, or sibling; at other times, the researcher observes how the child names the doll and plays with it, and what the child has the dolls say to one another.

6. Figure-drawing techniques include those in which the subject is given paper and pencil with instructions to "draw a man" or "draw a tree." Each technique has standardized methods of administration, scoring, and interpretation, although like all of the projective techniques, questions are raised about the validity of the evidence.

7. Psychodramas and sociodramas are as much observation technique as they are an interview situation. However, the researcher does suggest to the subject that he or she act the part in a play—either playing the subject's own part, as if it were a life situation in the psychodrama, or the part of a designated other, such as wife, father, brother in the sociodrama. The researcher may then encourage the subject to tell why he or she played the part in a particular way.

The Telephone Interview
The telephone interview relies totally upon oral questions and responses, with little other interaction between the interviewer and the respondent. The major advantages are its low cost, the rapid completion of the interview, and the high response rates. In addition, large scale telephone surveys may be conducted within a few hours of an occurrence that the researcher wishes to study, for example, an epidemic or a massive influenza innoculation. The interviewer is not required to travel to unfamiliar or dangerous neighborhoods, in order to conduct a telephone survey.

However, there are several disadvantages in using the telephone interview. The chief of these is the problem of representativeness. Not everyone has a telephone; moreover, only those with listed telephones may be reached. But, the telephone interview may be used in conjunction with other techniques to be representative. In such cases, the telephone survey is useful when speed is important or when data is otherwise unobtainable.

Other Methods of Data Collecting

Less frequently used methods of data collecting include: 1) the critical incident, 2) content analysis, and 3) the Q methodology. These combine various methods of getting information.

1. *The critical incident requires a respondent to write an account of a particular situation.* For example, the researcher may ask the respondent to record a stressful incident that occurred in the past several months. The researcher then analyzes the content of the report. A large number of reports are necessary; 2000 is the recommended number. This limits the method to those with sufficient time both to collect the data and to analyze it by content analysis.

2. *Content analysis uses communications as units of analysis.* Verbal or behavioral data is classified, summarized, and tabulated in order to understand: a) the communication process itself, b) the intentions behind the communication, and c) the effect of the communication upon the audience. Simply put, content analysis investigates one or more of the following: 1) the sender (who), 2) the message (what), 3) the means of transmission (how), 4) the audience (to whom), 5) why (encoding the intention of the sender), and 6) the effect (decoding responses to the message). The encoding and decoding process requires inference, or reasoning, to analyze the data, and thus may be the most intellectually demanding of all techniques of data analysis (Fox, 1976, p. 259).

The steps in content analysis include: 1) selecting the unit of content to be analyzed; 2) selecting theory to guide the formulation of categories and coding rules; 3) developing the categories; 4) collecting the observations; and 5) analyzing and interpreting the findings.

Content analysis may consist only of counting words, for example, the number of times a particular word is used to describe a depressed patient. Or the analysis may consist of inferring the intentions of the sender and/or the effect on the audience. The sampling process may include random sampling to select words, phrases, sentences, paragraphs, sections, chapters, books writers, or contexts to be studied.

The system of classification or coding used must be carefully established and tested before data collection begins, and the system must anticipate a quantitative analysis, especially if data will be processed by computer. Content analysis is useful to measure attitudes, such as those of politicians toward health care, as well as to identify patterns of communication between health personnel and clients.

3. *The Q methodology is a method of collecting data in which the subject sorts a deck of cards on which words, phrases, or messages are written. The Q sort,* as the procedure is called, requires the subject to sort the cards according to a particular characteristic that the researcher has identified—approve/disapprove, high priority/low priority. The characteristics are usually placed on a continuum with several categories: category one indicates greatest approval; category five indicates disapproval; categories between one and five indicate less approval and more disapproval. The number of cards to be sorted ranges from over fifty to one hundred. Q sorts can be applied to a wide variety of problems and are helpful to study individual attitudes objectively. However, to use large samples is time consuming. But, without a fairly large sample, it is not possible to generalize.

Examples from Nursing Research

Interviews are often used in nursing research. For example, White and Maguire (1973) studied job satisfaction among hospital nursing supervisors, using 34 interviews ranging in time from fifteen to ninety minutes. Each respondent was asked to describe a time when she or he felt satisfied with the job and a time when she or he felt dissatisfied. The total number of stories related was sixty-two, thirty-one satisfying and thirty-one dissatisfying. The interview was focused by the two questions but otherwise was unstructured, allowing the nurses to comment as long as they wished.

Davis and Underwood (1976) used a semistructured focused interview to study the role of, function of, and decision-making process in a community mental health center. Four areas of focus included role, function, decision making, and demographic data.

Downs (1964) used a semistructured interview to study maternal stress in primigravidas. She memorized the interview guide to preserve a more natural atmosphere. The average time per interview was 15 to 20 minutes.

In addition to their use in the interview, projective techniques are used many other ways. Christensen et al (1979) used a version of the Thematic Apperception Test to devise a form to assess the need for achievement, affiliation, and power in nurse practitioners' professional development. Valadez and Anderson (1972) used ten captioned-line-drawn pictures with a nurse and patient to ascertain the effect of a rehabilitation workshop on the attitudes of sixty nurses, before and after completion of the workshop. Porter (1974) used projective techniques to determine how grade school children perceived their internal body parts.

Hurwitz and Eadie (1977) used three methods of research in their study of the psychologic impact of participation in abortion on nursing students: a series of questionnaires that were administered weekly; reports of dreams written by the student, either at the time of completing the questionnaires or not long afterward; and content analysis of the dream reports. The researchers were able to develop classification systems for dream subjects that included emotional states represented in the classifiable dreams; characters other than the dreamer mentioned in the reports; settings of the dreams; and primary themes of the dreams.

Freihofer and Felton (1976) used the Q method of data collection to study the nursing behaviors that family members or significant others desired most or least in the care of dying patients. Eighty-eight typed cards were given to a sample of 25 relatives or friends who sorted the statements on the cards into nine piles that indicated most to least desired nursing behaviors.

Comparison of the Interview and the Questionnaire: Advantages and Disadvantages

In comparison with the interview, the questionnaire is likely to cover a wider geographical area; to reach a larger number of people; to insure respondents' anonymity, thereby eliciting more frank answers; and to require less skill and funds to administer. With careful pretesting, the questionnaire may provide more uniform responses than the interview, especially if it is necessary to have several interviewers, each of whom may affect the measurement situation differently. Questionnaires are especially useful to describe the characteristics of a large population, such as a student body, a hospital, or a community. Using a carefully selected probability sample, the questionnaires offer the possibility of making refined descriptive statements about existing behavior or conditions. No other method of obervation can reach as large a population as rapidly with comparable accuracy. Many questions may be asked respondents on a given topic in the natural and presumably less stressful environment.

Yet, questionnaires, and surveys in general, are subject to serious weaknesses. Questionnaires can collect only self-reports of recalled past action or of prospective hypothetical action. What people do and what they say may differ, especially in cases where recall is selective. People likewise may not understand themselves, that is, they may not be able or willing to express unconscious attitudes and beliefs. Also, the requirement for standardization means that the least common denominator is represented. And response may be low—under fifty percent of the queries. Finally, the researcher cannot deal with context or social life, the "feel" of the situation, as one can in the interview where observation plays a part.

Interviews may be the only way to reach a large proportion of the American population, especially if a long and complex set of questions is necessary. A mailed questionnaire may be risky, because the respondents may not be able to read or understand the questions. Not only can the skilled interviewer maintain interest, she or he can ask and, if permissible, can explain the questions of a complex schedule. Since the interviewer is also an observer, a much better picture of the respondents is obtained during the interview. Many people are willing to cooperate if all they have to do is talk. In addition, interviews may be granted by persons who would not be reached by questionnaire—the rich and secluded, the executive whose mail is screened by secretaries, or the very poor. Nevertheless, disadvantages of the interview technique are considerable: the method requires the time and money to train interviewers, transportation to move them to the point of the interview, and the ability to interpret the copious notes that may be taken in an unstructured interview.

Bias in the Questionnaire and Interview

Bias, the tendency to obtain data that differs from the "true" data, may creep into both questionnaires and interviews. For example, the content of a question may be loaded in one direction; that is, it may be more likely to obtain answers in one direction than another. In addition, timing may introduce a bias; for example, publicity on abortion may affect attitudes reported on questions about abortion.

Bias may also be introduced by interviewers. Systematic differences may exist from one interviewer to another. Training and careful selection of interviewers helps minimize bias, but the interviewer's perception of the subject being interviewed may unwittingly influence responses. Such biasing factors may never be completely overcome, but they may be reduced with highly structured interviews and carefully trained interviewers.

The *halo effect* is a type of bias that may enter into the use of rating scales. Generalized impressions may carry over from one rating to the next, or the rater may attempt to make ratings consistent. Halo effects may be reduced by having different raters rate the subject or process, or by having the same raters do the rating at different times, without being aware they are rating the same subject or process as before.

SUMMARY

When it is not possible to observe directly, questionnaires and interviews are useful means for collecting data. The *questionnaire* obtains information from respondents who answer a list of fixed questions with little or no assistance from the researcher, while the interview always involves interaction. The construction of a questionnaire includes writing a covering letter; formulating the questionnaire proper, beginning with instructions to respondents, then the questions and response categories; precoding, and inducements to respond.

Questions are the heart of the data collecting procedure. Questions must be appropriate; the content must be related to the research proposal; and the wording must be clear, brief, simple, and applicable. Negative characteristics, such as double-barreled questions or leading questions, must be avoided. The ordering of questions must be logical, proceeding from the general to the specific. The response categories must be mutually exclusive and exhaustive, and the instructions must be clearly written. Usually placed at the conclusion of the questionnaire, demographic data should include questions that may be used as a criterion measure. Many inducements to respond are available, the most effective being an appeal to the respondent's altruistic nature. The physical appearance of the questionnaire is also important, as is any factor that helps motivate the respondent. What a sufficient number of questionnaire returns is has not been agreed upon, although fifty percent may be regarded as adequate.

Various data collecting techniques use questionnaires in special ways. The Delphi technique uses successive but different waves, or rounds, of questionnaires to elicit particular responses from a panel of experts. Questionnaires are also used by persons seeking sociometric data, although the questions presumably could be asked in an interview.

The *interview* is a method of data collecting in which the interviewer asks the respondent questions, either face-to-face or by telephone. The interview may be highly structured, semistructured, or totally unstructured. Highly structured and formal interviews require carefully trained interviewers who must transmit questions and answers in a neutral manner. The partially structured interview includes the focused interview, which covers topics but also leaves the interviewer free to pursue the data as he or she thinks best. The clinical interview is also partially structured and deals with patients or clients, nursing needs or nursing diagnoses. It combines observation and questioning. The unstructured interview allows both the interviewer and the respondent to pursue topics freely. The interviewer often attempts to get inside the private world of the respondent to discover influences in the respondent's daily life. Projective techniques, such as the Rorschach test or the Thematic Apperception test, are at times used in conjunction with unstructured interviews.

The telephone interview relies totally upon oral questions and responses, with little other interaction between interviewer and respondent. The major advantage of the telephone interview is speed; also, costs are low and response rates high. Yet, the telephone interview may not be representative, because of factors such as unlisted telephones or persons without access to telephones.

The *critical incident* is a technique that gathers data either by interview or by questionnaire. Respondents recall an incident that has occurred in the past three months, then they write an account that the researcher analyzes. The large number of incidents necessary—some 2000—limits this technique to those with enough time and expertise to collect and analyze the data.

Questionnaires and interviews both have their place in the data-collecting process. Generally, questionnaires reach a larger population at a lower cost, while interviews reach those who can neither read nor write and combine both questioning methods and observations. However, disadvantages accrue to each method, including questions of validity and reliability.

Content analysis is a method of data collection and analysis that uses communications as units of analysis. The researcher may count words in a communication process or use a sampling process to select words, phrases, or chapters of a book to be studied. The researcher uses this method to classify, summarize, and tabulate who the sender was, what the message was, how the message was transmitted, the audience to whom the message was sent, why the message was sent, and the effect of the message upon the receiver. The *Q methodology* uses subjects to sort piles of cards with specific statements into categories that indicate attitude. Subjects place characteristics on a continuum, with various categories representing from greatest approval (first category) to disapproval (last category). The number of cards to be sorted ranges from over fifty to one hundred. Q sorts are especially helpful to study attitudes objectively.

Bias in questionnaires and interviews may arise from the way a question is asked, the time a question is asked, or by a systematic difference in interviewers. Bias may also be introduced by the respondent. The *halo effect* arises when raters carry over the rating from one item to the next. Halo effects may be reduced by having different raters rate the same subject, or by having the same raters do the rating at different times.

STUDY QUESTIONS

1. You wish to study teenage obesity. Construct a ten-question questionnaire to examine what the teenager eats between meals. Include instructions to respondents, questions, response categories, and demographic data you wish to collect. How would you encourage the teenager to respond?
2. Examine the following questions, and identify what if anything is wrong:

   • Do you prefer to lose weight by diet, or would you rather use medication?
   • Have you ever thought of killing yourself?
   • How often do you have intercourse in one week?
   • Don't you think it is not right for a nurse to wear street clothes on the job?

3. Construct a five-question questionnaire, using a Likert-type scale to obtain information on the attitudes of student nurses toward dying patients.
4. Construct a five-question interview schedule for a telephone interview to examine knowledge of sickle cell anemia.
5. You would like to study how children perceive nurses and doctors. Write a brief sentence-completion test that would collect such data.
6. Select a page from your nursing or research text. Use content analysis to identify words associated with health care on the page. What is the message the writer is attempting to transmit?

REFERENCES AND SUGGESTED READINGS

Aamodt, A. (1972): The child's view of health and healing. In Batey, M. (ed.), Communicating Nursing Research (Vol. 5). Boulder, Colo.: WICHE, pp. 38–54. *Draw a picture and tell a story about it. Projective techniques to get at the meaning of health and sickness cross-culturally.*

Babbie, E. (1975): The Practice of Social Research. Belmont, Calif.: Wadsworth. *Chapter 5, "Questionnaire Construction," and Chapter 11, "Surveys."*

Beard, M. and Scott, P. (1975): The efficacy of group therapy by nurses for hospitalized patients. *Nursing Research 24*, 120–124. *Sociometric techniques.*

Christensen, M. et al (1979): Professional development of nurse practitioners. *Nursing Research 28, 51–56. Version of the Thematic Apperception Test used to assess needs for achievement, affiliation, and power.*

Davis, A. and Underwood, P. (1976): Role, function, and decision making in community mental health. *Nursing Research 25, 256–259. Semistructured focused interview.*

Downs, F. (1964): Maternal stress in primigravidas as a factor in the production of neonatal pathology. *Nursing Science 2, 348–367. Semistructured interview.*

DuBois, C. (1944): The People of Alor. Minneapolis: University of Minnesota Press. *An anthropologist cooperates with a psychiatrist. Projective testing.*

Fox, D. (1976): Fundamentals of Research in Nursing (3rd ed.). New York: Appleton, Chapter 10.

Freihofer, P. and Felton, G. (1976): Nursing behaviors in bereavement. *Nursing Research 25, 332–337. Use of the Q-sort.*

Habenstein, R. (ed.) (1970): Pathways to Data. Chicago: Aldine. *Thirteen articles by various scholars report methods of data collecting.*

Holsti, O. (1969): Content Analysis for the Social Sciences and Humanities. Reading, Mass. *Content analysis.*

Hurwitz, A. and Eadie, R. (1977): Psychologic impact on nursing students of participation in abortion. *Nursing Research 26, 112–120. Content analysis of dreams; questionnaire.*

Lin, N. (1976): Foundations of Social Research. New York: McGraw-Hill. *Chapter 13: questionnaire and survey.*

Lindeman, C. (1975): Delphi survey of priorities in clinical nursing research. *Nursing Research 24, 434–441. Special type of survey.*

Parten, M. (1950): Surveys, Polls and Samples, New York: Harper and Row. *Surveys.*

Porter, C. (1974): Grade school children's perception of their internal body parts. *Nursing Research 23, 384–391. Projective techniques.*

Rose, M. (1972): The effects of hospitalization on the coping behaviors of children. In Batey, M. (ed.), Communicating Nursing Research (Vol. 5). Boulder, Colo.: WICHE. *Naturalistic observations at home; interviews.*

Schmitt, F. and Wooldridge, P. (1981): Psychological preparation of surgical patients. In Fox, D. and Leeser, I. (eds.), Readings on the Research Process in Nursing. New York: Appleton, pp. 126–137. *Questionnaires.*

Valadez, A. and Anderson, E. (1972): Rehabilitation workshops: change in attitude of nurses. *Nursing Research 21, 132–137. Projective techniques: captioned line-drawn pictures.*

Walizer, M. and Wiener, P. (1978): Research Methods and Analysis. New York: Harper and Row. *Chapter 10 describes question constructions, responses, questionnaires, interviews.*

White, C. and Maguire, M. (1973): Job satisfaction and dissatisfaction among hospital nursing supervisors. *Nursing Research 22, 25–31. Pilot study; interviews, thought-unit category analysis.*

Williams, M. (1972): A comparative study of post-surgical convalescence among women of two ethnic groups: Anglo and Mexican-American. In Batey, M. (ed.), Communicating Nursing Research (Vol. 5). Boulder, Colo.: WICHE, pp. 58–73. *Interviews of 50 minutes each with 64 persons, using interpreter in two cases.*

CHAPTER **12**

MEASUREMENT, SCALING, VALIDITY, AND RELIABILITY

All research aspires to produce accurate answers to scientific questions. However, accuracy must be proved. To prove accuracy of research, the scientist must specify the method of observation, how observations were measured, the kind of scale used, and the means by which data were analyzed. The researcher must also evaluate how good various elements were, such as scales and instruments. To judge the worth and accuracy of such elements of research, the researcher uses various assessments of validity and reliability.

Upon completion of this chapter, the student should be able to: 1) define measurement; 2) describe and give examples of the four types of measurement scales; 3) define and identify types of validity; 4) discuss factors that jeopardize internal and external validity; 5) identify and define ways of assessing reliability.

MEASUREMENT

Measurement is the assignment of numerals to objects or events, according to rules (Stevens, 1959, p. 25). Measurements determine relationships, such as quantities, degrees, or extent of observations. Measurement assumes comparison. The symbols of the observations—but not the observations themselves—can be added and subtracted, and the sums and quotients can be compared with one another, according to the rules. Measurement allows the symbols of measurement to be represented economically in tables, graphs, and diagrams. Observations in such forms tend to be rather awkward, if possible at all.

Measurement is a central process in scientific research. Without measurement, hypotheses cannot be tested, and observations cannot be summarized. Thus, measurement is crucial to theory. Without measurement, theory would remain speculation. Ways of measuring include: 1) counting, 2) comparing, and 3) ranking.

1. *Counting is the oldest way of measuring.* Fingers and toes were counted; knots placed on a length of string were counted; and rocks were used to stand for individuals or events, and counted. The symbols, even the fingers and toes, could be manipulated more easily than the observations themselves.

Counted items are considered to belong to the same class of events. For example, men, women, and children, may differ from one another by sex and age, but all may be put into the same category—human population—and counted collectively. Therefore, counting frequencies transforms qualitative variables such as sex into quantities, that is, numbers of people. Direct enumeration of this kind is measurement at the simplest level.

2. *Comparing requires a standard unit of measure.* In fact, official standards for comparing measures, such as length and weight, are preserved in national capitols such as Washington, D.C. Comparative units of measure, such as the second, the hour, and the day, or the ounce, the pound, and the ton, are used daily and, in cases of commercial exchange, are monitored by the government.

Comparison of measures found in research tend to be of several different kinds: 1) The researcher may measure a single unit at a single point in time. An example of this is the case study. 2) The researcher may also measure and compare a single unit at two or more points in time. An example of this is the longitudinal study of change in a patient, a community, or a culture. The basis of comparison here is the same unit at different times. 3) The researcher may measure and compare several units at one point in time. An example of this is the survey, which collects data by questionnaire or interview from a number of units in a short span of time. 4) The researcher may measure and compare several units at two or more points in time. An example of this is the experiment that examines both the experimental and the control group at two points in time—before and after the independent variable is introduced into the experimental group.

3. *Ranking observations as larger or smaller, higher or lower, or better or worse requires a scale.* For example, quantitative scales measure height, weight, and temperature, while qualitative scales may measure variables, such as quality of nursing cares, as poor, fair, good, better, or best.

SCALING

A *scale* is a device for measuring the magnitude or quantity of a variable. The scale may be a series of steps or degrees, a scheme of graded amounts from highest to lowest, an indicator of relative size, or a scale may designate the appropriate category, such as age or sex, into which units of observation may be placed. Four types of scales commonly used as levels of measurement are: 1) nominal, 2) ordinal, 3) interval, and 4) ratio. The nominal and ordinal are qualitative scales, while the interval and ratio are quantitative scales (see Table 12–1).

1. *The nominal scale consists of a number of discrete, mutually exclusive and exhaustive, named categories.* Nominal scales are used to put qualitative attributes of nursing diagnosis, such as occupation, marital status, blood type, or sex, into named categories. For example, sex may be classified as either male or female but not both. Study subjects can be put into one and only one sexual category. Neither is there a continuum from one category to the other. Thus, the nominal scale is discrete, not continuous.

The data derived from a nominal scale can only be counted to determine frequency: how many are the same and how many are different. Data from questionnaires and demographic surveys often use the nominal scale. Descriptive and exploratory designs that seek to answer the question, "What is this?" use the nominal scale to put things into categories and name the categories.

Nominal scales may be used *after* the data are collected. The researcher examines the observations and uses the nominal scale to organize qualitative descriptive data into categories. Nominal scales are also used *before* observation to establish and organize categories of data that the researcher expects to observe. In her study of nursing therapeutics in body positioning of spinal-cord-injured patients, Rottkamp (1976) used a nominal scale to "measure" body position: supine; prone; right side lying; and sitting. Some experts would not agree that this is measurement, but would point out that we can know when such objects or subjects are "approximately equal" (Kerlinger, 1974, p. 436). However, nominal measurement is the lowest level of measurement. Quantification consists of counting the number of objects or subjects that fall into the various categories.

TABLE 12–1. SUMMARY OF MEASUREMENT SCALES

Scales and Statistics to Measure	Basic Definition	Examples
Nominal The mode percentages chi-square	A noninterval scale that indicates "same" or "different" to permit the naming of the person, place, thing.	Male/female category Blood-type category Diagnosis Questionnaire data
Ordinal The mode percentages chi-square median percentile	A scale of "equal-appearing intervals"; however, size of intervals are not known; measures more or less.	Course grades of A, B, C, D Status of patient, such as critical/serious/satisfactory Graphic rating scales Thurstone-type scales Likert-type scales and numerous others
Interval All statistical tests	A scale of equal intervals, with an arbitrary zero point.	Temperature measured by centigrade or Fahrenheit scale
Ratio All statistical tests	A scale of equal intervals, with an absolute zero point.	Kelvin temperature scale; time; length; weight; certain types of test scores

2. The ordinal scale is a qualitative scale comprised of "equal-appearing intervals" that rank observations from large to small. However, ordinal numbers indicate rank order only; they do not indicate that the intervals between the ranks are equal. Observations such as the cheerfulness of patients may be divided into "equal-appearing intervals," such as "cheerful," "more cheerful," and "most cheerful." In order to be observed and measured, each of these ranks may be operationally defined, but the distance between the units cannot be calculated as equal in the same way that time or weight can. Nevertheless, there is more of a continuity between categories of cheerfulness, as measured by the ordinal scale, than between categories of the nominal scale.

The grading or ranking of the ordinal scale may be according to some underlying continuum of intensity (most to least); distance (nearest to farthest); or preference (love to hate). The ordinal scale is capable of rank-ordering subjects or objects on a particular characteristic, although it cannot distinguish the exact degree to which one differs from the others. Ordinal scales commonly have only three to five categories, since it is usually difficult to make fine distinctions beyond this point.

A large number of ordinal scales may be found in the literature. Three commonly used in nursing research are: a) graphic rating scale; b) differential scales, such as the Thurstone scale; and c) summated scales, such as the Likert scale.

The *graphic rating scale* is an evaluation scale in which the researcher develops a continuum from highest to lowest, and the respondent ranks the variables by placing a check at the appropriate point. The disadvantage of this scale is the tendency to avoid marking either extreme (highest quality care or very poor care), causing a pile-up of scores in the central categories. Nonetheless, the scale is a simple one to use and shows the relationship of one category to the others.

☐	☐	☐	☐	☐
Highest quality care	Very good care	Average care	Below average care	Very poor care

Figure 12–1. Nursing care assessment by a graphic rating scale.

The *Thurstone scale* is a differential scale for the measurement of attitudes. With a differential scale, the respondent who agrees with one statement will likely disagree with those on either side. Twenty to twenty-five statements are selected, whose scale value has previously been established by judges. Sample statements are similar to those below:

    _____ 1. This ward is so busy I seldom see a nurse.

    _____ 2. The nursing care I have received has been good.

    _____ 3. The meals are usually late and poorly prepared.

The Thurstone scale attempts to go a step beyond the rank-order scale to develop equal-appearing intervals. It is more refined than the graphic scale.

The *Likert scale* is a summated scale in which the respondents indicate their agreement or disagreement with statements. The researcher first formulates a number of statements clearly favorable or clearly unfavorable to the attitudes being studied. Five categories express approval or disapproval. Below is an example of a Likert scale:

	STRONGLY AGREE	AGREE	NO OPINION	DIS- AGREE	STRONGLY DISAGREE
1. I receive good nursing care on this ward.	☐	☐	☐	☐	☐
2. The food is always good.	☐	☐	☐	☐	☐

The remaining two scales are quantitative rather than qualitative.

3. The interval scale measures the distance between points on a quantitative measuring instrument. The intervals on this scale are known and are equal. The distances between the intervals can be added and subtracted, and the summaries may be subjected to all statistical tests appropriate to the type of sampling used. The interval scale does not have an absolute zero point. For example, the centigrade thermometer is an interval scale with an arbitrary zero point of 0, while the Fahrenheit scale has an arbitrary zero point of 32.

4. The ratio scale is the highest level of measurement among the scales. In addition to having equal intervals quantitatively measured, the ratio scale has an absolute zero point. Examples include time, length, weight, and the Kelvin temperature scale.

To be useful, all measures and scales must be valid and reliable. Both validity and reliability judge how good the various components and processes of research are. However, they differ in that *validity* refers to the extent to which various research elements—design, scales, instruments, methods, definitions—measure what each purports to measure, while *reliability* refers to the consistency with which the scale or instrument measures. A reliable instrument may not always be valid. For example, a merchant's scale may weigh a steel ball exactly the same each time it is weighed by the same researcher or by different researchers, but the scale may be weighing ten pounds short each time. The scale is consistent and dependable, but it is neither accurate nor valid. It is not weighing what the researcher wants it to weigh. Reliability can never be substituted for validity. The researcher must be sure the scores reflect the "true" differences among the particular variables she or he wants to measure.

Bias in Measurement and Other Errors

A major factor that influences measurement is constant error, or biasing, that systematically affects the characteristic being measured. Bias may be caused by "social desirability" influence or the "acquiescent response set" (Selltiz, 1976, p. 153). The *social desirability* influence is the tendency of respondents to give a favorable picture of themselves, to agree or disagree with a question to the extent that they think responses are socially desirable rather than to respond how they truly feel. The *acquiescent response set* is the tendency of respondents to agree or disagree with statements regardless of their content, especially when presented with a series of statements.

In addition to systematic or biasing errors of measurement, other factors may cause measurements to vary from one act of measurement to the next. These include the following: 1) transient personal factors: fatigue, health, attention; 2) a situational factor: someone is listening to the interview; 3) variations in administering the measure: bored researchers, tired observers; 4) differences in sampling of the items: questions or observations include only a few items from the total number possible; 5) lack of clarity of the measuring instrument: instrument may be too complex, or instructions may be ambiguous; 6) mechanical failures: pencils break in answering questionnaires, or machines break down; and 7) errors in processing and analysis: coding errors, errors in arithmetic, etc. (see Selltiz et al., Chapter 6, for explication).

VALIDITY

Validity is a judgment of the extent to which a component of research—method, scale, instrument, or measure—reflects the theory, concept, or variable the researcher intends it should. A valid instrument measures what it purports to measure. Some methods of judging validity are: 1) content validity, 2) face validity, 3) predictive validity, 4) concurrent validity, and 5) construct validity.

1. Content validity is concerned with the study's sampling adequacy. It intends to judge whether or not all possible observations were sampled for use in a questionnaire, interview schedule, or check-list. It requires an examination of all possible questions, observations or tests that potentially could have been used to measure the characteristics under study. This is seldom possible. However, the researcher can give careful consideration to exactly what is to be measured and how. Questions on a questionnaire should be as representative of as many appropriate questions as possible. Check-lists should properly sample the items to be observed, and systems of classification should be exhaustive. It is helpful to have a panel of judges who are experts in the content area to review such items. Careful consideration and judgment act together to evaluate the validity of content. No objective method assures it.

2. *Face validity is the extent to which the instrument (check-list, scale, system of classification, etc.) appears to be logically appropriate.* However, judging the validity of a scale or instrument by merely looking at it entails subjective judgment and is therefore weak. Its primary virtue is that it requires little time. An experienced researcher can quickly spot gross errors, by examining whether or not the scale seems to be actually measuring what the researcher intends it should, or whether or not the researcher has provided a relevant sample of the variable under study.

3. *Predictive validity, sometimes called empirical validity, is the ability of the instrument to measure and predict.* For example, an I.Q. test is valid if it predicts accurately which students will do well in academic work. Predictive validity may also be judged by comparing the results of one test or instrument with results of a test or instrument of known validity. For example, the age and sex distribution found in a research sample may be validated by comparing it with the findings of the U.S. Bureau of Census, which collects demographic variables from the total population and, therefore, measures what the researcher wants her or his instrument to measure. The predictive validity of an instrument designed to identify characteristics of neurotics or psychotics may be validated by comparing it with instruments that have examined these characteristics in known neurotics or psychotics. Projective tests, such as the Thematic Apperception Test or the Minnesota Multiphasic Personality Inventory, are validated in this way.

4. *Concurrent validity is derived from the ability of the instrument or design to measure present observable behavior.* It distinguishes those who differ in their present state. However, certain states may not be directly observable; instead, these may be examined by finding visible factors that are logically linked to the state. For example, the amount of support a mental patient has from kin and friends may be determined by how many visitors, letters, cards, or phone calls the patient has. However, for many characteristics, such as attitudes, few such methods have been identified. In such cases, the researcher uses construct validity to judge the extent to which the research tool is valid.

5. *Construct validity, the validity of concepts (constructs), judges the extent to which the research tool measures the concept or variable the researcher wants it to measure.* Construct validation is an indirect approach that estimates the extent to which a subject actually possesses the characteristic presumed to be reflected by a particular scale or test. In such cases, multiple measures of the same concept are often used. For example, attitudes toward euthanasia may be first measured by giving respondents a questionnaire; later, an interviewer may question the same respondents. Then, the researcher may examine the behavior of the respondent: how the respondent acts when asked to sign a petition for or against euthanasia. Thus, construct validity may be established by using multiple measures.

Factors Jeopardizing Internal and External Validity

Validity may be judged as internal or external. *Internal validity* refers to judgments of the measures or designs within the study sample; *external validity* refers to the researcher's ability to generalize from the study sample to the larger population from which the sample was drawn.

For example, the internal validity of an experimental design deals with the question of whether the independent variable (the experimental treatment, or stimulus) actually made a difference to the research findings. Internal validity is the basic minimum for every experiment—its reason for being. Without the assurance that the experimental treatment made a difference in the observed effect, there is no way to interpret the findings of the experiment. On the other hand, external validity deals with the extent to which the study subjects or objects were representative of the larger population from which they were drawn, that is, the extent to which the findings of the small sample may be generalized to the larger population.

The selection of a research design or tool that is internally and externally valid is every researcher's ideal. Yet, this goal is not always reached. For example, Campbell and Stanley (1966) identify a number of extraneous variables that jeopardize the internal validity of the experimental design: 1) history, 2) maturation, 3) testing, 4) instrumentation, 5) statistical regression, 6) differential selection bias, and 7) experimental mortality, and interaction among these factors.

History refers to specific events that occur between the first and second measurement of the experimental group. A lapse of time may allow for events to occur that influence the second measurement. An exciting afternoon, emotional disturbances, or drinking lots of coffee could change the response from the first measurement to the second, thereby interfering with the action of the independent variable. A control group that undergoes all of the experiences (except the independent variable) helps control the effects of history.

Maturation is the process that occurs within the respondent as time passes. Biological and psychological processes may cause the respondent to become tired, hungry, or bored. Or, the problem under study may go into a stage of remission or cure itself independently of the experimental treatment, thus confusing the effect of the independent variable. These effects are controlled by randomization and the use of control groups.

Testing refers to the effect that taking the first test has upon subsequent tests: respondents may do better on the second test because they have practiced by taking the first test, rather than because of the effect of the independent variable. This effect may be controlled by avoiding the first test.

Instrumentation refers both to the measuring instrument and to the researcher who uses the instrument. Instrument decay—autonomous changes in the measuring instrument, such as the stretching or fatiguing of a spring scale—may interfere with valid measurements. The researcher too may experience fatigue or a decline in efficiency. Changing researchers may also interfere with the validity of the instruments. Instrument error is controlled by pretesting before research and by using the same instrument for all measurements. Observer error is controlled by using equivalent random samples of interviewers. Using double blind studies that keep the interviewers ignorant of which is the experimental and which is the control group is also helpful.

Statistical regression is a process that occurs when groups have been selected for study on the basis of extreme scores. For example, students chosen because of their low scores tend to average higher on subsequent tests. The tendency to move closer to the average score is called *regression toward the mean*, a ubiquitous phenomenon. Random assignment from an extreme pool of scores to either the experimental or the control group controls regression.

Differential selection is the method by which subjects are chosen for the research groups. If random sampling is not used, a bias may be introduced into the study. *Matching*—the process of equating the subjects in terms of certain variables—may be used, although it should be used as an adjunct to and not instead of random sampling.

External validity is the ability to generalize from the study sample to the population. External validity is jeopardized by any factor that interferes with the representativeness of the sample. The effects of testing, selection biases, reactions to the unnatural environment of the laboratory, and prior experiments may jeopardize external validity. Another threat is the *Hawthorne effect*—the unnatural behavior that results when subjects know they are being observed.

RELIABILITY

Reliability is the extent to which a specified procedure, such as measurement, yields consistent observation of the same facts, from one time to another and from one situation to the other. Reliability refers to the stability, consistency, accuracy, and dependability of an instrument or measurement. If a test is reliable, repeating it will yield the same result. However, reliability has accrued a variety of meanings over time, due in part to the context in which it was developed and used. Reliability was developed in the context of various tests of ability at a time when extraneous variables received little attention (Selltiz et al., 1976, p. 182). Inconsistency in the results of repeated use of the same instrument was thought to represent errors of measurement rather than the influence of unrecognized and unknown extraneous variables. But, it began to be recognized that inconsistencies of results did not necessarily mean measurement error. New concepts and theories of reliability began to appear. Terms formerly lumped together under the concept *reliability* began to be differentiated. Some are not yet in wide usage. Characteristics of reliability that are examined today include: 1) stability, 2) equivalence, and 3) homogeneity.

Stability of Reliability

Stability is the extent to which repeated administrations of an instrument or measure give the same results. A stable instrument of measurement remains consistent on repeated applications.

To determine the stability of the measuring instrument, the researcher may compare repeated measurements: the same test may be given to a sample of study subjects on two or more occasions and the scores then compared. Such assessments are called *test-retest* reliability. Test scores are compared by computing a *reliability coefficent,* or *correlation coefficient,* between the two sets of scores. If the two scores are unrelated, the correlation is equal to zero; if the scores are perfectly correlated, the correlation coefficient would be $+1.00$; if negatively related, the score will lie between 0.0 and -1.00.

Internal Homogeneity

Internal homogeneity, or *consistency,* is the extent to which all of the subparts of an instrument or scale measure the same characteristic. To determine internal homogeneity, the items on a test are split into two parts, and each of the parts is scored independently. The scores on each of the two parts are then used to compute a correlation coefficient. If the instrument is internally homogeneous, the correlation should be high.

The test may be split in two ways: the first half of the test may be split from the second half. For example, a test of fifty questions may be split into one test comprised of questions 1–25 and a second test composed of questions 26–50. Another way the test may be split is by the number of the questions. For example, odd questions may comprise one test, and all even questions the second test. In the past, the split-half method was often used. It was soon noted that the first half of the test often contained items not found on the last half and vice versa. In addition, the subjects could become fatigued toward the end of the test or make guesses and perform less well. Therefore, the split-half method began to be replaced by splitting the test by odd- and even-numbered questions. If the test was internally homogeneous, every subject should get about the same score on both tests. The extent of internal homogeneity was measured by correlating the scores on the two tests.

Equivalence

Equivalence refers to two processes: inter-rater or inter-observer reliability; and the extent of agreement between the measurement of two instruments. Inter-rater or inter-observer reliability is estimated by having two or more researchers observe or measure the same study subjects at the same time. The coefficient of equivalence indicates the extent to which these measurements agree. Different instruments may attempt to measure the same thing. For example, a measure of anxiety may use a number of instruments: pulse rate, blood pressure, perspiration, etc. The extent to which these measures agree estimates the equivalence. The instruments could also be a test. In this case, two different forms of the test are required. One form of the test is administered to the study subjects, and the second form of the test is administered shortly thereafter to the same subjects. If the correlation coefficient between the scores is high, the instruments are estimated to have good reliability. The measurement procedure is considered reliable to the extent that consistent results are obtained from separate applications.

Examples from Nursing Research

O'Neil (1972) used simultaneous measurements of several behaviors to study the effect of behavior modification procedures on the motor problems of a child with cerebral palsy. Two observers recorded simultaneously for a total of 18 sessions. Percentage of agreement between observers' data was calculated using the formula:

$$\frac{\text{number of agreements}}{\text{total number of agreements} + \text{disagreements}}$$

Nakagawa (1972) reports an historical epidemiological investigation, using records of first admission to a state mental hospital to study the pattern of psychiatric symptom change. A detailed system of coding was developed to classify presenting complaints. To determine the level of intercoder agreement, 10 percent of the records were double-coded. A reliability test (Scott's) was then applied to the double-coded cases. The reliability of the coders was calculated to be 0.85, indicating reasonably good reliability.

Bullough (1974) used a Likert-type scale to measure the level of work-satisfaction among nurse practitioners. A five-item scale enabled respondents to rate their jobs in terms of creativity, importance, use of their skills, autonomy, and interest.

SUMMARY

Measurement is a procedure whereby rules assign symbols and numerals to objects or events, in order to determine relationships such as quantities, degrees, or extent of observation. Ways of measuring include counting frequencies, comparing measurements against a known standard, and ranking observations as larger or smaller or better or worse, using quantitative or qualitative scales.

A *scale* is a device for measuring the magnitude or quantity of a variable. Four types of scales commonly used as levels of measurement include the nominal, the ordinal, the interval, and the ratio. The nominal scale, the lowest level of measurement, consists of a number of discrete, mutually exclusive and exhaustive, named categories. The data derived from a nominal scale can only be counted to determine frequency. The ordinal scale is a qualitative scale comprised of equal-appearing intervals. Ordinal numbers indicate rank order only, not that the intervals between the ranks are equal. Some ordinal scales are the graphic rating scale, the differential scale, and the summated scale. The graphic rating scale is a simple scale in which the researcher develops a continuum from highest to lowest, and the respondent ranks the variables by placing a check at the appropriate point. The Thurstone scale is a differential scale to measure attitudes. Respondents who agree with one statement will likely disagree with those on either side. The Likert scale is a summated scale in which the respondents indicate their agreement or disagreement with statements. The interval scale measures the distance between equal intervals on a quantitative measuring instrument. However, the instrument does not have an absolute zero point. The ratio scale, the highest level of measurement, has both an absolute zero point and equal intervals. To be useful, all scales must be valid and reliable.

Validity is the extent to which a component of research, such as a scale, method, instrument, design, or measure, reflects and measures what the researcher intends it should measure. Methods of judging validity include content validity, face validity, predictive validity, concurrent validity, and construct validity. Content validity is concerned with the sampling adequacy of the study, that is, whether or not all possible observations were included. The researcher strives for content validity by using representative measures where posssible. Face validity is the extent to which the element of research, such as the scale, questionnaire, etc., appears to be logically appropriate on examination. It is a weak judgment, due to the subjective element and limited time of study. Predictive validity is the ability of the instrument to measure and predict: accurate predictions tend to validate the measure. Concurrent validity is the ability of the instrument or scale to measure present observable behavior. When certain states are not directly observable, visible factors may be found to measure the factor logically. Construct validity judges the extent to which the research tool measures the concept, variable, or construct the researcher wants it to measure. Multiple measures of the same concept are often used to establish validity.

A number of factors may jeopardize internal validity (validity within the sample) and external validity (the ability to generalize from the sample to the population from which the sample was drawn). Internal validity is jeopardized by history, maturation, testing, instrumentation, statistical regression, differential selection bias, and experimental mortality. Using randomization, control groups, and double-blind experiments helps control these factors.

Reliability is the extent to which a specified measurement yields consistent observations of the same facts, from one time to another and from one situation to another. Characteristics of reliability include stability, equivalence, and homogeneity. A stable instrument or measure remains consistent on repeated applications. To determine stability, the researcher may use a test-retest, giving the same test to the same study subjects on two or more occasions. The scores are then compared by computing a reliability coefficient. Internal homogeneity is the extent to which all subparts of an instrument or scale measure the same characteristic. To determine internal homogeneity, the items on a test may be split, either by dividing the test into half (first half and last half) or by using all odd questions for one test and all even questions for another. The extent of internal homogeneity is measured by correlating the scores on the two tests. Equivalence refers to inter-rater reliability, and the extent of reliability between two different instruments. Inter-rater reliability is estimated by having two or more researchers observe the same study subjects at the same time; the coefficient of equivalence indicates the extent of agreement. Instruments such as tests are examined by developing two different forms of the test, which are given one after the other to the same subjects. If the correlation coefficient between the scores is high, the instrument is estimated to have good reliability.

STUDY QUESTIONS

1. Give examples of measurements you have used in nursing: counting, comparing, and ranking.
2. Name a nominal scale used in nursing practice or research.
3. Develop a Likert-type scale of ten questions to measure an attitude important in nursing care.
4. Identify ratio scales used in nursing when a patient is first admitted to the hospital.
5. What does judgment have to do with validity of measures?
6. Distinguish between *content validity* and *construct validity*.
7. Differentiate between *internal validity* and *external validity*.
8. How would you control for the effects of history in an experiment?
9. What are the characteristics of *reliability?*
10. Give examples of *stability, internal homogeneity,* and *equivalence.*

REFERENCES AND SUGGESTED READINGS

Bullough, B. (1974): Is the nurse practitioner role a source of increased work satisfaction? *Nursing Research 23,* 14–19. *Likert scale used.*

Campbell,, D. and Stanley, J. (1963): Experimental and Quasi-experimental Designs for Research. Chicago: Rand McNally, pp. 5–12. *Factors jeopardizing internal and external validity.*

Fos, D. (1976): Fundamentals of Research in Nursing (3rd ed.). New York: Appleton. *Chapter 11 examines reliability and validity.*

Kerlinger, F. (1974): Foundations of Behavioral Research (2nd ed.). New York: Holt, Rinehart, and Winston. *Part 8, "Measurement."*

Lin, N. (1976): Foundations of Social Research. New York: McGraw-Hill. *Chapter 10 includes validity, reliability, scales.*

Nakagawa, H. (1972): An epidemiological study of psychiatric symptom pattern change. In Batey, M. (ed.), Communicating Nursing Research. Boulder, Colo.: WICHE. *Measures of intercoder agreement using Scott's reliability test.*

O'Neil, S. (1972): The application and methodological implications of behavior modification in nursing research. In Batey, M. (ed.), Communicating Nursing Research. Boulder, Colo.: WICHE, pp. 179–191. *Measures of behavior.*

Rottkamp, F. (1976): A behavior modification approach to nursing therapeutics in body positioning of spinal cord injured patients. *Nursing Research 25,* 181–185. *Nominal scale of body positioning behaviors.*

Selltiz, C. et al (1976): Research Methods in Social Relations. New York: Holt, Rinehart, and Winston. *Chapter 5 discusses general problems of measurement.*

Simon, J. (1978): Basic Research Methods in Social Science (2nd ed.). New York: Random House. *Chapter 15 examines measuring.*

Stevens, S. (1959): Measurement, psychophysics, and utility. In Churchman, C. and Ratoosh, P. (eds.), Measurement: Definitions and Theories. New York: Wiley, pp. 18–63. *Defines measurement.*

Walizer, M. and Wienir, P. (1978): Research Methods and Analysis. New York: Harper and Row. *Chapter 14 discusses reliability and validity.*

PART 6

Analyzing Data

CHAPTER **13**

DATA ANALYSIS

Data analysis is the process by which the researcher summarizes and describes data and, if possible, makes inferences from the study sample to the population from which the sample was drawn. Using descriptive statistics enables the researcher to summarize and describe data. Using inferential statistics allows the researcher to estimate the probability that findings from the study sample may be generalized to the target population.

This chapter examines descriptive statistics used by nearly all researchers: rates, ratios, proportions, percentages, averages, and ranges. The next chapter describes the use of inferential statistics.

Upon completion of this chapter, the student should be able to: 1) state how to convert raw data into organized summaries; 2) explain how to calculate simple descriptive statistics, such as rates, ratios, proportions, and percentages; 3) describe how to tabulate data; 4) state how to summarize data in tables and graphs; 5) describe how to calculate measures of central tendency and variation; and 6) explain how to interpret data summaries.

CODING THE DATA

Often, the first step to convert raw data into organized summaries is coding. *Coding* is the process by which data are put into categories, transformed into symbols, and counted. The data can usually be represented in a *matrix*, a grid with intersecting rows and columns:

Respondent	Sex	Race
001	m	w
002	f	w
003	m	b

where m = male, f = female, w = white, and b = black.

To transform data into symbols, various types of codes are used. The code needed to machine tabulate data differs from the code needed to sort and count data by hand. For hand tabulation, word description of the categories is satisfactory, such as single, married, widowed, or divorced for marital status. On the other hand, machine tabulation requires that the categories be expressed in numerical symbols. For example, coding numerically for marital status may be as follows: single—1, married—2, widowed—3, divorced—4, and so on. Coding instructions employed in the United States census may often be obtained upon request, thereby enabling the researcher to use standardized codes. At times, the researcher may use the outside margin of pages of questionnaires or interview schedules to write in the code appropriate for each question. This method, called *edge coding*, saves considerable work in processing data. If the data are to be processed by machine, the edge-coded source is used for keypunching and verification. This saves the time necessary to develop code sheets.

RATIOS, PROPORTIONS, PERCENTAGES, AND RATES

Data obtained from qualitative scales, such as the nominal and the ordinal, is summarized as ratios, proportions, percentages, and rates.

Ratios
The *ratio* between two quantities is the number of times that one number contains the other.

$$\text{Ratio} = \frac{\text{frequency of A}}{\text{frequency of B}}$$

A is one category of observations and *B* is another category, or the total of all such similar events. For example, to find the sex ratio, of a category containing 150 males and 250 females, divide the number of males by the number of females, and multiply by 100 to remove partials.

$$\text{Ratio} = \frac{150}{250} = 0.6 \text{ males per female}$$

Multiplying by 100 to remove partial fractions equals 60 males in the group for every 100 females.

Proportions and Percents

A *proportion* is the relation in size of one thing compared to another, an equality of ratios. (It is also a method of finding the fourth term of such a proportion, when three are known). A *percent* is a convenient way to express many proportions; for example, ten percent of the children were absent because of illness. Percent is the parts in each hundred: ten percent is 10 parts in each 100, or 10/100 of the whole. In the example above, where a category contained 150 males and 250 females, the portion and percent of males to the total population is:

$$\frac{\text{males}}{\text{total people}} = \frac{150}{400} = 0.375;$$

or, expressed as parts per 100: $0.375 \times 100 = 37.5\%$ of the total population is male.

$$\text{Proportion} = \frac{\text{category frequency}}{\text{total number}}$$

$$\text{Percent} = \frac{\text{category frequency}}{\text{total number}} \times 100$$

Rates

A *rate* is a quantity, amount, or degree measured in proportion to something else. For example, the standard population is a norm or standard of reference based on a particular actual census of a living population, in proportion to which the distribution of age, sex, and race may be measured.

$$\text{Rate} = \frac{NA}{NA + NB} \times \text{base}$$

In the formula above, NA equals the number of times event A occurs; NB equals the number of times the event might have occurred but did not; and the base is a standard preselected number, such as 100, 1,000, all of which are related to a given period of time.

INDEX NUMBERS

An *index number* is an average that indicates changes between sets of data over time. It is often used to report economic trends; for example, the value of the dollar is often expressed as an index, with the value of the dollar during a particular year serving as the base.

$$\text{Index Number} = \frac{\text{value in period A}}{\text{value in base period}} \times 100$$

Period *A* above is any period for which an index is desired, while the base period is a point in time during which the value is set equal to 100. The problem in making an index is selecting an appropriate base period, preferably one of relative stability and not depression, recession, or inflation.

TABULATING THE DATA

Tabulation of data is the process of arranging the material in a concise and logical order. The classification procedure that forms categories and groups is commonly begun before the data are gathered but seldom actually completed until all data have been collected. Following this process, the data may be organized in various ways: constructing an array of the material is a common way.

An *array* is a list of the observations in which the data are ranked from lowest to highest. For example, if the observations have been collected on the ages of persons in the sample, there may be a number of different ages in the age category that may be ordered by listing each one from the youngest to the oldest: 18, 19, 20, 21, 22, 24, 29, 29, and so on. Thus, the array organizes data in a form that may be easily described and summarized.

The next essential process is to count the number of cases that belong to the various categories. The result of such a count is called a *frequency* (designated by the letter f). The frequency tells how often a characteristic occurs, such as age "20" or sex "female." At times, a frequency count is the only kind of quantitative data that is possible to obtain. At other times, it is the first step toward a more complicated analysis of the observations.

A *frequency distribution* indicates how certain characteristics are spread across different locations or categories. For example, if we wish to know how age is distributed among males in the sample—how many men are under 21 years of age, how many are between 21 and 40, between 41 and 60, between 61 and 80, and between 81 and 100—a count of the men in each age group will give the frequency distribution, which may then be depicted by a figure, chart, or table.

To make a frequency distribution, it is necessary first to establish the set of categories into which the data will be grouped. The categories must be exhaustive, mutually exclusive, homogeneous, logical, and consistent. All of the categories must be the same size, spanning the same number of units of measurement. The categories of age for adult males noted above span 20 years each, beginning at 21 years of age, a fairly universal definition of adulthood in Western society.

Groups of scores (weights, ages, lengths, etc.) placed into categories of particular units are called *class intervals* (designated by the lower case letter *i*). *Class* is the category, such as "age," while *interval* is the standard size of each category (20 years in the example above).

Frequency distributions using class intervals are helpful to analyze ordinal and interval data, which may then be depicted in a table or a graph.

Tables

After the data have been tabulated, the next step may be to arrange the data in tables. The purpose of a table is to:

1. Conserve space, by presenting the data in such a way that the narrative may be reduced.
2. Aid in the visualization of relations among the data and facilitate the process of data comparison.
3. Help forward the process of summation and detect errors and omissions in the categories.
4. Make the tabulated data easier to remember.
5. Put together statistical tables as a basis for computation.

Tables are of several different kinds. The first tables used in the research analysis summarize raw data. These *general purpose tables* are the original, primary tables, designed to include large amounts of source data that will supply information for later tables and graphs. *Special purpose tables* are secondary tables, designed to analyze, summarize, or interpret material; or to illustrate or demonstrate certain points or significant relationships found in the primary data.

Every table has both a *title*, which is placed above the body of the table, and a *number*, Arabic or Roman, which is either centered above the title or placed on the first line with the title.

The parts of a table include the columns (vertical data), rows (horizontal data), and cells (small space defined by the intersection of a column and a row). The line headings of the rows comprise the stub, which is at the left margin of the table; the column headings are at the top of the table, as well as over the stub. A box heading may extend over more than one column; if so, the headings under a box are called *subheadings* (see Table 13–1).

TABLE 13–1. A MODEL OF A TABLE

---

(1) TABLE. (2) A MODEL OF A TABLE AND
ITS COMPONENTS* (3) A SUGGESTED
LAYOUT OF A SECONDARY TABLE, TO BE
INCORPORATED INTO THE TEXT OR THE
REPORT.

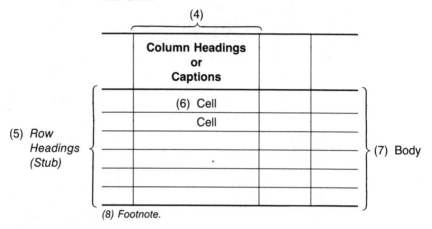

Key to the elements of the above table:

(1) Table number—center above title or place on line with title; may be Arabic or Roman.
(2) Table title—describes the data contained in the table.
(3) Headnote—infrequently used; this further describes the data referred to in the title.
(4) Column—shows data for one category, according to categories contained in the rows or stubs.
(5) Row—shows data for a category, according to data contained in column head.
(6) Cell—intersection of a row and a column.
(7) Body—all of the cells in a table.
(8) *—explanatory footnotes concerning the table itself, using asterisk or dagger to alleviate confusion with textual footnotes.

In statistics, the size of a table depends upon the number of individual frequencies, or cells, contained in it. Size is usually determined by first noting the number of horizontal cells or rows, and then the number of vertical cells or columns. Where the table contains a single row or frequency, that row equals one.

Graphs

A *graph* is a diagram or line that shows how one quantity depends on or changes with another. Commonly used graphs are the pie graph, bar graph, histogram, and frequency polygon, and the pie graph.

The *pie graph* is a circle (360 degrees) which represents 100 percent of the sample—the various parts of the sample being converted to degrees, i.e., angle values of the circle. It is used to represent frequencies for categories which are discontinuous, such as those formed by a nominal scale (see Figure 13–1).

The bar graph, histogram, and frequency polygon utilize the vertical scale or axis of a graph (called the ordinate) to record frequency, and the horizontal scale or axis of a graph (called the abscissa) to record categories.

The *bar graph* like the pie graph represents frequencies for discontinuous categories which arise from the nominal scale. The bar graph utilizes the X or Y axis of a graph to record its data, the frequencies being recorded on the ordinate Y axis and the categories on the abscissa. The bars are discrete and nontouching (see Figure 13–2) reflecting the nature of nominal data.

The *histogram* is a *frequency distribution graph* which records continuous data from ordinal and interval scales. Assuming equal class inter-

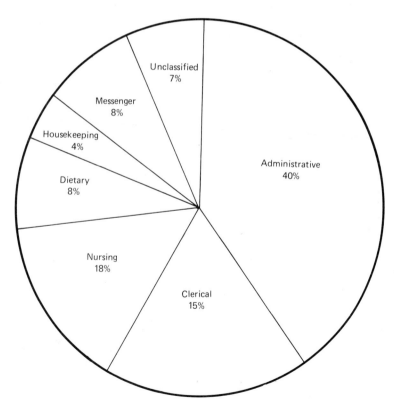

Figure 13–1. Pie graph showing percentage of activities performed by the staff nurse by skill level.

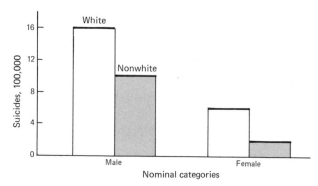

Figure 13–2. Bar graph depicting suicides by race and sex.

vals, the frequency of a class is represented by the height of the bars and the class interval by the width of the bar. Thus to construct a histogram, bars of equal width should be made to stand for the size of the class interval. The height of the bars represents the frequency with which the occurrence in each category takes place. The frequency always goes on the vertical axis or the ordinate while the categories or class intervals go on the horizontal axis or abscissa.

The bars of a histogram touch one another, indicating continuous data. A space, however, should be left between the ordinate and the first bar. Frequencies should start at zero and the proportions of the

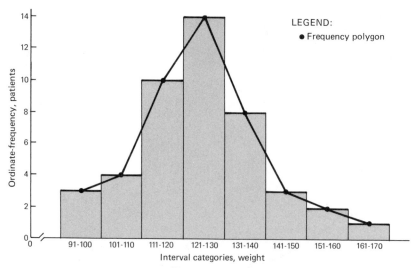

Figure 13–3. Histogram and frequency polygon.

graph should be reasonable, having the frequency units and the class intervals properly divided (see Figure 13–3). A narrow abscissa with tall ordinates or a wide abscissa with short ordinates form misleading graphs.

A *frequency distribution polygon* may be made from a histogram by putting a dot in the center of the top of each column and connecting the dots with a line.

MEASURES OF CENTRAL TENDENCY AND VARIANCE

Data from quantitative scales may be described by two summary measures: the measure of central tendency (mean, median, and mode), and the measures of variance (range and standard deviation).

Central Tendency
The most typical, common, or average value for all of the subjects studied is called the *central tendency*. *Central* refers to a middle value, while *tendency* refers to the general trend of the numbers, in terms of their central or middle value. For example, if all of the ages in a sample were being studied, an observation of one age may be compared with all ages, i.e., with the distribution of the variable *age* in the population. Once all of the ages were listed, the array organized and the data were summarized, then the age that is most frequently found in the sample (the mode) may be determined, along with the average age of the sample (the mean) and the middle age in the sample (the median).

The Mean. A simple descriptive statistic and the most widely used is the *mean* or *average*. It is obtained by adding together all of the values or scores and dividing this number by the total number of scores. The mean is symbolized by $\overline{X}$; the formula for calculating the mean is:

$$\overline{X} = \frac{X}{N}$$

where $\overline{X}$ = mean or average, Σ = the sum of (the Greek letter *sigma*), X = the individual scores, and N = the total number of the observations or scores. The mean is affected by the value of every case; thus, the extreme and erratic items may be given undue weight. For example, if the researcher wished to calculate the average monthly salaries of ten persons who made $280, 300, 310, 320, 330, 340, 350, 370, and 10,000, respectively, to get the mean $\overline{X}$, the researcher would add up or take the sum Σ of all of the individual scores X and divide by the total number of scores N. The mean $\overline{X}$ would be \$12,920 divided by 10, or a monthly average of \$1,292.

However, the mean should not be used if the distribution of scores is very skewed, i.e., unsymmetrical or distorted. In the example used above, the one large income has pulled the mean income far above what it would have been if the scores were symmetrical. If the sample of scores has a reasonably symmetrical distribution, the mean is a good measure of central tendency.

The mean is often advantageous to use, merely because it is so well known and understood. If there are fewer observations than 30, the items may be treated individually. However, if a larger number exists, the data should be arranged in a frequency distribution first, then the mean of the distribution calculated.

The Median. The *median* is the middle score that divides a set of scores into two equal parts. The median is the measure of central tendency most commonly used with a skewed distribution of scores. It is also used with scores based on an ordinal measurement scale, which ranks scores from largest to smallest, with intervals not exactly determinable. For example, if a researcher wished to have the patients on a ward rank the efficiency of nursing care with the categories "excellent," "good," "fair," "poor," and "terrible," each of these categories could be assigned a code number from one for "terrible" to five for "excellent." However, it is important to remember that these are not scores in the usual sense, but simply numerical codes or guides to the categories. If fifteen patients were to rank the nursing care, the scores might look something like this:

$$5,5,5, \quad 4,4,4,4,4, \quad 3,3,3,3, \quad 2,2, \quad 1$$

In these scores listed above, the median score is a four, which stands for the category "good." The median is the middle score. It lies between the two middle scores, if the total number of scores is even, or it is the middle score, if the total number of scores is odd.

Based on values lying immediately on either side of it, the median is not as influenced by the size of extreme items as is the mean; thus, it may be used effectively where individual values are extreme and atypical.

The Mode. The *mode* X is the simplest measure of central tendency to calculate, defined as the most frequent score. The mode may be used with any scale, but it is the only measure of central tendency usable with the nominal scale. Like the median, the mode is useful in cases where it is desirable to eliminate the effects of extreme variations. In a frequency distribution, the mode is that point on the scale of the variable where the frequency is the greatest. At times, there may be one mode (unimodal), or two modes (bimodal), or three modes (trimodal), unless there is a distinct central tendency. In a large sample, the mode may have little significance.

Thus, if the nominal scale is used, the best measure of central tendency is the mode; if the measurement scale is ordinal, the best measure of central tendency is the median; with equal interval scales, when scores have reasonable symmetry, the best measure is the mean. Where the measurement is equal intervals but the scores are skewed or asymmetrical, the best measure of central tendency is the median.

Variance

The purpose of describing the central tendencies of the data is to provide a single value to represent a group of unlike values. For example, averages accent the best single representative of a set of scores or numerical values. On the other hand, the variance examines dispersion, or how observations are spread out. The variability of the scores may be of as much interest as the central tendency, since the actual observations are not totally concentrated but instead are spread out or distributed among many values or categories. The extent to which these observations are dispersed around the central values, whether clustered close around the average or widely scattered, may be measured. The three principle measures of variance are the total range, the interquartile range, and the standard deviation.

The Range. The simplest measure of the dispersion of data is the total *range,* a relatively crude and unstable measure of dispersion that defines the difference between the largest and smallest observations in a set. Therefore, the total range is limited, taking into account only these two specific observations—the largest and the smallest. In spite of this, the range, like the mode, is useful to read tables or quickly scan data for a rough picture of the scope of observations and their tendency to be dispersed. The formula for obtaining the total range is as follows:

$$\text{Total Range} = (\text{the largest } X) - (\text{the smallest } X)$$

where X is an individual score.

Knowing the total range is sometimes a better indicator of the nature of the data than knowing the mean. For example, examine the grades below that two groups of eight students each made on a test:

Group A	Group B
100	60
80	55
60	50
50	50
50	50
40	50
15	45
5	40
400	400

where Group A $\overline{X} = \dfrac{400}{8} = 50$ and Group B $\overline{X} = \dfrac{400}{8} = 50$.

Adding the individual test scores X together and dividing by the total number of test scores, eight in each case, the mean $\overline{X}$ (50) for each group is found to be identical. Yet, the scores for each group vary considerably. If the total range for the two groups were known, more useful information would be in hand about the variation among the scores than knowing the mean alone. The total range for Group A is 95 (100 − 5 = 95), while for Group B it is only 20 (60 − 40 = 20). This means that a greater variation exists within the scores of Group A than within Group B, although the mean of both is identical. Therefore, the range gives a better understanding of the variability of ten scores.

The range does have limitations. For example, a change in one individual score, the lowest or the highest, can alter the total range drastically. If Group B had one score of 100, the entire range would change. In addition, the range fails to give the overall variability within the group of scores. To correct this problem somewhat, another measure of range, the interquartile range, is often employed.

The Interquartile Range. The *interquartile range* is a positional value found by making an array of values, i.e., lining up the values in order of size, and dividing the array into quarters. The range of categories or scores that includes the middle 50 percent of the scores is the interquartile range, the range *between the scores* comprising the lowest quartile, or quarter, and the highest quartile, or quarter. The formula for obtaining the interquartile range is:

$$\text{Interquartile range} = Q_3 - Q_1$$

where Q_3 is the category in and below which are ¾ of the scores, and Q_1 is the category in and below which are ¼ of the scores. Q is the symbol for quartile.

Using the test scores of Group A above, the interquartile range may be identified:

Group A	
100	
80	Q_4
60	Q_3
50	
50	Q_2
40	
15	
5	Q_1

where $Q_3 - Q_1 =$ the interquartile range.

Normal Frequency Distribution and Standard Deviation. The *normal frequency distribution curve,* also called the *bell-shaped curve,* the *normal curve,* or the *Gaussian curve* (after its inventor), has properties that are valuable in the statistical analysis of data. The curve indicates that most of the values of the measurements of a variable under study cluster together and possess about the same scale value, forming the mode, the median, and the mean. A much smaller number of the variables or study subjects possess more extreme or deviant values on either extreme of the curve (see Figure 13–4). In the normal curve, 68 percent of all values fall within one standard deviation on either side of the mean (± one SD), 95 percent of all values fall within two standard deviations from the mean (±2 SD), and 99.87 percent fall within three standard deviations from the mean (±3 SD).

To understand standard deviation and its relationship to dispersion, it is helpful to consider a simple example of how individual scores deviate from the mean, and how they are dispersed around the central tendency represented by the average score of the group, i.e., the mean (see Table 13–2).

With the calculation of the mean for the group, it is now possible to calculate how much each individual deviates from the mean score (see Table 13–3).

Having averaged all of the scores, the deviations of each individual score from the mean fall one-half on the positive side and one-half on

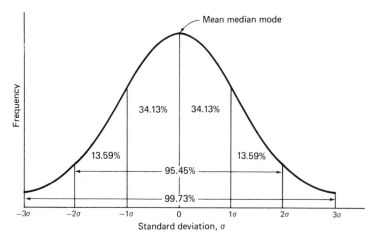

Figure 13–4. The Normal Frequency Distribution Curve and Standard Deviation.

the negative, resulting in a summated score of zero. Therefore, this method cannot be used to find an average deviation or variance.

To solve this problem, each number may be squared to eliminate the negative signs. This procedure gives the following: the average variability of the squared deviation scores may be obtained by dividing 6600

**TABLE 13–2. AN ARRAY
OF WEIGHTS OF TEN
CHILDREN**

Individual Weights (X) (in pounds)
20
50
60
60
70
70
70
80
100
120

Where $\Sigma X = 700$ pounds, $N = 10$ individual weights, $\bar{X} = \dfrac{\Sigma X}{N} = 70$, $\bar{X} = 70$ pounds.

TABLE 13–3. WEIGHTS OF CHILDREN EXPRESSED AS DEVIATION FROM THEIR MEAN

Original Weights (X)	Deviation Scores $(X - \bar{X})$
20	−50
50	−20
60	−10
60	−10
70	0
70	0
70	0
80	+10
100	+30
120	+50

Σ of all deviation scores = 0

by N, or 6600 ÷ 10 = 660 (see Table 13–4). This average squared deviation is in units of the pounds squared; therefore, to return the measure to the original units, the square root of the average squared deviation must be calculated: 660 = 25.69 pounds—the standard deviation SD. To sum up:

$$SD = \sqrt{\frac{\Sigma(X - \bar{X})^2}{N}} = \sqrt{\frac{6600}{10}} = \sqrt{660} = 25.69 \text{ pounds (see Fig. 13–5).}$$

TABLE 13–4. SQUARED DEVIATION SCORES WEIGHTS OF CHILDREN

Individual Scores (X)	Deviation Scores $(X - \bar{X})$	Squared Deviation Scores $(X - \bar{X})^2$
20	−50	2500
50	−20	400
60	−10	100
60	−10	100
70	0	0
70	0	0
70	0	0
80	+10	100
100	+30	900
120	+50	2500
		6600

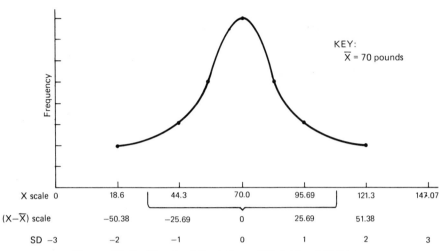

Figure 13–5. Standard Deviation of Weights of Children.

Thus, to calculate the standard deviation, the following procedure is followed: (1) determine the mean $\overline{X}$ of all of the values; (2) find the difference between each individual value X and the mean $\overline{X}$; (3) square each deviation; (4) find the sum of the squared deviations and divide by the total number of values, to get the mean or average squared deviation; (5) take the square root of the average squared deviations to obtain the standard deviation SD, or the average of the extent to which each score deviates from the mean.

Complementary to the arithmetic mean, the standard deviation is the most widely used measure of variability. It is used when the frequency distribution approximates a normal curve relatively well. *Standard* comes from the fact that the standard deviation indicates a group average spread of scores or values around their mean. *Deviation*, indicating the spread of scores around the mean, is measured by how much each score deviates, or is scattered, from the mean.

Standard Scores. Symbolized by the small letter z, *standard scores* tell how many standard deviations away from the mean the particular raw score is. The formula for standard score is:

$$z = \frac{(X - \overline{X})}{\text{SD}}$$

where z = standard score, X = individual score, $\overline{X}$ = mean, and SD = standard deviation.

For example, standard scores with a mean set at 500 and a standard deviation set at 100 are used by Medical College Aptitude Tests. Many intelligence and achievement tests use standard scores with a pre-established mean and standard deviation.

Interpretation of Data Summaries

Interpretation of the data summaries consists of extracting meaning and conclusions from the data. The method of interpretation is reasoning, from data summaries, tables, graphs, tests, and comparisons. The researcher summarizes what was found; draws conclusions about the significance and importance of the data findings for nursing; compares findings to other studies; and relates findings to the research problem, assumptions, hypotheses, or existing theory. The researcher states the extent to which it is possible to generalize from the findings of the study sample to a larger population. The researcher also identifies gaps in knowledge that need to be filled by future research; suggests specific areas for additional research; and criticizes his or her own work, pointing out strengths and weaknesses. When possible, the researcher makes recommendations for using the findings in practice, or suggests the extent to which it is possible to prescribe, given the current level of knowledge.

SUMMARY

The summary, analysis, and interpretation of data begin when all the data are collected, although the researcher plans for this step from the beginning of the project. Qualitative data are summarized as rate, ratios, proportions, and percentages, quantitative data are summarized by additional measures, including mean, median, mode (central tendency), and standard deviation (variation).

The first step in summarizing data is to code the data: to transform it into symbols and count it. The codes for hand tabulation may be words that describe the various categories, but codes for machine tabulation must be numerical symbols. Edge coding, in which the researcher uses the outside margin of data-collecting sheets to write codes, speeds up the work of data processing.

Qualitative data are summarized as ratios, proportions, percentages, and rates. A *ratio* between two quantities is the number of times that one number contains the other. A *proportion* is the relation in size of one thing compared to another—an equality of ratios. A *percent* is the parts in a hundred that a portion of the whole represents. A *rate* is the quantity, amount, or degree measured in proportion to something else.

Data may be tabulated—arranged in a concise and logical order—by using an array, a frequency, or a frequency distribution. An *array* ranks the observation from lowest to highest. A *frequency* counts the number of cases that belong to various categories. A *frequency distribution* indicates how certain characteristics are spread across different categories.

Tables and graphs are helpful ways to depict data summaries. Tables may take many forms but all include basic information, including title, stub, box head, line, column, cell, body, and source of data.

A *graph* is a diagram or line that shows how one quantity depends on or changes with another. Commonly used graphs are the pie graph, bar graph, histogram, and frequency polygon. The *pie graph* is a circle that represents 100 percent of the sample. It is used to represent discontinuous frequencies, such as those measured by the nominal scale. The *bar graph* is also used to depict data measured by the nominal scale, but it uses the X or Y axis of a graph to record its data. The histogram is a frequency distribution graph that records continuous data from ordinal and interval scales. The frequency of a class of data is represented by the height of the bars; the interval by the width of the bars. A frequency distribution polygon may be made from a histogram by putting a dot in the center of each column and connecting the dots with a line.

Measures of central tendency include the mean or average score, the median or middle score, and the mode or most frequent score. The *mode* is the only measure of central tendency usable with the nominal scale; the *median* is useful if the distribution of the scores is skewed; and the *mean* is the most widely used measure and represents the average score.

The *variance* examines the dispersion of scores around the central values. The *range* is the simplest measure of dispersion; it defines the difference between the largest and the smallest observations. The *interquartile range* includes the scores between the lowest quarter of an array of scores and the highest quarter. The *standard deviation* is an index that measures the extent that individual scores on the average deviate from the mean.

Interpretation of data summaries is extracting the meaning from the data. The researcher uses reasoning and comparison to draw conclusions or to relate findings to the research problem's hypotheses or theory. The researcher must determine the following: the extent to which it is possible to generalize; the gaps in knowledge that continue to exist; and the research needed to fill those gaps. In addition, the researcher criticizes the research, noting its strengths and weaknesses. When possible, the researcher makes recommendations for the use of the research findings in practice. The current level of knowledge must be noted in making such recommendations.

The function of data analysis is to provide a summarization of completed observations, in order that research questions may be answered. The function of interpretations of data is to bring the intellectual focus of the researcher to bear upon the data, in order to elucidate the meanings of the research findings.

STUDY QUESTIONS

1. You are studying all personnel in the hospitals of Central City who are involved with bedside nursing care. Make a list of the categories you would expect to find. How could the categories be transformed into numerical symbols?
2. You have a category (race) that contains 400 persons, 150 of whom are black. What proportion and what percent of the category are not black?
3. Construct an array for the following set of blood pressure scores, with attention first to the systolic and then to the diastolic:

    130/60   190/100   110/50   240/120   120/80   90/40   185/100

4. Below are a set of test scores. What is the median? the mean? the mode?

100, 100, 40, 60, 70, 70, 70, 65, 65, 65, 65, 80, 95, 85, 30, 70, 70, 80, 80

5. Below are a group of weights. Construct a frequency distribution.

105	120	138	155	161	170	178	181
110	123	150	157	165	173	179	185
118	130	151	160	169	175	179	189

6. With the data from above, construct a histogram.
7. Drawing on the data in question five, construct a table indicating a relationship between weight, sex, and race. Columns one and two are white women; columns three and four are black women; columns five and six are black men; and columns seven and eight are white men.
8. Construct a bar graph showing the relationship between the weight of black men and white men, compared with black women and white women.
9. Compare measures of central tendency with those at variance.

REFERENCES AND SUGGESTED READINGS

Abdellah, F. and Levine, E. (1965): Better Patient Care Through Research. New York: Macmillan. *Chapters 8 and 9 examine processing data, and analysis and interpretation of research findings.*

Brink, P. and Wood, M. (1978): Basic Steps in Planning Nursing Research. North Scituate, Mass.: Duxbury Press. *Chapter XIV, "Planning for Analysis of Data."*

Dempsey, P. and Dempsey, R. (1981): The Research Process in Nursing. New York: D. Van Nostrand. *Chapter 5, "Data Analysis."*

Fox, D. (1976): Fundamentals of Research in Nursing (3rd ed.). New York: Appleton. *Chapter 5, "Descriptive Statistics."*

Lin, N. (1976): Foundations of Social Research. New York: McGraw-Hill. *Chapter 5, "Describing One Variable," and Chapter 7, "Statistical Inference."*

Maxwell, A. (1961): Analysing Qualitative Data. New York: Barnes & Noble. *Chapter X, "Classification Procedures."*

Selltiz, C. et al (1976): Research Methods in Social Relations (3rd ed.). New York: Holt, Rinehart, and Winston. *Chapter 13, "Data Processing," Chapter 14, "Analysis and Interpretation."*

Wandelt, M. (1970): Guide for the Beginning Researcher. New York: Appleton. *Step 10, "Organization of Data."*

CHAPTER 14

STATISTICAL INFERENCE

Statistical inference is a combination of mathematical processes and logical principles that allows the researcher to test inferences and statistical hypotheses (null hypotheses) against actual data. The researcher uses statistical inference for two purposes: to estimate the probability that data found in the randomly drawn sample accurately reflects the target population or universe from which it was drawn; and to test the null hypotheses formulated from the research hypothesis.

Upon completion of this chapter, the student should be able to: 1) define concepts used in the study of inferential statistics; 2) compare descriptive and inferential statistics; 3) describe *samples, populations,* and *chance factors;* 4) describe how to estimate population parameters; 5) compare the estimation of population parameters with the testing of statistical hypotheses; 6) describe the relationship between the research hypothesis and the null hypothesis; 7) explain how to formulate a null hypothesis; and 8) describe Type I and Type II errors. No formulas will be used in this chapter. Interested students are referred to suggested readings at the end of the chapter.

CONCEPTS USED IN THE STUDY OF INFERENTIAL STATISTICS

Like research in general, inferential statistics has a language of its own. Learning the concepts used in the study of inferential statistics enables the student not only to read research reports with better understanding but also to understand the general process associated with the ability to generalize from a sample to the target population from which it was drawn. Table 14–1 summarizes very briefly some of the concepts used in this chapter.

A COMPARISON OF DESCRIPTIVE AND INFERENTIAL STATISTICS

A *statistic* is both a summary value, such as the mean, that is calculated from a sample of observations and an estimator of some population parameter (i.e., *true value*). A statistic is both the factual data and the use of such data to infer or estimate population parameters from sample statistics.

Descriptive statistics, such as the mean, summarize research data from a *sample*, while *inferential statistics* use the data from randomly drawn samples, both to infer characteristics of the *population* from which the sample was drawn and to test statistical hypotheses. Descriptive statistics may be used whether or not random sampling has been used, but inferential statistics requires random sampling and other processes based on the principles of probability. Researchers in the clinical area often use random assignment alone rather than in combination with random selection, but base their inference to the larger population— that is, the external validity of their study, or the ability to generalize— on the findings of repeated study of samples. Descriptive statistics summarize the unwieldy mass of raw data, transforming it into frequencies, means, and other summaries that point out the characteristics of the sample. While of basic importance, such findings are usually limited to the sample under study, unless the process of random sampling has been used.

Inferential statistics allows the researcher to go beyond the description and summary of data. Inferential statistics is a tool that enables the researcher to use findings summarized from randomly collected samples to make judgments about a population, and to test a statistical hypothesis about the characteristics of a population. The researcher can infer or estimate the extent to which relationships observed in the study sample would occur in the population from which the study sample was drawn by random sampling.

TABLE 14–1. DEFINITIONS OF SELECTED CONCEPTS

Chance Factors—the residual, unknown factors that affect events after the factors that determine events have been isolated.

Hypothesis

    null—likewise known as H_0, the *statistical hypothesis,* the *test hypothesis,* and the *benchmark hypothesis;* refers to any hypothesis that is subject to nullification by a sample statistic; an hypothesis formulated to state no relationship between specified variables and populations.

    statistical—same as null hypothesis.

    research—likewise known as the *scientific, experimental,* or *theoretical hypothesis,* and H_1, a statement of the predicted interrelationships among a number of variables that the researcher expects to find in the sample data.

Level of Significance—the probability that an observed relationship or value could be attributed to the tendency for the sample statistic to fluctuate from one sample to the other. The probability of rejecting the null hypothesis when it is true. In research involving human subjects, often set at .001, but no lower than .01.

Mean—the average value.

Population—any set of persons, things, or measurements having an observable characteristic in common. A universe.

    parameter—a hypothetical *true* value for a population; any measurable characteristic of the population, such as the population mean.

    target population—the specified subjects or cases from which the study sample was drawn and about which the researcher intends to generalize. May be distinguished from the accessible population, which refers to that population actually available for a study.

Sample—any subset of a population.

    sample statistic—a value computed entirely from the sample, such as the mean or average, that the researcher computes from observations.

Sampling—the process of selecting a subset of a population for inclusion in a study.

    random sampling—affording each unit in the population an equal chance or probability of being chosen for the study sample.

    sampling distribution—data that represent characteristics of samples.

Statistic—both a summary value, such as the mean, that is calculated from a sample of observations, and an estimator of some population parameter, i.e., the *true value* of a population.

Statistics—*descriptive*—summary measures such as means, medians, modes, percentages, ratios, and standard deviations calculated from measurements of samples units.

    inferential—the process by which the researcher is able to generalize from the sample data to the target population.

Tests of Statistical Significance—a technique of testing that allows the researcher to determine whether or not summary measures could be independent estimates of the same population parameter.

Populations, Samples, and Chance Factors

Central to the study of statistical inference is the relationship among the concepts of population, sample, and chance.

Any set of persons, things, or measurements having an observable characteristic in common constitutes a *population*, or, as it is sometimes called, a *universe*. A *population parameter* is a hypothetical *true* value for a population—any measurable characteristic of the population, such as the population mean or variance. A population may be finite, for example, all patients who come to City Clinic for the treatment of cancer. Or the population may be infinite, for example, all persons who have or ever will have cancer. Population parameters are usually designated in the literature by Greek letters such as *mu* (μ), which stands for the population mean; or small *sigma* (σ), which stands for the population standard deviation.

A *sample* is any subset of a population, symbolized as a rule by English letters, such as $\overline{X}$ (the mean), and X (a single score). A *sample statistic* is a value computed entirely from the sample, a numerical descriptive measure, such as the mean or average, that the researcher summarizes and computes from observations. Samples may be variously collected, but to be used to infer, a sample must have been selected by random sampling.

Chance factors are the residual, unknown factors that affect events, after the factors that determine events have been isolated. The observable world is not a world of complete certainty; there is always uncertainty. But, neither is the world one of chance alone. The researcher attempts to reduce factors of which he or she is ignorant. Where uncertainty remains, the researcher tries to calculate the extent of such factors and the risk of error they introduce. The laws of probability provide the basic ingredient in inferential statistics and enable the researcher to calculate the element of risk as inference is made from sample to population.

Estimation of Population Parameters

To estimate a population parameter, such as the population mean, the researcher begins after the data are collected. As the researcher knows, the data found in the sample may differ from that of the "parent" population. For example, one hundred different samples randomly drawn from the same population may differ somewhat in statistics such as the mean, both from one another and from the population. Yet, sampling is the most economical way in most instances to study a population. The size of the population, the cost in time and money necessary to observe all elements, and the difficulty of being able to observe all of the subjects make the study of the total population prohibitive. Moreover, measuring the total population could destroy or change the units, or affect the subsequent state. To determine the characteristics of the total universe of a person's blood, it is not necessary to take all the blood from the body. Therefore, the researcher takes a sample, and from this sample estimates or infers the parameters of the population. However, a number of problems are inherent in such an approach. First, the researcher in all likelihood has data from only one sample, which contains about thirty subjects. Due to the vagaries of chance sampling, there is the probability that a discrepancy may exist between the sample statistic and the population parameter. A *sampling error*— the deviations of all sample means drawn from a population from the true mean of the population—may have occurred as a result of random sampling. The sample statistic, such as the mean, may deviate from the true mean of the population. Second, the researcher determines how close the mean of the sample is to the mean of the population that may be unknown. How is the mean of an unknown population estimated?

It is possible to demonstrate that the mean of samples not only tends to gravitate toward and to cluster around the population means, but that the pattern of distribution of a large number of sample means drawn from the same population tends to assume a shape approaching that of the normal (the bell-shaped) curve.

To examine these assertions, it is necessary to understand the process of obtaining a sampling distribution, although few researchers will actually go through this time-consuming and tedious process.

Sampling distributions are data that represent characteristics of *samples*, not individual cases. For example, individual cases may be put into various categories whose mode, median, and mean may be calculated, revealing the characteristic of *one sample*. But, a sampling distribution of the mean uses an infinite number of samples drawn from the same population. For example, to construct a sampling distribution of the means of a large number of samples, the researcher would take the following steps:

1. Designate the target population.
2. From this population, draw by random sampling a very large number of samples (for example, thousands of samples); each of these samples must be of equal size and must contain no less than 30 subjects.
3. Compute the mean for each of the samples.
4. Put all of the sample means into a frequency distribution graph.
5. Calculate the means of the sample means.

According to the "central limit theorem," the mean of this distribution will probably approach the population mean, and the shape of the frequency distribution graph will probably fit the characteristics of the normal, bell-shaped (Gaussian) curve. Thus, the researcher can be assured that the statistic from the sample will always bear a relationship to the corresponding population parameter that may be unknown. The sample statistic tends to cluster around the population parameter in a recognizable manner. The researcher with data from a single randomly drawn sample may feel assured that, while the data may vary from the population parameter, they usually will not vary far, especially if the number of observations in the sample is large. In addition, the variance of the sample can be calculated with techniques of inferential statistics. Should the researcher be able to increase the size of the sample, the average sampling errors will decrease, although the researcher must quadruple the sample size to cut errors in half. The fact that the sampling distribution of means approaches a normal curve allows the researcher to treat the distribution much the same way he or she treats any normal distribution.

Estimation of Population Parameters and Testing of Statistical Hypotheses

The two general types of statistical inference include the estimation of population parameters, which have just been examined, and the testing of statistical hypotheses, which will be examined now. The estimation of a population parameter begins *after* the data are collected. On the other hand, the testing of statistical hypothesis begins *before* the data are collected: the researcher formulates the statistical (null) hypothesis from the research hypothesis,* specifies the "level of significance" at which the null hypothesis is to be rejected, and then collects the data that he or she will analyze to test the hypothesis.

Both estimating population parameters and testing statistical hypotheses are based upon probability theory and the use of random sampling. Both are concerned with population parameters, as these are related to sample statistics; both must deal with sampling error; and both must rely upon the sampling distribution of a statistic. However, the estimation of a population parameter begins with the sample data and ends with a range of values (the confidence interval and its accompanying confidence level), within which the population parameter probably lies. On the other hand, testing of the statistical hypothesis begins with the null hypothesis, which predicts that the relationship between variables stated in the research hypothesis is probably only due to

---

*The *research hypothesis* is a statement of the *expected relationships* among phenomena being studied; the *null hypothesis* states that the differences obtained in the values between the groups being compared could have occurred by chance alone.

chance. It ends with a decision to accept or reject the null hypothesis, on the basis of sample data. The use of inferential statistics in testing the null hypothesis, to arrive at a decision to accept or reject it, will now be examined.

The Null Hypothesis and Related Concepts

A *null hypothesis* is formulated in order to be rejected. The researcher uses principles of probability to test the statement that observed effects are only chance occurrences. Data that fail to support the null hypothesis indicate to the researcher that the findings probably are *not* due to chance alone, a crucial point in the interpretation of the data. However, the researcher can make two types of errors in deciding to accept or reject the null hypothesis (see Table 14–2). A *Type I* error arises when the researcher decides to reject the null hypothesis when it is actually true. A *Type II* error is made when the researcher decides to accept the null hypothesis when it is actually false. The researcher controls the risk of making a Type I error (rejecting a true null hypothesis) by selecting a level of significance. The *level of significance* is simply a phrase used to designate the probability of rejecting a null hypothesis when it is true. It does *not* indicate the findings' importance or meaning.

TABLE 14–2. ERRORS IN HYPOTHESIS TESTING

The Decision of the Researcher Is To:	The Null Hypothesis Is Actually:	
	True	False
1. Reject the null hypothesis	Type I error, with a given probability of alpha*	Correct decision
2. Accept the null hypothesis	Correct decision	Type II error with a given probability of beta†

*Alpha: the level of significance or the degree of risk involved in rejecting the null hypothesis.
†Beta: the degree of risk involved in failing to reject the null hypothesis.

Steps to follow in the formulation and testing of a null hypothesis include the following, each of which will be discussed:

1. Formulate the research hypothesis.
2. Formulate the null hypothesis, which states that the results observed are due to chance alone.

3. Specify the level of significance at which the null hypothesis is to be rejected. The level of significance is usually set at .05 or at .01. A level of significance of .05 means that a true null hypothesis would be rejected in only 5 samples out of 100. A level of significance of .01 means that a true null hypothesis would be rejected in only 1 sample out of 100.
4. Complete all steps in the planning phase of the research project.
5. Obtain the study sample by random sampling.
6. Collect and summarize the numerical data.
7. Complete analysis of data, using appropriate statistical tests to calculate the probability that the null hypothesis is true.
8. Make a decision to accept or reject the null hypothesis at the given level of significance.

Step One: Formulate the Research Hypothesis. The *research hypothesis,* likewise known as the *scientific hypothesis,* the *experimental hypothesis, H_1,* or the *theoretical hypothesis,* is a statement of the predicted interrelationships among a number of variables (at least two) that the researcher expects to find in the sample data. The research hypothesis is formulated during the planning period, with reference to theories or empirical generalization from which it is deduced. The purpose of hypothesis testing is to ascertain the extent to which the relationships observed in the sample statistics may be generalized to the population from which the sample was drawn. Ultimately, the researcher hopes the data will support or clarify theories designed to explain what is present in the empirical world; how phenomena change; how things remain the same; and/or how events or variables are interrelated.

For example, the experimental hypothesis is tested by observing the specified variables before and after an independent variable has been introduced; comparing the changes in the experimental group with any changes in the control group; and inferring whether the hypothesis should be rejected or accepted on the basis of the findings. However the researcher does not know whether the findings are the result of his or her manipulation of the independent variable or of sampling error. Therefore, the researcher formulates a statistical (null) hypothesis, in order to test statistically the probability that the findings are due to chance alone. Rejection of the null hypothesis tends to strengthen the research hypothesis.

Step Two: Formulate the Null Hypothesis. The null hypothesis, likewise known as H_0, the *statistical hypothesis,* the test hypothesis, and the *benchmark hypothesis,* was conceived to refer originally to any hypothesis that is subject to nullification by a sample statistic (Fisher, 1960). However, it is often used in a more restricted sense to refer to a hypothesis for-mulated to state no relationship—no correlation or causality—between specified variables or specified populations.* The formulation of a null hypothesis from an experimental hypothesis is illustrated with the fol-lowing example modified from Simon (1978, p. 406).

Simon formulates a null hypothesis (which he calls a *benchmark hypothesis*) to examine whether an independent variable "removes" a sample under study from the original population. In this case, the orig-inal population consists of patients who have cancer. The researcher proposes to test the experimental hypothesis that a drug (drug *A*) cures cancer, using a sample of twelve patients who are selected from the population of cancer victims. The researcher first randomly divides the sample of twelve into two groups: the experimental group who will get drug *A*, and the control group who will not. He then introduces the drug, the independent variable, into the experimental group. After the drug is given, five of the six patients in the experimental group are said to be well, while two of the six in the control group who did not receive the drug are likewise pronounced well. Did the drug affect the rate of recovery from cancer? Will patients who take the drug in the future have a higher rate of recovery than they would have had if they had not taken the drug? Specifically, did drug *A* remove the patients in the experimental group from the original population of cancer victims with its original chances to get well?

In this case, the null hypothesis states, "Patients who take drug *A* still belong to the original population of cancer victims with its original chances to get well." That is, the patients have the same chance to get well as if they had never taken the drug. According to the null hypoth-esis, the drug will make no difference: any differences observed are due to chance alone. If the researcher can test this null hypothesis and find evidence that leads him *not* to accept it, the researcher thereby strength-ens the hypothesis that drug *A* is related to the rate of recovery: that

---

*The formulation of the null hypothesis is complex, involving not only the hypothesis but a number of related statements included in the following steps:

1. The null hypothesis is formulated from the research hypothesis before data are collected.
2. The null hypothesis states that the statistics observed are due to chance alone.
3. A statement that accompanies the null hypothesis specifies *alpha*—the "level of significance" (Type I error)
4. If possible, the statement specifies the number of observations *N* that will minimize *beta* (Type II error).
5. The statement identifies statistical tests to be used to analyze the data.

All of these steps are taken in Phase I—the planning phase of the research.

drug *A* removed the experimental group from the original population, with its original probability of recovery, and provided the patients with a different (and better) probability of recovery.

To formulate the null hypothesis, the researcher first states the experimental hypothesis: "A patient who takes drug *A* will be cured." Second, he or she rephrases the statement, introducing the concept of chance: "Patients who take drug *A* have the same chance to get well as those who do not take drug *A*." Third, he or she formulates the null hypothesis with reference to specific populations: Patients who take drug *A* still belong to the same population as patients who do not take drug *A*, i.e., any difference observed between those who took the drug and those who did not is due to chance. The experimental hypothesis has now been translated into the null hypothesis that can be tested by statistical inference.

Where the research hypothesis states that a difference will be found, the null hypothesis states that no difference will be found; where an effect is expected, the null hypothesis states no effect will be found; where the researcher looks for correlation, the null hypothesis states no correlation will be found and so on.

Once the null hypothesis is formulated, the next step is to specify the alpha-level of significance involved in rejecting the null hypothesis.

Step Three: Specify the Level of Significance and Related Concepts. The 'level-of-significance' is the probability of rejecting the null hypothesis when it is true. The level of significance, however, means different things depending upon whether 'one-tail' or 'two-tails' of the sampling distribution curve are to be used to test the null hypothesis. The 'region of rejection' is likewise related to the level of significance, since the 'regions' consist of the sample values which are located in one or both tails whose combined probability is equal to the level of significance.

The level of significance is the probability that an observed relationship or value could be attributed to the sampling error, the tendency for the sample statistic to fluctuate from one sample to the other as well as from the population. The *level of significance* is often defined as the probability of rejecting the null hypothesis when it is true, since the selection of the level of significance determines whether or not a null hypothesis will be rejected. The researcher may make an error when he or she makes a decision to reject the null hypothesis—the null hypothesis may be true. The researcher can estimate how often he or she is likely to make such an error. This kind of error is called a *Type I* error and is intimately tied to the level of significance set by the researcher. The level of significance (set at .05, .01, .001, etc.) is set by the researcher as the maximum risk or error he or she is willing to run when he or she rejects the null hypothesis. The researcher uses the level of significance to evaluate the probability that the sample statistic was obtained due to chance. Statistical tests reported to be significant at the .05 or .01 level indicate that the findings would occur by chance only 5 times in 100 (.05), or 1 time in 100 (.01). If the result is likely to occur by chance and the researcher rejects the null hypothesis, he or she is betting that the findings are not one of the 5 in 100. However, 5 percent of the time the researcher will probably be wrong. The level of significance is set at what the researcher believes to be an appropriate level, given the nature of the study and its consequences; but another researcher may set the level of significance at a different level, thereby arriving at a different decision to reject the null hypothesis. Studies that deal with vital issues of human health and welfare usually require the researcher to set the level of significance high (.01, .001, or higher). Less concern about the consequences of rejecting the null hypothesis allows the researcher to set the level of significance lower, for example, .05 is often employed in sociological research. It should be clear that level of significance has nothing to do with the importance or meaning of the research, only with the probability of chance occurrences. Moreover, rejection of the null hypothesis does not indicate what the nonchance factor is. It is the research hypothesis that specifies alternatives to the null hypothesis.

Step Four. Complete all steps in the Planning Phase of the research project (see Chapter 3, Phase I).

Step Five: Draw the Sample. Reliance on a sample is the factor that makes the data and inferences probabilistic. Studies that do not employ random sampling, both in the selection of subjects from the population and in the assignment of subjects to the experimental and control groups, should not use tests of significance designated as parametric tests. Therefore, the sample must be drawn by one of the several methods of random sampling. Such sampling is not only scientific but may yield more valid data than those collected by other methods. Sampling size is also important. The larger the size N of the sample, the smaller the probability of making a Type II error, or accepting the null hypothesis when it is actually false. However, it is important to distinguish between error of sampling and error of measurement caused by a defective instrument. Whether measuring blood pressure or attitudes, a defective instrument will not be corrected by increasing the number of observations. Such errors, called *systematic errors,* are corrected only by selecting a valid and reliable instrument.

Step Six: Collect and Summarize the Numerical Data. Data may be collected in many ways, including observation, questioning, and measurement. Data summaries are obtained by the use of descriptive statistics that calculate frequency, percentages, ratios, central tendencies, and variance.

Step Seven: Use Appropriate Statistical Tests. Statistical tests are classified as nonparametric or parametric tests of statistical significance. *Nonparametric tests,* such as the Mann–Whitney U test, median test, or the chi square test, are not as rigorous as parametric tests and are used when the measurement scale has been nominal or ordinal, when the sample size is small, and when a normal distribution of data cannot be assumed. Nonparametric tests require only that random sampling has been used to select the study sample and that the measurements are independent. *Parametric tests,* such as the t-test and the analysis of variance (ANOVA), require random sampling, measurement on a quantitative scale such as an interval or ratio scale, and a normal distribution of data.

Step Eight: Make a Decision to Accept or Reject the Null Hypothesis. It is not possible to say, without question, that the null hypothesis is true or false. The researcher makes a decision to accept or reject the null hypothesis based upon judgment—how probable it is that observed differences were due to chance, rather than to factors proposed by the research hypothesis. Since the entire population was not examined, but only a sample randomly selected from that population, the estimations are based on incomplete information and may not be accurate.

SUMMARY

Statistical inference is a combination of mathematical processes and logical principles that allows the researcher to test inferences and statistical or null hypotheses against actual data. Statistical inference is used to estimate the probability that data found in a randomly drawn sample accurately reflects the target population and to test null hypotheses formulated from research hypotheses.

Descriptive statistics differs from inferential statistics in that descriptive statistics summarize data from a sample, while *inferential statistics* infer characteristics of the population from which the sample was randomly drawn. Inferential statistics test statistical hypotheses as well. The major difference between the two is related to the use of randomization in inferential statistics, which allows the researcher to generalize from the sample to the target population; descriptive statistics summarize data from a sample and cannot be generalized beyond that sample.

A *sample* is any subset of a population, while a *population* is any set of persons, things, or measurements having an observable characteristic in common. *Chance* factors are the residual, unknown factors that affect events after the factors that determine the events have been isolated. The laws of probability upon which inferential statistics are based provide the basic ingredients to calculate the chances the researcher takes as he or she infers from sample to population.

A *population parameter* is estimated from randomly drawn samples. However, the researcher needs to determine how close the mean of the sample is to the mean of the population, which may be unknown. Population means may be calculated through the use of sampling distributions, which calculate the means of many samples' means. The estimation of a population parameter begins after the data are collected.

The testing of a statistical hypothesis begins before the data are collected, when the researcher formulates the statistical hypothesis from the research hypothesis. The research hypothesis is tested by observing the specified variables before and after an independent variable has been introduced. The researcher does not know whether the findings are the result of his or her manipulation of the independent variable or whether they occurred by chance. The statistical hypothesis is formulated to test statistically the probability that findings are due to chance alone. If the research hypothesis states that a difference will be found in the experimental and control groups, the statistical hypothesis states that no difference will be found. After testing, the researcher must make a decision to accept or reject the null hypothesis. If the null hypothesis is rejected when it is true, the researcher commits a Type I error. If the null hypothesis is accepted when it is false, the researcher makes a Type II error.

STUDY QUESTIONS

1. Why is it important for nurses in research to understand what *statistical inference* means?
2. Can statistical inference allow the researcher to make completely accurate tests or estimates? Why or why not?
3. What is the basis for inference in research?
4. If a nurse has made a descriptive study, is it possible to use inference?

5. What is a *statistic?* What is *descriptive statistics?* Can a nurse who has data from a sample that was not drawn by random sampling use descriptive statistics? Why or why not?

6. What is *random assignment?* Can a nurse infer from one sample?

7. What is a *population* or *universe?* What is a *population parameter?*

8. What is the difference between a *finite* and an *infinite population?*

9. What is a *sample?*

10. What is *chance?* Why is it important for the nurse researcher to understand this concept?

11. What is the difference between a *sampling distribution* and the *distribution of cases (frequency distribution)?*

12. What is a *null (statistical) hypothesis?*

13. What is the difference between inferring from a sample to a population, and testing a statistical (null) hypothesis?

14. Discuss the relationship between the research hypothesis and the null hypothesis.

15. Use the research hypothesis, "Patients who take drug *A* will be cured of cancer," and state a null hypothesis.

16. Distinguish between a *Type I* error and a *Type II* error.

REFERENCES AND SUGGESTED READINGS

Bullough, B. (1981): Is the nurse practitioner role a source of increased work satisfaction? In Fox, D. and Leeser, I (eds.), Readings on the Research Process in Nursing. New York: Appleton, pp. 215–223. *Chi-square.*

Chase, C. (1976): Elementary Statistical Procedures. New York: McGraw-Hill. *Chapter 8, "Probability and statistical inference."*

Dixon, W. and Massey, F. (1957): Introduction to Statistical Analysis. New York: McGraw-Hill. *Chapter 4, "Universe and sample"; Chapter 7, "Statistical inference."*

Duncan, R., Knapp, R., and Miller, M. (1977): Introductory Biostatistics for the Health Sciences. New York: Wiley. *Chapter 3, "Populations, samples, and the normal distribution."*

Fox, D. (1976): Fundamentals of Research in Nursing. New York: Appleton. *Chapter 7, "Inferential statistical concepts and procedures."*

Gerber, R. and Van Ort, S. (1979): Topical application of insulin in decubitus ulcers. *Nursing Research 28,* 16–19. *Pearson Product Moment Correlation Coefficients, analysis of variance, frequency distribution, central tendency.*

Lin, N. (1976): Foundation of Social Research. New York: McGraw-Hill. *Chapter 7, "Statistical inference: an introduction."*

Mueller, J1, Schuessler, K., and Costner, H. (1970): Statistical Reasoning in Sociology. New York: Houghton Mifflin. *Chapter 13, "Parameter estimation."*

Phillips, J. and Thompson, R. (1967): Statistics for Nurses. New York: Macmillan. *Part II deals with the bases for inference; Part III examines inferences, using frequency and ranked data; Part IV discusses inferences, using means and variances.*

Rodgers, J. (1977) Relationship between sociability and personal space preference at two different times of day. In Downs, F. and Newman, M. (eds.), A Source Book of Nursing Research (2nd ed.), pp. 171–177. *Means, standard deviations, and F values; Pearson Product moment correlation coefficients.*

Rottkamp, B. (1981): A behavior modification approach to nursing therapeutics in body positioning of spinal cord injured patients. In Fox, D. and Leeser, I., *Readings on the Research Process in Nursing.* New York: Appleton, pp. 107–114. *Mann-Whitney U test.*

Simon, J. (1978): Basic Research Methods in Social Science. New York: Random House (2nd ed.). *Chapter 27, "Inferential statistics: introduction."*

Walizer, M. and Wienir, P. (1978): Research Methods and Analysis (2nd ed.). New York: Harper and Row, Chapter 16, p. 466.

CHAPTER 15

THE USE OF THE COMPUTER IN RESEARCH

The *computer* is an electronic device that adds, subtracts, multiplies, and divides at tremendous speeds. Research has been completely revolutionized by computers that analyze data at a rate of speed inconceivable in previous decades, when each calculation was done by hand. The student can use a computer, and should learn to use a computer, if one is available. Hand calculators range in complexity from the simple and inexpensive to expensive machines that can be programmed. Hand calculators that compute mean, standard deviation, and variance are quite helpful in analyzing data. The savings in time alone is worth the investment.

The student who plans to use a computer must consult with computer experts early in the planning process to determine costs, availability of the computer, and the form in which data must be presented. The student does not need to know the inner workings of a computer in order to use one, but the student should know the limitations of the computer and the role of the researcher. Upon completion of this chapter, the student should be able to: 1) describe in simple terms how the computer works; 2) define selected data processing terminology; 3) discuss what the computer can and cannot do; 4) identify the components and functions of a computer system; and 5) describe steps to take in using the computer.

HOW A COMPUTER WORKS

To understand how a digital computer works, it is helpful to compare its operations with that of a student with only a hand calculator. To analyze the data, the student using a hand calculator would use four kinds of equipment: 1) the calculator to solve individual arithmetic problems; 2) a work sheet to write down the order in which the individual calculations were performed, and the intermediate and final totals; 3) mathematical tables for reference; and 4) the student's mind, which would control the entire operation.

The corresponding parts of the computer include: 1) a high speed arithmetic unit that can execute millions of operations in one second—corresponds to the desk calculator; 2) a storage unit or memory unit—corresponds to both the work sheets and the mathematical tables; and 3) a control unit—corresponds to the mind of the human operator, and causes the computer to take the proper steps in the proper order.

The storage unit or memory unit of the computer includes the instructions for the problem to be solved, the numbers needed, and the intermediate results. The storage unit takes a number of forms: magnetic tape, magnetic drum, or magnetic core. Magnetic core memories, the most widely used type, are so fast that any part of the stored information can be selected and consulted in less than ten-millionths of a second.

Computer arithmetic is often binary arithmetic—a numbering system that used two digits, 0 and 1. Combinations of 0 and 1 can represent any number, letter, or symbol to be used by the computer. Each of the thousands of individual circuits are like electric light-switches that can be turned on or off. The binary arithmetic systems enable the computer to work on this simple on-off principle.

To solve a problem on the computer, the operator gives the computer a complete set of instructions called a *program*. The program, which can be selected in consultation with a computer expert, includes a list of operations to be performed. The computer center at a university usually has both a professional staff for consultation and a set of computer programs that can deal with the kind of data analysis that most nurse researchers need, such as the Biomedical Data (BMDD), or the Statistical Package for the Social Sciences. The student does not need to know the various languages computers use—FORTRAN, BASIC, COBOL—but must be able to identify what variables are being used and the methods of data analysis necessary.

The SPSS is widely used for several reasons: the manual contains detailed and clearly written instructions, and the package offers a range of statistical procedures with explicit instructions.

Many researchers think we are reaching a time when students will be able to have their own minicomputer. These computers are not only becoming more readily available, they are growing cheaper and cheaper. The decreasing cost, together with increasing knowledge, forecasts a vast increase of computer use, even at the undergraduate level.

What the Computer Can and Cannot Do

What the computer can do is perform more arithmetic in one second than the student could do in months and months. And the computer is accurate. Whereas we students can make an error, the computer can perform highly complex calculations without making any errors at all, and it doesn't get tired. It can calculate for hour after hour without making mistakes from overwork or boredom. However, computers do break down, and when they do, it takes an expert to repair them. A burned out wire or an electrical surge may shut the computer down for hours. But, the most severe limitation of the computer is its inability to think. It cannot reason; it cannot infer. It can only perform those operations that it has instructions to perform. Any extraneous material, such as a misplaced period or comma, can interfere with calculations. The instructions, or programs, must be in detail, one step at a time. However, programming is the task of computer experts. Students can rely on the consultants at the computer center or computer statisticians to recommend the proper program for the research data. This should be done early.

Since computer time is costly, the student must investigate whether or not there is computer-time for his or her school and class. Most nursing schools have computer time alloted, and some of this may be designated for undergraduate students. Computer costs, often reckoned in terms of minutes, may nonetheless be a bargain if we consider the time and effort that hand calculations require.

Data-Processing Terminology

A number of terms used in data-processing are commonly heard but have a particular meaning only to computer experts. These include the following: *field, file, deck, code, record, byte,* and *record length.*

A *field* refers to the specific columns of a data card to which a variable is assigned. For example, a subject's age may be assigned to two columns, column one and column two. A subject who was 43 years old would have the 4 punched in column one and the 3 punched in column two. A *file* is all the data obtained from a given case: all the data describing the experiences and behavior of a patient who was intensively observed is in that patient's file. A file is comprised of *records,* or *data cards,* although this term sometimes refers to magnetic tapes or discs when these are used.

A *deck* is a set of records that contain the same bits of information for all subjects. A *byte* generally refers to a data card column, specifying a location within a record. But, it is more appropriate to refer to data as being stored on magnetic tapes or discs than it is to use the term *column*, which specifically refers to cards. *Code* is also a technical term used with tapes or discs to refer to the same item that a *punch* would refer to, if a card were being used. The *record length* of a card refers to the eighty columns or eighty bytes of the card. However, in cases where tapes and discs are being used, the eighty-column format is no longer accurate— the tape or disc may be 240 columns, or bytes, in length.

The traditional wording that grew up around the data processing cards that were first used, and are still used, often carried over into the use of tapes or discs, where the wording was no longer actually appropriate. Therefore, new words came into being to describe more precisely what the researcher meant.

Components and Functions of Computer Systems

The components of a computer system include both the machines *(hardware)* and the programs *(software)* that specify what the computer is to do. The hardware consists of a number of machines, such as the key punch, card reader, central processing unit, control panel or console, card punch printer, and tape unit. Not all systems use all the hardware available; some are basic. The student tends to become familiar with the hardware and software connected with the *input* devices that convert raw data into a form the computer can read and store, and the *output* elements that anlayze the data.

For example, research data may be punched onto a data processing card by means of a *keypunch machine* and verified by a *verifier*. Both of these are similar to a typewriter. Using a keypunch machine, the operator types onto a keyboard that activates a punching device, which makes holes in the proper columns of the data processing card. The card contains eighty columns and twelve rows for storing both research data and program instructions. A separate card is used for each instruction in the program or each separate case. The verifier looks very much like a keypunch machine, except it does not punch holes. It is used to make sure that the information originally punched is accurate. The verifier operator punches the same information that the keypunch operator should have punched. If the two do not agree, a light comes on to indicate the error. Verification is an important process that is integrated into many steps of the computer operation, although the method of verification varies from one stage of the process to another.

Once the data processing card is punched and verified, it is put through a card reader that records the information and returns the card

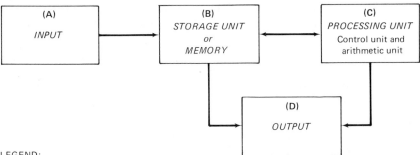

LEGEND:
(A) The program — a set of complete instructions to solve problems — is fed into computer. The raw
     data is fed into the computer. Program and data comprise the *INPUT*.
(B) The information is stored in the *MEMORY UNIT*: each cell can store either one instruction or
     one numerical value. The memory unit can store large amounts of information and allow rapid
     access to any portion of that information.
(C) Instructions stored in the memory are sent to the control unit, which interprets instructions,
     determines sequence of operations, and controls the processing of information. The control unit,
     together with the arithmetic unit (which does the arithmetic calculation), form the *DATA
     PROCESSING UNIT*.
(D) Information that results from the calculations of the computer comes out in an understandable
     form such as a printout — a verbal and numerical description of the findings — the *OUTPUT*.

Figure 15–1. Input, memory, processing, and output.

to the operator. Punched and verified data may be stored on magnetic
tapes, on computer discs, or in their original format. Unless the cards
are properly stored, they may become warped and useless for computer
operations.

The card reader may transfer the research data to magnetic tapes
that feed information to a memory core in the central processing unit.
The central processing unit, containing both the control unit and the
arithmetic unit, uses data from the memory core to perform the calculations that the control unit directs.

Once calculations are complete, the output devices translate the
answers into a form the researcher can understand. This is usually a
printout copy, although a card punch may reconvert what is in the
memory back onto eighty-column data processing cards (see Figure
15–1).

STEPS TO TAKE IN USING THE COMPUTER

To use the computer to analyze data, the student begins early to take
the first of several steps. Each shall be examined briefly.

1. Define what you wish the computer to analyze. This information comes directly from the research proposal. The variables identify exactly what is to be studied and analyzed. For example, a nursing problem may be concerned with the number of persons in a community who have elevated blood pressure. The research proposal is to document by interview and instrumentation the blood pressure of a randomly selected sample of 100 adults in a specified community, to discover how many blacks and how many whites have an elevated blood pressure. The variables to be analyzed are blood pressure and race. The researcher can develop the interview schedule and blood pressure records to indicate that race will be put in column one—*1* for black, and *2* for white. Columns 2 through 8 can denote blood pressure.

2. Consult a professional at the computing center. The second step is to find an appropriate person to advise you throughout the project. The student in particular needs to know what program should be used. Canned programs, such as the Statistical Program for the Social Sciences (SPSS), are usually readily available in most university centers. However, in order to give the computer full instructions, the programmer must speak to the machine in programming languages, such as FORTRAN (an acronym for *for*mula *trans*lation) or BASIC (*B*eginners *A*ll-purpose *S*ymbolic *I*nstruction *C*ode). Fortunately, it is not necessary for the student to learn either the computer language or how to program the computer. Expert advise is usually forthcoming from those at the computing center, providing the student has contacted a person early in the research process and has located the funds to pay for computer time.

3. Transform the raw data into a medium that the computer can read. The third step occurs after the data are collected. The student must now transform the data from the interview schedule and accompanying records to a medium that the computer can "read." A common form is the data processing card, or punch card (see Figure 15–2). These cards contain eighty vertical columns and twelve horizontal rows into which coded data are punched. For example, the person's race in the study above may be punched in column one, while the blood pressure data will need more columns—2 through 8. For example, a blood pressure of 150/102 is punched as follows: *1* in column two; *5* in column three; *0* in column four; */* in column five; *1* in column six; *0* in column seven; and *2* in column eight. The card would still have seventy-two columns left, if the researcher wished to add additional information such as age, sex, marital status, or state of health. One-hundred cards must be punched and verified, one for each subject.

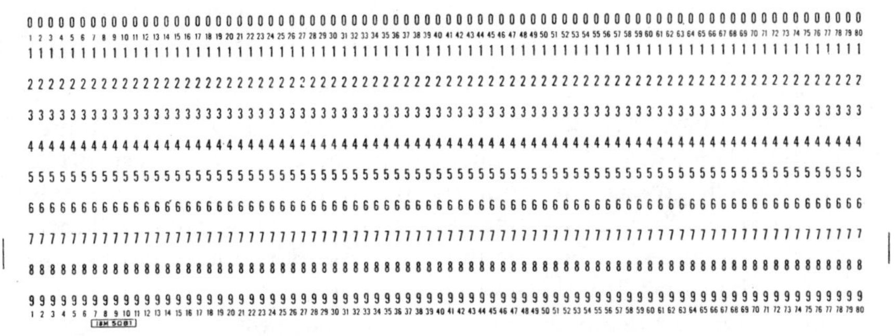

Figure 15-2. The data processing card.

4. *Inform the computer.* The fourth step is to inform the computer how the data have been set up on the data processing cards. For example, the student who uses the SPSS program precedes it with the following instructions. On the first card, a list of the variables—race and blood pressure—is punched. On the second card, the fixed location of each variable is noted—race takes up one column, while blood pressure takes up the next seven. On the third card, the computer is informed of the type of input medium being used—in this case, *card.* On the fourth card, the number of cases in the study—100—is punched. The fifth card contains the information concerning the frequencies the computer is to count—how many blacks and whites had a blood pressure of 150/100. The sixth card tells the computer which statistics to compute—the mean, the variance, and so on. The final card, number seven, instructs the computer to begin to read the input data. The cards containing all research data now follow. It is clear from these instructions how the researcher must carefully inform the computer as to what it must do and how. If the computer operation is to go forward accurately or at all, no step can be skipped.

5. *Examine the output of the computer.* The fifth step is to examine the analyzed data carefully for errors. For example, row 1 is punched for the column on sex of respondent, and only the numbers 1 for female, 2 for male, and 3 for not reported were used. A 4 appears in the data, so the researcher should return to the original source to look for errors in keypunching. Once errors are cleared up, the researcher must plan to store the data so that analysis is simple and access to the contents is easy. Analysis of the computed data requires comparison of the values in the columns or rows, or in various conbinations of the columns and rows.

SUMMARY

The *computer* is an electronic device that has revolutionized the research process, because it can add, subtract, multiply, and divide at tremendous rates of speed. With assistance in the planning and analysis phases of the research project, the student can use the computer in her or his work: the researcher does not need to understand the inner working of the computer to use it, but she or he must understand what the computer has the capability of doing.

The computer needs *input*—a program and raw data—to begin its operations. The memory unit or storage unit includes both the instructions for the problem to be solved, the numbers or data needed, and the intermediate results. From the memory unit, information goes to the processing unit, which is comprised of the control unit and the arithmetic unit. The control unit interprets the instructions, determines the sequence of operation, and controls the processing of information. The arithmetic unit does the arithmetic calculation. The control unit, together with the arithmetic unit, form the data processing unit. Information, or *output*, comes out of the computer in an understandable form such as a printout. The data processing terminology uses many common words to stand for particular computer operations. Many terms refer specifically to the data computer cards, although magnetic tapes and discs now in use contain neither column nor rows.

The computer system is comprised both of *hardware*—the various machines that process data—and *software*—the programs that specify what the computer is to do and how. The student may learn to use the keypunch machine and verifier, although this takes practice to produce an error-free result. The keypunch machine makes holes in the proper columns of the data processing card, so the computer may electronically read the information. The verifier is similar to the keypunch machine but, instead of punching holes, it verifies the holes already punched, lighting up when an error is detected.

In planning and executing a research project that includes use of the computer, the student must be acquainted with several important steps. The student must define with the computer is to analyze; consult a professional early in the planning stages; transform raw data into a medium that the computer can read; inform the computer how the data are set up; carefully examine the output of the computer for errors; and plan for the permanent storage of the data.

STUDY QUESTIONS

1. What is a *computer?* Compare the operations of a computer with those of the researcher who uses a desk calculator to analyze data.
2. What are the advantages and disadvantages of using a computer?
3. What *hardware* is the student apt to use in computer operations?
4. What *software* is available in most university centers?
5. If you were to use the computer in a research project of your own planning, what steps would you take?
6. What are the interrelationships among *input, memory, processing,* and *output?*
7. Describe a *data processing card.* What do the numbers mean? How are they used?
8. Locate the nearest computer center. Call to find the cost of using the computer for five minutes. Are there grants available for you to use the computer?

REFERENCES AND SUGGESTED READINGS

Babbie, E. (1973): Survey Research Methods. Belmont, Cal.: Wadsworth Publishing. *See Chapter 10.* (1975): The Practice of Social Research. Belmont, Cal.: Wadsworth Publishing. *See Chapter 13 for selected data-processing terminology.*

Nie, N. et al. (1975): Statistical Package for the Social Sciences. New York: McGraw-Hill. *Includes a number of major programs.*

Polit D. and Hungler, B. (1978): Nursing Research. New York: J. B. Lippincott, Chapters 22 and 23.

Simon, J. (1978): Basic Research Methods in Social Science (2nd ed.). New York: Random House, pp. 245–246; Chapter 26.

Selltiz, C., Wrightsman, L., And Cook, S. (1976): Research Methods in Social Relations (3rd ed.). New York: Holt, Rinehart, and Winston, Chapter 13.

CHAPTER 16

THE STUDENT'S REPORT: ORGANIZATION AND SELF-EVALUATION

The *research report* is a written or spoken communication that informs a selected audience about a research project. The objective of the report is to present what the audience wants or needs to know as clearly and succinctly as possible. The researchers extract the relevant material from their working papers, organize the content in logical order, and document each step with care, taking the needs of the audience into consideration.

Upon completion of this chapter, the student should be able to: 1) identify various audiences who read or hear nursing research reports; 2) state how to organize the content of the research report in a logical manner; 3) ask and answer questions that help self-critique the student's report; 4) identify various media in which reports may appear; and 5) identify sources helpful to develop styles of writing suitable for reports.

THE AUDIENCE

Effective communication of the research findings begins with the identification of the audience. The first audience reached by the student is usually the supervising professors and classmates. The student should also plan to submit the paper, with the approval of the supervising professor, to professional meetings and suitable journals, in order to receive a wider review. The first meeting of professionals may be members of the faculty who hear brief oral reports of the completed research. In addition many nursing organizations have sections for student papers in their meetings, in order to encourage research among the rising generation of professionals. If such sections do not exist, it may be possible to initiate one. The supervising professor may join with the student to prepare the paper for submission to a professional meeting or journal.

The audience at professional meetings or for nursing journals may be diverse, including nursing researchers, practitioners, policy makers, sponsors of research or interested members of the general public. Each of these may look for different information in a research report. Nurses engaged in basic or applied research may look for information that contributes to the body of nursing knowledge or to the practice of nursing. Practitioners may seek information helpful in the assessment, intervention, or evaluation of nursing care. Policy-makers in nursing may look for information to improve or change existing policies or administrative structures. Nursing professors may examine in particular the theories, concepts and methods of data collection and analysis used in the study. Students must carefully consider the primary audience they intend to reach, although secondary audiences also may be kept in mind.

To evaluate this element of their report, the student must answer the following questions: Who is the primary audience I am trying to reach? What is it they want or need to know?

ORGANIZATION OF THE CONTENT OF THE REPORT

The organization of the research report varies from one scholar to another. Usually, the report follows the outline of activity pursued by the students, as they planned and carried out the research activity: 1) introduction; 2) research statement (drawn from the research proposal); 3) review of the literature; 4) research design; 5) method of sampling; 6) research methods; 7) description of the pilot study, if any; 8) analysis and interpretation of data; 9) conclusions; 10) bibliography and appendices; and 11) abstract (see Table 16–1).

The main heading of the research report often follows rather faithfully the major steps of research depicted in Chapter 3. Each main head of the research report will be examined briefly, with accompanying questions for self-evaluation. The student may also wish to review the section on how to criticize a research report for assistance.

TABLE 16–1. SUGGESTED OUTLINE FOR A RESEARCH REPORT

I. Introduction
   A. Importance of the general problem to nursing
   B. Specific problem
II. Research statement
   A. Statement of what the researcher studied and how
   B. Definition of concepts/variables
   C. Hypotheses, if any
   D. Objectives of the study; purpose
   E. Ethical implications of the research
III. Review of the literature
   A. Review of related and competing theories
   B. Review of relevant research
   C. Specification of theory and research used in study
   D. Review of observations to formulate theory, if applicable
IV. Research design
   A. Description of the particular design used
   B. Description of control used, if any
   C. Discussion of the validity and reliability of the design
V. Sampling
   A. Description of the target population
      1. Discussion of how the sample was drawn, sample size,
         response rate
      2. Discussion of bias, if any
VI. A. Description of the method of data collection used
   B. Description of categories, instruments, scales, operational
      definitions
   C. Discussion of the reliability and validity of methods, instruments
VII. Pilot study
   A. Description of findings
   B. Subsequent revisions
VIII. Analysis and interpretation of data
   A. Description of statistics used and how the data was analyzed
   B. Summary of data in graphs and tables, with narrative explanation
   C. Interpretation of findings
IX. Conclusion
   A. Implication of findings for nursing
   B. Recommendations, suggestions for future research
X. Bibliography and appendices
XI. Abstract

Introduction to the Report

The introduction to the report is not always easy to write. Sometimes the final version of the introduction is written after other parts of the report are complete. It is often helpful to examine how other researchers have introduced the general and specific problem in their report. For example, McCorkle (1974) began her report on the effect of touch on seriously ill patients by noting the importance of verbal interaction in meeting the emotional needs of patients. Hays and Larson's (1963) *Interacting with Patients* was cited as a reference. Nonverbal communication was introduced in the next sentence as a second mode by which nurses can respond to patients' emotional needs. In the third sentence, the specific kind of nonverbal communication—"touch"—was introduced. In the fourth sentence, McCorkle cited a reference, Clark's (1968) article on loneliness and nursing intervention, to establish the importance of touch in communicating with the patient. Therefore, in the space of four sentences, McCorkle introduced the reader to the general problem, the specific problem, its importance to nursing, and studies reported in the literature that establish the significance to nursing. Upon completion of the introductory paragraph(s), the student should ask: Have I stated the general problem and the specific problem in terms of the importance to nursing? Are one or two references cited to establish this? Do the major concepts stand out? Does the reader know precisely what was studied, after reading the introduction? Is the introduction clear, yet concise?

The Research Statement

The *research statement* is drawn from the research proposal. The proposal is forward looking, defining what will be studied. The research proposal is converted into the research statement, which informs the audience precisely what *was* studied and how. Having informed the audience of the general and specific problem to be studied, the student now communicates in summary form all the elements of the research: how the sample was drawn, how the data were collected, the time and site of the study, and any other pertinent information that sets the stage for the information that follows. The audience should not have to go searching through the report to discover whether or not the research design was experimental or a survey; or whether or not the sample was randomly selected. The following research statement summarizes what was studied, who was studied, and how:

> This study investigated the relationship between stressful environmental conditions in pregnancy and the subsequent pathology seen in the newborn. The data were collected by interview and record review

from 100 subjects. The subjects were selected by systematic sampling from a target population of pregnant women who attended pre-natal clinics in Central City during the months of September and October. Those who gave informed consent were included in the study sample.

After writing the research statement, the student may go in one of two directions. If the researcher conducted an exploratory or descriptive study that did not use hypotheses, the report may next include definitions of concepts and objectives of the study. If the researchers did use hypotheses, these may be stated, followed by definitions of variables and, if desired, objectives.

The definition of concepts, a subheading of the research statement, informs the audience exactly what the researcher means by a particular term. Since a clear consensus does not exist on the definition of concepts, this is necessary. The student should not only define the concept, but also give the source in the literature from which the definition was drawn. Next, the student gives the objectives that were set—what was planned to be accomplished by the research.

If *hypotheses are used,* they should be stated as a subhead of the research statement, followed by operational definitions of the variables used. Like the definition of all major concepts, operational definitions should be accompanied by reference to the literature from which these were drawn.

Upon completion of the research statement, students should ask: Does the audience now know *what* I studied, *how* I collected the data, *who* the study subjects were, *how* I collected the sample from the population, *when,* and *where* the study took place? Have I noted here, or will I note later, the ethical implications of the study? Have I disguised the name and place of the study to insure anonymity of agencies and subjects? Are concepts defined with reference to the nursing literature? Are the concepts observable and measurable, or have I referred the audience to an instrument, such as an operational definition, that makes the concept observable and measurable? Are the hypotheses clear and succinct? Is the source or sources of the hypotheses clearly stated, with reference to the theoretical literature? Does an operational definition of each variable follow each hypothesis, to clarify how I observed and measured the variables? Have I clearly stated the objectives, or the intentions, with which I began the study? Have I explained why I chose such objectives?

The Review of the Literature
The *review of the literature* informs the audience of several factors: 1) the extent to which the student researcher is familiar with current and clas-

sic publication; 2) the competing theories in the literature that propose to explain the phenomena under study; 3) the research that supports or refutes these theories; and 4) the theoretical viewpoint or assumptions from which the research proceeded deductively that best explains what has been observed.

A brief critical review of the literature is preferable to a long, rambling description. However, the entire report may be a review of the literature, in which case the organization of the content takes this into consideration.

When the review of the literature has been written, the student should ask these questions: Does the review include primary sources, rather than secondary sources? Does the review relate to the problem studied? Does the review include the most recent works, as well as the classics? Does the review contain a succinct report of different theories and the research designed to test hypotheses formulated from these? Has the researcher made it clear which theory was used? Is the review written in such a way that the researcher can use it to interpret data? Are concepts that are identified in the literature clearly indicated? Are instruments that are located in the literature and used in research clearly documented? Are all citations included in the reference or bibliography? If the research is designed to formulate theory, are the observations of others clearly developed and reported?

The Research Design

The *research design* informs the audience about the plan of research—it describes the design (experimental, survey, historical-documentary, etc.) and the controls used, and notes any problems with validity or reliability. The researcher may want to inform the audience why this design was used rather than another, and note ethical implications or design problems that were experienced. Questions to be answered include the following: If an *experimental design* was used, has the method for sampling been clearly explained? Has the method of assigning subjects to the control or the experimental groups been explained? Have the independent variable and the dependent variable been designated? Is it clearly explained how the researcher manipulated the variables? Is the control of extraneous variables explained? If a *survey* was used, does the report explain all elements of the research design? Is it clear whether a questionnaire or an interview was used? Are variations on these designs explained? Is it clear what the design intends to accomplish? If an *historical* design was used, does the researcher explain what records were used, how access was obtained, how the researcher determined whether the records were complete and accurate? In each of these cases, is the validity and reliability of the research design assessed and explained?

The Sampling Process

If the researcher has not reported about the sampling process, this should be next. The sampling process is one of the most crucial areas in the research process. The audience will want a clear description of exactly how the target population was identified and precisely how a sample was selected from the population. Subsequent analysis of data is dependent upon this account; therefore, the audience will scrutinize the sampling process closely. The researcher should make it clear exactly how the subjects were selected, as well as any problems that arose. This part of the report must be carefully examined to answer the following questions: What was the nature of the population: was it homogeneous or heterogeneous? Were members of the population accessible, or was it necessary to identify a population from which study subjects could be drawn? Did the researcher take the subjects as they arrived in the hospital or clinic? Was random sampling replaced with random assignment only? What was the size of the sample? Was it large enough to reflect the characteristics of a heterogeneous population? If probability sampling was not used, did the researcher identify possible biases? How many of the potential study subjects declined to take part in the research? What was the response rate to the questionnaire? Were any randomly selected patients' charts or other documents unavailable? Since subsequent data are dependent upon sampling, the student should scrutinize this part of the report.

Research Methods

The researcher must tell the audience exactly how he or she collected the data from the sample, whether by observation, questioning, measurement, or a combination of these. If observation was used, the researcher must explain the means used to observe: the operational definitions, the systems of classification and categorization, the instruments, as well as the reliability and validity of each. The researcher must explain to the audience the kind of observation used—participant or nonparticipant—and describe how many observers took part in the study and how they were trained. The audience must be informed of all behaviors observed and how all observers were able to observe the same behavior.

If an interview was used, the interview schedule should be described or attached to the report in the appendix. The researcher should also describe how interviewers were selected and trained. In cases where an unstructured interview was used, the researcher must explain how data were recorded.

The use of a questionnaire requires that the researcher describe and/or attach the questionnaire, together with the covering letter, to the research report. The source of the questions on the questionnaire may need explanation, and the researcher should describe how the questionnaire was formulated or obtained.

Upon completion of this portion of the report, the researcher should make certain the following questions were answered: Is the method of data collection clearly described? Are all instruments, scales, and measures reported, together with the reliability and validity of each? If used, is the observational process carefully explained, including any steps to protect the subjects? If interviews were used, was the interview schedule well developed and tested? Was a proper place for the interview arranged, in order to protect the privacy and confidentiality of the respondent? Does the report describe whether or not the interview was highly structured, or the degree of probing that may have occurred in an unstructured interview? Is the length of the interview reported?

The Pilot Study

The researcher reports the development of the pilot study in as much detail as the consideration of space allows. The audience should be informed who was in the sample, what the findings were, how the instruments performed, what problems emerged, and how the researcher coped with these. Any elements of the research design that were revised as a result of the pilot study should be recorded.

Analysis and Interpretation of Data

The analysis, summary, and report of the findings are the heart of the research report. The researcher must inform the audience how the data were handled, whether by hand or by computer. Relevant coding procedures should be reported and summaries depicted in tables and graphs. The reader should be informed of statistical analysis.

To interpret the findings, the researcher should discuss the statistical results in the light of the problem, the research proposal, and/or the hypotheses. Results should be compared with those discussed in the review of the literature and, where appropriate, the relationship between the findings and the theoretical orientation or assumptions should be discussed. If the study began with observations, the researcher should report whether these relate to known concepts or whether new concepts must be invented to stand for the observations. If possible, the researcher should attempt to integrate the findings or suggest tentative relationships among them. Upon completion of this part of the report, the student should ask the following questions: Have I discussed the objectives I set at the beginning of the study? Have I met these objectives? Are all the results carefully discussed? Have I organized and interpreted the data in the best possible fashion? Should further interpretation of tables and graphs be made? Have I worked in an unbiased way, reporting what was found rather than what I had hoped would be found?

Writing Style

The student who seeks to present a paper in a conference or submit it to a journal of publication should study the rules that govern participation or publications. A careful examination of the format used in research reports in a current journal may also be helpful.

Students wishing to improve their writing styles will benefit from an examination of a number of publications devoted to this purpose. Barzun and Graff (1970) include six chapters on *writing:* how to organize paragraphs, chapters, and parts; the use of *plain words;* how to write clear sentences; the art of quoting; the rules of citing; and how to revise for printer and public. Cordasco and Gatner (1979) published the brief *Research and Report Writing* that includes techniques of composition and specimen papers. Strunk and White's (1972) second edition of *The Elements of Style* include elementary rules of usage, principles of composition, and an approach to style that is often recommended. The *Manual of Style,* published by the University of Chicago Press, includes an extensive section on style; and a popular book is Turabian's (1973) *A Manual for Writers of Term Papers, Theses, and Dissertations.* In addition to these aids, the most valuable assistance is from the supervising professor or colleague who reads the paper, suggesting areas that need improvement.

The Media

Oral presentations are common in the classroom; in local, state, or national professional meetings; and in nonprofessional clubs and associations that use health personnel as speakers.

Research reports may appear in nursing journals or in journals of allied disciplines. Technical reports are often printed within the school or university, and, at times, professors use reports to accompany other teaching aids. Once the report appears in one medium, opportunities may arise to include it in edited books, conferences, or workshops. The student may also use a good report as a proposal for a grant, in job applications, or in application to graduate school.

SUMMARY

The *research report* is a written or spoken communication that informs an audience about the research findings and procedures. The researcher draws relevant material from the work, which he or she relays to an audience, beginning with a problem and ending with conclusions and recommendations.

The audience who is to hear the report or read the paper influences both the form and the content. Specific audiences will expect to hear selected portions of the research findings.

To write the report, the student begins with an organization of the data. The most helpful form of organization is an outline, which may be as informal or formal as desired. A carefully developed formal outline greatly assists in writing the report. The main heads of the report and the subdivisions lead both the writer and the reader into a logical discussion of the research process. Beginning with the introduction, the student may develop the report by following much the same organization proposed in the research design. A researchable problem is identified and the research proposal records what the researcher studied and how it was studied. The identification and definition of significant concepts then follows, after which the hypothesis and the objects of the study are stated. Ethical implications of the study may be reported here or in conjunction with the research design. In either case, the third part of the report includes the review of the literature, or a summary of relevant theoretical and research reports. The research design, main heading number four, describes the plan of the research and what design was used, experimental, survey, or historical. The sampling process is then described in detail, followed by the research methods. Most readers scrutinize the research methods closely, requiring the researcher to write a careful and accurate account. The researcher follows this report with an account of the pilot study, if one was undertaken. The analysis and interpretation of data is the heart of the research report. The researcher informs the reader in this section how the data were analyzed and summarized, and what the results of the study were.

The researcher uses the findings to draw implications for nursing practice. The research may suggest action in the assessment, intervention, or evaluation of nursing practice, or the researcher may recommend further refinement of the instruments or scales, in order to assure more valid findings.

The media in which the research report may appear includes nursing conferences, workshops, meetings, journals, or books. The writing style in each of these may vary according to the nature of the audience.

STUDY QUESTIONS

1. Identify an audience for a research report you are writing or would like to write.

2. Formulate an outline that is helpful in writing your own report, or that can be a guide for future reports.
3. Write a one-paragraph introduction to your research report and evaluate it.
4. What is the value of the *research statement* to the audience?
5. Write a research statement for your own project.
6. What are the major criteria in defining concepts or formulating hypotheses?
7. Discuss how a review of the literature is helpful to both the audience and the researcher.
8. In the section of the report entitled *research design,* what elements of research does the student inform the audience about?
9. Discuss the crucial elements to document in the *sampling process.*
10. Discuss the questions that the student should ask to evaluate the research methods.
11. Describe what should be included in the report concerning the pilot project.
12. Why is the analysis and interpretation of data often called the *heart* of the research report?
13. Locate at least one source that is helpful in improving the writing style of a research report.
14. Identify one medium you could use to present your report.

REFERENCES AND SUGGESTED READINGS

Barzun, J. and Graff, H. (1970): The Modern Researcher (rev. ed.). New York: Harcourt, Brace, and World, Part III.

Clark, E. (1968): Aspects of loneliness: toward a framework of nursing intervention. In Zderad, L. (ed.), Developing Behavioral Concepts in Nursing. Atlanta, Ga.: Southern Regional Education Board, pp. 33–40. *Communication and loneliness.*

Cordasco, F. and Gatner, E. (1963): Research and Report Writing. New York: Barnes & Noble. *A College Outline Series primarily for college undergraduates, but generally useful. Includes specimen papers.*

Fox, D. (1976): Fundamentals of Research in Nursing (3rd ed.). New York: Appleton. *Chapter 13, "Critically Evaluating the Written Research Report."*

Goode, W. and Hatt, P. Methods in Social Research. New York: McGraw-Hill. *Chapter 21, "Preparing the Report."*

Hays, J. and Larson, K. (1963): Interacting with Patients. New York: Macmillan. *Communication with patients.*

Manual of Style (1969): Chicago: The University of Chicago Press. *Part 2, "Style."*

McCorkle, R. (1974): Effects of touch on seriously ill patients. *Nursing Research* 23, 125–133. *Example of good introduction to research report.*

Polit, D. and Hungler, B. (1978): Nursing Research. New York: J. B. Lippincott, Chapters 28 and 29.

Strunk, W. and White, E. (1972): The Elements of Style (2nd ed.). New York: Macmillan. *Short book of 78 pages, with helpful information.*

Treece, E. and Treece, J. (1973): Elements of Research in Nursing. Part V. St. Louis: C. V. Mosby.

Turabian, K. (1973): A Manual for Writers of Term Papers, Theses and Dissertations. Chicago: University of Chicago Press. *Useful throughout.*

Webster's Dictionary of Synonyms (1951): Springfield, Mass.: G. & C. Merriam Co. *Helpful to find a particular word.*

GLOSSARY

Abstract: short statement that gives the main ideas of an article or book.

Analysis: examination of data to identify parts and their relationship to the whole; separation of a whole into its constituent parts.

    Computer analysis: use of computers to process data and perform statistical operations.

    Content analysis: procedure for analyzing oral, written, visual, or behavioral data.

    Secondary analysis: use of large-scale data sets in one's own research.

Applied research: process in which the researcher scientifically collects data to be used in the clinical, administrative, or instructional area, in order to find solutions to nursing problems; evaluate nursing practices, procedures, policies, or curricula; assess the needs of patients, staff, or students; and/or make decisions to change or continue various nursing processes.

Array: list of observations in which data are ranked from lowest to highest.

Art: skill or craft; nursing art is the ability to practically apply nursing knowledge with proficiency and expertise.

Assumption: basic principles often documented and assumed to be true but not proved.

Basic research: process in which data are scientifically collected to advance knowledge without particular reference to its immediate or practical use.

Bias: to prejudice, slant, influence, or improperly affect research data.
   Experimenter bias: expectancies of the researcher that may affect outcomes.
   Hawthorne effect: knowledge of being included in a study may change the behavior of study subjects.
   Interviewer bias: tendency of the interviewer to influence the respondent's reply.
   Measurement bias: use of inappropriate, invalid, or unreliable instruments to measure data.
   Observer bias: tendency of the observer to see, hear, and remember what he or she wants to see, hear, and remember.
      Halo effect: observer is influenced by characteristics not related to the variable under study.
   Rater bias: rater may be influenced by the halo effect, or may rate too positively or too harshly.
   Record bias: distortions introduced due to selective deposit, retrieval, survival, and recording of data.
   Respondent bias: tendency of the respondent to distort verbal self-report, because of unwillingness or inability to answer correctly.
   Response-set bias: factors that interfere with measurement of attitudes or answers to questions such as the wish to project a favorable self-image.
   Sampling bias: use of study subjects that are not representative of the target population; loss of study subjects during research; nonresponse of study subjects to questionnaires or queries.

Bibliography: alphabetical list of writings related to topic under study; includes dates of printing, editions, author, title, etc.
   Annotated bibliography: bibliography with notes added to comment or explain.

Case study: research design involving the in-depth study of an individual, group, community, institution, whole society, incident, or situation. The case study may be descriptive or analytical. It may examine changes that have occurred in a social unit, after nature has introduced a stimulus. A case study that seeks to explain change rather than describe characteristics has been called a *pre-experimental design* by Campbell and Stanley (1963).

Category: class or division for the purpose of organizing observations.

Causation: process in which an event or phenomenon, called the *caus-*

ative agent, precedes, leads to, produces, or results in a change in another factor.

Central tendency: statistical summary measure that is representative of a series of measures; includes the mean or average score, the median or middle score, and the mode or the most frequent score.

Chi-square test (x^2): nonparametric statistical test, used to determine if observed values differ from expected values; compares groups in terms of qualitative variables.

Class interval: subdivision of the total range of a quantitative variable that is divided into intervals of equal size.

Classification studies: studies that place observations into named categories.

Coding: transforming research data into the symbols used in computer analysis.

Cohort: study subjects who are grouped together on the basis of a common characteristic, such as age.

Comparative studies: studies of more than one group to compare and contrast data.

Concept: complex observations or symbols that the mind organizes into a single word or idea.

Concept-formulation studies: studies that organize the researcher's observations and experiences into a meaningful whole, expressed by a word or concept.

Conceptual framework: interrelationships among the concepts that underlie the research proposal or theory.

Conceptualization: process by which data are arranged according to concepts.

Concomitant variation: consistent and persistent manner in which phenomena vary or change together, because either a causal connection exists between the two, or both are caused by a common factor.

Confidentiality: element of ethical research that is the researcher's ability to keep data sources protected, by using numbers instead of names, and locked records that reveal code names/numbers.

Constructs: concepts.

Control: to rule, regulate, restrain, check, correct, or limit error or distortion of knowledge.

> **Experimental control:** process of randomization, manipulation, and modification of experimental conditions by the researcher.

Control group: group of study subjects who are similar or equivalent to the experimental group in every way possible, except that the control group is not exposed to the experimental variable.

Correlational studies: studies of how variables change in terms of one another; an increase in the magnitude of one is associated with a change (either increase or decrease) in the other.

Cross-sectional study: collection and analysis of data from one point in time.

Data: units of information.

Data analysis: summary of completed observation to answer the research question; a study of the relationships between the parts and the whole.

Data tabulation: process of arranging data in a concise and logical order, such as in tables.

Deductive reasoning: logical thought that moves from theory to fact, by means of propositions stated as hypotheses.

Delphi technique: research technique in which successive waves of questionnaires elicit responses from a panel.

Demography: study of population variables, such as fertility, mortality, age, sex, and migration.

Descriptive research: research to recount, characterize, narrate, describe, or classify observations.

Dispersion of scores: range and standard deviation that summarize how scores are spread out.

Documentary-historical design: plan to collect research data by using documents, records, and oral history.

Edge coding: use of the margin of data sources, such as questionnaires, to write a code that is a symbol for the answer, for example, 1 for female, 2 for male, etc.

Effect: event that follows the action of a causal agent; response to the action of an independent variable, as manifested in the dependent variable.

Empirical: data obtained from using human senses.

Empirical generalization: statement of the observed relationship between concepts.

Error: mistake or inaccuracy.
  Measurement error: inaccuracies that arise from the measurement process.
  Observer error: mistakes the observer makes due to inadequate training or psychological bias.
  Response error: inaccurate or incomplete answers given by respondents.

Sampling error: tendency for statistics from different samples drawn from the same population to fluctuate. Type I error: rejection of a true null hypothesis. Type II error: acceptance of a false null hypothesis.

Ethics: study and evaluation of human conduct.

Applied ethics: actual human conduct in real situations, such as research.

Evaluation research: research to judge the characteristics (good or poor) of an entity, such as nursing practices or policies.

Ex-post-facto research: research done "from after the fact"—after nature or life has introduced the stimulus whose effect the researcher wishes to study.

Experiment: research to examine cause and effect, or correlations.

Experimental design: plan of research that includes randomization, manipulation, and control.

Solomon four group experimental design: combination of the "true," or "classic" design and the two after-group control design.

True, or classic experimental design: four-cell design in which study subjects or objects are randomly selected from the total population, randomly assigned to either the experimental or the control group, and measured both before and after the researcher manipulates the independent variable by introducing it into the experimental group and withholding it from the control group.

Two after-group control design: two-cell design in which a randomly selected group of study subjects is randomly divided into an experimental group and a control group, neither of which is measured or tested before the researcher introduces the independent variable into the experimental group.

Experimental group: group of study subjects or objects into which the researcher introduces the independent variable.

Explanatory design: plan of research that seeks to explain and predict.

Exploratory design: form of descriptive research that is specifically focused.

External criticism: examination of the validity of historical data.

Fact: empirically verifiable observation that the mind orders into a concept.

Field study: research that uses a natural site for study, such as a community.

Frequency distribution: summarization of research data by enumeration.

Generalization: application of findings from the study sample to the broader population from which the sample was drawn; application of findings to a broader situation.

Halo effect: generalization of one characteristic of a subject or object to other characteristics that may influence the observer or rater.

Hawthorne effect: response of subjects who know they are being watched or studied, which tends to influence their behavior.

Heterogeneous: mixture of unlike subjects, objects, or elements of research.

Histogram: frequency distribution graph.

Homogeneous: category or grouping of like characteristics, subjects, or objects.

Hypothesis: proposition that states the expected relationships to be found.

    Null hypothesis: statement predicting that the differences to be obtained in the values between the groups being compared could have occurred by chance alone.

    Research hypothesis: proposition that states what the expected relationships among variables will be upon observation.

    Working hypothesis: predictions that lie close to observed data.

Index: alphabetical listing of references, often by both subject and author.

Inductive reasoning: process in which the researcher begins with observations and facts and moves toward generalizations.

Inference: estimations and judgments based on data other than direct observation; generalization from a sample to the population from which the sample was drawn.

Inferential statistics: theory and method of analyzing quantitative data that allows the researcher to attach probability estimates to the generalizations drawn from data.

Informed consent: ethical approach to research in which the study subjects are given full knowledge about the research project in which they are being asked to participate.

Instrumentation: construction and use of instruments by the researcher to observe, measure, and analyze data.

Interpretation of data: researcher's reasoning that gives meaning to the data.

Interview: interaction between researcher and respondent in which questioning elicits verbal data.

    Partially structured interview: use of an interview schedule that also allows the interviewer latitude to move in interesting and productive directions.

Clinical interview: use of an interview schedule that combines observation with free questioning.

Focused interview: use of an interview schedule that focuses on questions and topics to be covered during the interview but allows the researcher freedom to deviate from the schedule.

Structured interview: use of a standardized interview schedule by an interviewer who asks the same question, with the same wording, in the same order, using identical procedures as all other interviewers in the research project.

Telephone interview: questioning by telephone.

Unstructured interview: general approach in which the interviewer encourages the respondent to broach and explore topics as long as he or she wishes; includes projective techniques.

Interview schedule: series of questions that the interviewer asks.

Level of significance: probability level that states the risk of rejecting the null hypothesis when it is true.

Manipulation: process by which the researcher treats or manages the independent variable, in order to study its effect on the dependent variable.

Measurement: procedure whereby rules assign symbols and numerals to objects or events, in order to determine relationships such as quantities, degrees, or extent of observations; includes counting, comparing, and ranking.

MEDLARS: *Medical Literature Analysis and Retrieval System,* a computer-based literature retrieval system available at libraries; it retrieves specialized bibliographical information from the National Library, at Bethesda, Md.

Model: symbolic or physical representation of an idea; an analogy of the actual phenomenon.

Methodological design: plan to develop or evaluate tools for research.

Nominal data: observation and facts that can only be separated into mutually exclusive categories.

Normal curve: bell-shaped curve in which the mean (average), median (middle), and mode (most frequent) scores are clustered about the curve's center with few values or measurements at either extreme end.

Nursing: profession based on the art and science of caring for persons in sickness and health.

Nursing research: scientific process for collecting observable, verifiable data, in order to describe, explain, or predict nursing phenomena.

Nursing science: both the body of knowledge and the scientific method of approach to the empirical world of nursing.

Observation: method of collecting data in which the researcher scientifically watches and records pertinent information.

Nonparticipant observation: observer watches and records but does not participate as a member of the group of study subjects being observed.

Participant observartion; observer watches, collects, and records data, while interacting with the group of study subjects as a member of the group.

Unobtrusive observation: simple observation of exterior signs, expressive movements, physical positioning, language, or time usage in which the researcher does not intrude.

Observation methods: means of observation devised before the researcher begins to observe, including systems of classification, operational definitions, instrumentation, scaling, and measurements.

Operational definition: set of directions or procedures that designate precisely how to observe, measure, and record the phenomena to be observed.

Phenomenon: observed datum.

Pilot study: study carried out at the end of the planning phase of research, in order to explore and test the research elements.

Population: total category of persons or objects that meets the criteria for study established by the researcher; any set of persons, objects, or measurements having an observable characteristic in common; a universe.

Accessible population: that category of persons or objects available to the researcher.

Target population: total category of persons or objects from which the study sample was drawn and about which the researcher wishes to generalize.

Probability theory: explanation of the possibility that events occurred by chance.

Proposition: statement of the interrelationships observed among concepts (empirical generalization) or predicted between variables (hypothesis).

Prospective design: plan of research beginning with the collection of data and proceeding forward in time.

Purpose: end or aim; the purposes of nursing research are to observe in order to know; to know in order to predict; to predict in order to control, practice, and prescribe in a professional manner.

Q-sort: method of collecting data in which the subject sorts cards, with written words, phrases, or messages, in terms of a particular characteristic, such as approve-disapprove; or high priority–low priority.

Questionnaire: technique of collecting data by means of written questions that subjects answer in writing, with little if any help from the researcher.

Random sampling: method of sampling that allows every member of the population an equal chance of being selected for the study sample.

Random start: selecting numbers or names from a list, by closing the eyes and touching the list blindly for a starting point.

Randomization: process that affords each member of the target population an equal chance of being chosen for the study sample, or for assignment to either the experimental or the control group.

Reliability: extent to which data are consistent, accurate, and precise; extent to which procedures such as measurement yield consistent data; stability, equivalence, and internal homogeneity of instruments.

Research: systematic, careful collection, analysis, and interpretation of data to obtain new knowledge, to add to existing knowledge, or to solve problems.

    Applied nursing research: process whereby the researcher collects data to be used in the clinical, administrative, or instructional areas. Designed to find solutions to nursing problems; evaluate nursing practices, procedures, policies, or curricula; assess needs of patients, staff, students; and/or make decisions to change or continue aspects of nursing.

    Basic nursing research: process whereby the researcher collects data to advance nursing knowledge, whether or not this knowledge is immediately usable in nursing.

    Scientific research: process in which observable, verifiable data are systematically collected from the empirical world we know through our senses, in order to describe, explain, or predict events.

Research designs: plan and structure that guides the research process. Includes descriptive-exploratory designs; experimental, quasi-experimental, and pre-experimental designs; surveys; documentary-historical designs; methodological designs; ex-post-facto designs; correlational designs; and various mixtures and modifications of these.

Research methods: ways and means by which the researcher collects data; primarily observation, questioning, and measurement.

Research model: symbolic or physical representation of the research plan; may represent steps to take in a temporal framework.

Research problem: question or dilemma that the researcher wishes to investigate.

Research proposal: written statement that summarizes what the researcher plans to do, how, and why it is important to nursing.

Review of the literature: extensive, exhaustive, and systematic examination of publications relevant to a research project.

  Critical review: process by which the strengths and weaknesses of publications are assessed.

Sample: portion of a larger population of subjects or objects.

Sampling: process of selecting a portion of a target population for study.

  Accidental sampling: study subjects are chosen solely by convenience.

  Cluster sampling: process in which the target population is first divided into categories or clusters, often geographic; then, the unit for study is selected from each cluster by random sampling.

  Nonprobability sampling: process whereby subjects or objects are selected for study by other than probability sampling.

  Probability sampling: process in which each element of the population is given an equal chance of being included in the study sample.

  Purposive sampling: study subjects are chosen that are judged to be typical of the population.

  Quota sampling: study subjects are chosen to reflect the characteristics of the population being studied.

  Simple random sampling: basic probability design that gives each element in the population an equal chance of being chosen.

  Systematic sampling: process by which every *nth* element is drawn from a list of the entire target population.

  Stratified random sampling: process by which units of a population are first grouped with respect to a significant characteristic into homogeneous strata, prior to sampling; then, a sample is drawn by simple, systematic, or cluster sampling.

Scale: device for measuring quantitative or qualitative variables.

  Interval scale: quantitative scale, with equal intervals and an arbitrary zero point; for example, the Fahrenheit scale.

  Nominal scale: qualitative scale that enables the researcher to place variables in discrete, mutually exclusive and exhaustive, named categories; for example, sex, race, diagnosis.

  Ordinal scale: qualitative scale in which categories may be ranked; for example, Likert-type scales.

  Ratio scale: quantitative scale, with equal intervals and an absolute zero point; for example, Kelvin temperature scale, length, weight, etc.

Science: way of thinking and method of studying the empirical world.

Statistics: *Singular:* the science of classifying relative numbers of occurrences as a ground for induction; *plural:* classified facts that can be expressed in numbers.

Descriptive statistics: process of summarizing and synthesizing data from a sample.

Inferential statistics: process that uses data from randomly drawn samples to infer characteristics of the population from which the sample was drawn and to test statistical hypotheses.

Statistic: summary value calculated from a sample of observations and an estimator of some population value (parameter).

Summary measures: mode, median, means, range, standard deviation, percentages, and similar summations computed from measurements of sample units.

Survey: collection of data by questionnaire or interview.

Theory: general statement that explains the relationships among propositions, concepts, or facts; summarizes existing knowledge, and predicts observations, if fruitful.

Time factors: research that occurs in different time frameworks.

Cross-sectional studies: collecting data at one point in time.

Longitudinal studies: collecting data over a period of time, to study population changes or changes in the characteristics of study subjects.

Panel studies: interviewing the same subjects at two or more points in time.

Trend studies: repeatedly asking the same question of equivalent samples of different individuals.

Validity: the extent to which a component of research, such as method, scale, instrument, or measure, reflects the theory, concept, or variable the researcher intends it should. A valid instrument measures what it purports to measure.

Concurrent validity: extent to which an instrument or design measures present observable behavior.

Construct validity: extent to which a research tool measures the concept or variable the researcher wants it to measure; whether or not the subject possesses the characteristic presumed to be reflected by the scale or test.

Content validity: concerned with sampling adequacy; it judges whether the content of the questionnaire, interview schedule, or check-list is representative of all possible questions or observations; a panel of judges in the content area is helpful to review the adequacy of the instrument.

External validity: extent to which the researcher is able to generalize from the study sample to the larger population from which the sample was drawn.

Face validity: extent to which the instrument is judged appropriate by an experienced researcher.

Internal validity: judgment of measures or designs within the study sample; for example, whether or not the independent variable actually made a difference to the research findings of an experimental study.

Predictive validity: sometimes called *empirical validity;* ability of the instrument, such as an I.Q. test, to measure and predict performance accurately.

Values: ideas and evaluations that members of a group share about what is important; the standards by which means and ends are judged.

Variable: concept defined by operational definition in such a way that changes or variations can be observed and measured.

Attribute variable: pre-existing characteristics of study subjects, such as age, income, occupation.

Dependent variable: also called the *effect,* the *response,* the *criterion measure;* behavior or outcome that the researcher wishes to predict, study, explain. It is observed to determine the effect of the independent variable upon it.

Extraneous variable: those variables present in large numbers in the research environment—especially in research involving human subjects—that may interfere with the research findings, by acting as unwanted independent variables and confusing the results of the research.

Independent variable: also called the *cause, stimulus, experimental variable,* or *treatment;* the variable that is manipulated by the researcher, in order to study its effect upon the dependent variable.

BIBLIOGRAPHY

Aamodt, A. (1972): The child's view of health and healing. In Batey, M. (ed.), Communicating Nursing Research. Boulder, Colo.: WICHE, pp. 38–56.

Abbey, J. (1980): FANCAP: what is it? In Riehl, J. and Roy, C. (eds.), Conceptual Models for Nursing Practice (2nd ed.). New York: Appleton.

Abdellah, F. et al (1960): Patient-Centered Approaches to Nursing. New York: Macmillan.

Abdellah, F. (1971): Forward. In Murphy, F. (ed.), Theoretical Issues in Professional Nursing. New York: Appleton.

Abdellah, F. and Levine, E. (1979): Better Patient Care Through Nursing Research (2nd ed.). New York: Macmillan.

Adorno, T. et al (1950): The Authoritarian Personality. New York: Harper and Row.

Akutagawa, D. (1965): A Study in Construct Validity of the Psychoanalytic Concept of Latent Anxiety and a Test of Projection Distance Hypothesis. Unpublished Ph.D. dissertation, Univ. of Pittsburgh.

Alderson, M. (1974): Effects of increased body temperature on the perception of time. *Nursing Research 23,* 43–49.

Amborn, S. (1976): Clinical signs associated with the amount of tracheobronchial secretions. *Nursing Research 25,* 121–126.

American Nurses' Association (1968): The nurse in research: ANA guidelines on ethical values. In *Nursing Research 17,* 104–107. (1975): Human Rights Guidelines for Nurses in Clinical and Other Research. Code No. D–465M. Kansas City: The Association. (1976): Preparation of Nurses for Participation in Research. Code No. D–54 2500. Kansas City: The Association. (1976): Research in Nursing. Kansas City: The Association.

Ammon, K. (1969): The effects of music on children in respiratory distress. In ANA Clinical Sessions. New York: Appleton, 127–133.

Annas, G. et al (1977): The Subject's Dilemma. Cambridge: Ballinger.

Arminger, B. (1977): Ethics of nursing research: profile, principles, perspective. *Nursing Research 26,* 330–336.

Auger, J. (1976): Behavioral Systems and Nursing. Englewood Cliffs, N.J.: Prentice-Hall.

Babbie, E. (1975): The Practice of Social Research. Belmont, Calif.: Wadsworth.

Barnard, K. (1973): The effect of stimulation on the sleep behavior of the premature infant. In Batey, M. (ed.), Communicating Nursing Research. Boulder, Colo.: WICHE, pp. 12–33.

Barnard, K. and Neal, M. (1977): Maternal-child nursing research: review of the past and strategies for the future. *Nursing Research 26,* 193–200.

Barzun, J. and Graff, H. (1970): The Modern Researcher (rev.). New York: Harcourt, Brace, & World.

Batey, M. (ed.) (1968–1978): Communicating Nursing Research. Boulder, Colo.: WICHE. Eleven volumes.

Baziak, A. and Denton, R. (1965): The language of the hospital and its effect on the patient. In Skipper, J. and Leonard, R. (eds.), Social Interaction and Patient Care. Philadelphia: J. B. Lippincott.

Beard, M. and Scott, P. (1975): The efficacy of group therapy by nurses for hospitalized patients. *Nursing Research 24,* 120–124.

Bell, J. (1977): Stressful life events and coping methods in mental-illness-and-wellness behavior. In *Nursing Research 26,* 136–141.

Benne, D. and Bennis, W. (1959): The role of the professional nurse. *American Journal of Nursing* (May), 837–882.

Benoliel, J. (1975): Research related to death and the dying patient. In Verhonick, P. (ed.), Nursing Research I. Boston: Little, Brown, pp. 189–227.

Bensberg, G. et al (1965): Teaching the profoundly retarded self-help activities by behavior shaping techniques. *American Journal of Mental Deficiency 69,* 674–679.

Blake, M. (1980): The Peplau development model for nursing practice. In Riehl, J. and Roy, C. (eds.), Conceptual Models for Nursing Practice (2nd ed.). New York: Appleton.

Bloch, D. (1974): Some crucial terms in nursing: what do they really mean? *Nursing Outlook 22,* 689–694.

Boggardus, E. (1959): Social Distance. Yellow Springs, Ohio: Antioch Press.

Bonjean, C., et al (1967): Sociological Measurement: An Inventory of Scales and Indices. San Francisco: Chandler.

Borg, W. and Gall, M. (1971): Educational Research. New York: David McKay.

Bowlby, J. (1956): Maternal-child separation. In Soddy, K. (ed.), Mental Health and Infant Development. New York: Basic Books.

Branch, H. (1979): Women in pain. In Kjervik, D. and Martinson, I. (eds.), Women in Stress: A Nursing Perspective. New York: Appleton, pp. 237–255.

Brill, E. and Kilts, D. (1980): Foundations for Nursing. New York: Appleton.

Brink, P. and Wood, M. (1978): Basic Steps in Planning Nursing Research: From Question to Proposal. North Scituate, Mass.: Duxbury Press.

Brown, E. (1948): Nursing for the Future. New York: Russell Sage. (1961): Newer Dimensions of Patient Care I. New York: Russell Sage. (1962): Newer Dimensions of Patient Care II. New York: Russell Sage.

Brown, M. et al (1977): Drug–drug interactions among residents in homes for the elderly. *Nursing Research 26*, 47–52.

Brown, M. and Grunfel, C. (1980): Taste preferences of infants for sweetened or unsweetened food. *Research in Nursing and Health 3*, 11–17.

Buckley, W. (1967): Sociology and Modern Systems Theory. Englewood Cliffs, N.J.: Prentice-Hall.

Bullough, B. (1974): Is the nurse practitioner role a source of increased work satisfaction? *Nursing Research 23*, 14–19. (1980): Factors contributing to role expansion for registered nurses. In Bullough, B. (ed.), Law and the Expanding Nursing Role (2nd ed.). New York: Appleton.

Bullough, B. (ed.) (1980): The Law and the Expanding Nursing Role (2nd ed.). New York: Appleton.

Burnside, J. (1973): Caring for the aged: touching is talking. *American Journal of Nursing 73*, 2060–2063.

Buros, O. (ed.) (1978): The Eighth Mental Measurement Yearbook. Highland Park, N.J.: Gryphon Press.

Calley, J. et al (1980): The Orem self-care nursing model. In Riehl, J. and Roy, C. (eds.), Conceptual Models for Nursing Practice (2nd ed.). New York: Appleton, pp. 53–59.

Campbell, D. and Stanley, J. (1963): Experimental and Quasi-Experimental Designs for Research. Chicago: Rand McNally.

Cannon, W. (1939): Wisdom of the Body (2nd ed. rev.). New York: W. W. Norton.

Caplow, T. (1971): Elementary Sociology. Englewood Cliffs, N.J.: Prentice-Hall.

Carlson, C. (ed.) (1970): Behavioral Concepts and Nursing Intervention. Philadelphia: J. B. Lippincott.

Carr-Saunders, A. and Wilson, P. (1933): Professions. In Seligman, E. (ed), Encyclopaedia of the Social Sciences. New York: Macmillan.

Cattell, R. and Scheier, I. (1961): Neuroticism and Anxiety. New York: Ronald.

Chapin, F. (1970): Social participation scale. In Miller, D. (ed.), Handbook of Research Design and Social Measurement (2nd ed.). New York: David McKay.

Chapman, J. (1977): Effects of different nursing approaches upon selected postoperative herniorrhaphy patients. In Downs, F. and Newman, M. (eds.), A Sourcebook of Nursing Research. Philadelphia: F. A. Davis, pp. 15–23.

Charter, S. (1975): Understanding Research in Nursing. Geneva: WHO Offset Pub. No. 14.

Chase, C. (1976): Elementary Statistical Procedures. New York: McGraw-Hill.

Chesney, M. and Tasto, D. (1975): The development of the menstrual symptom questionnaire. *Behavior Research and Therapy 13*, 237–244.

Christensen, M. et al (1979): Professional development of nurse practitioners. *Nursing Research 28*, 51–56.

Christy, T. (1975): The methodology of historical research. *Nursing Research 24*, 189–192.

Chun, K. et al (1975): Measures of Psychological Assessment. Ann Arbor: Survey Research Center.

Ciminero, A. et al (eds.) (1977): Handbook of Behavioral Assessment. New York: Wiley.

Cleland, V. (1977): Investigations in the clinical setting. In Verhonick, P. (ed.), Nursing Research II. Boston: Little, Brown, pp. 33–75.

Code for Nurses (1977): *American Journal of Nursing 77*, 876.

Coleman, L. (1980): Orem's self-care concept of nursing. In Riehl, J. and Roy, C. (eds.), Models for Nursing Practice (2nd ed.). New York: Appleton.

Conant, J. (1947): On Understanding Science. New Haven: Yale University Press.

Cooley, C. (1902): Human Nature and the Social Order. New York: Scribner's.

Davis, A. and Underwood, P. (1976): Role, function, and decision making in community mental health. *Nursing Research 25*, 256–259.

Dee, F. et al (1965): Self-acceptance of nurses and acceptance of patients: an exploratory investigation. *Nursing Research 14*, 345–350.

Dempsey, P. and Dempsey, R. (1981): The Research Process in Nursing. New York: D. Van Nostrand.

De Walt, E. and Haines, A. (1977): The effects of specified stressors on healthy oral mucosa. In Downs, F. and Newman, M. (eds.), A Sourcebook of Nursing Research (2nd ed.). Philadelphia: F. A. Davis.

Dickoff, J., and James, P. (1968): A theory of theories—a position paper. *Nursing Research 17*, 197–203. Researching research's role in theory development. *Nursing Research 17*, 204–206.

Diers, D. (1979): Research in Nursing Practice. Philadelphia: J. B. Lippincott.

Downs, F. (1967): Ethical inquiry in nursing research. *Nursing Forum 6*, 12–20. (1977): Maternal stress in primigravidas as a factor in the production of neonatal pathology. In Downs, F. and Newman, M. (eds.), A Sourcebook of Nursing Research (2nd ed.). Philadelphia: F. A. Davis.

Downs, F. and Fleming, J. (eds.) (1979): Issues in Nursing Research. New York: Appleton.

Downs, F. and Newman, M. (eds.) (1977): A Sourcebook of Nursing Research. Philadelphia: F. A. Davis.

Du Bois, C. (1944): The People of Alor. Minneapolis: University of Minnesota Press.

Dumas, R. and Leonard, R. (1963): The effect of nursing and the incidence of postoperative vomiting: a clinical experiment. *Nursing Research 12*, 12–15.

Duncan, R. et al (1977): Introductory Biostatistics for the Health Sciences. New York: Wiley.

Dunn, O. (1967): Basic Statistics. New York: Wiley.

Durand, B. (1975): Failure to thrive in a child with Down's syndrome. *Nursing Research 24*, 272–286.

Durkheim, E. (1951): Suicide (trans. Spaulding and Simpson). Glencoe, Ill.: The Free Press.

Eckland, B. (1965): Academic ability, higher education and occupational mobility. American Council on Education.

Elder, R. (1976): Orientation of senior nursing students toward access to contraception. *Nursing Research 25*, 338–345.

Erikson, E. (1950): Childhood and Society. New York: Norton.

Evans, et al (1968): A new measure of effects of persuasive communications: a chemical indicator of tooth brushing behavior. *Psychological Reports 23*, 731–736.

Felton, G. (1970): Effect of time cycle changes on blood pressure and temperature in young women. *Nursing Research 19*, 48–58.

Fessler, D. (1952): The development of a scale for measuring community solidarity. *Rural Sociology 17*, 144–152.

Festinger, L. (1957): A Theory of Cognitive Dissonance. Stanford, Calif.: Stanford University Press.

Fielo, S. (1975): A Summary of Integrated Nursing Theory (2nd ed.). New York: McGraw-Hill.

Fieve, R. et al (1971): A critical trial of methysergate and lithium in mania. In Kuper, D. (ed.), Lithium and Psychiatry Journal Articles. Medical Examination Pub.

Fleming, J. (1979): The future of nursing research. In Downs, F. and Fleming, J. (eds.), Issues in Nursing Research. New York: Appleton.

Fleming, J. and Hayter, J. (1974): Reading research reports critically. *Nursing Outlook 22*, 172–176.

Ford, V. (1973): Medicine among the Teton Dakota, Rosebud Indian Reservation, South Dakota. In Batey, M. (ed.), Communicating Nursing Research. Boulder, Colo.: WICHE.

Foster, G. and Anderson, B. (1978): Medical Anthropology. New York: Wiley.

Fox, D. (1976): Fundamentals of Research in Nursing (3rd ed.). New York: Appleton.

Fox, D. and Lesser, I. (1981): Readings on the Research Process in Nursing. New York: Appleton.

Freihofer, P. and Felton, G. (1976): Nursing behaviors in bereavement. *Nursing Research 25*, 332–337.

Freud, S. (1938): The Basic Writings of Sigmund Freud. New York: Random House.

Gebbie, K. (1976): Summary of the Second National Conference on Classification of Nursing Diagnoses. St. Louis: St. Lous University.

Geer, J. (1965): The development of a scale to measure fear. *Behavior Research and Therapy 3*, 45–53.

Gerber, R. and Van Ort, S. (1979): Topical application of insulin in decubitus ulcers. *Nursing Research 28*, 16–19.

Gesell, A. et al (1956): Youth: The Years from Ten to Sixteen. New York: Harper and Row.

Gibbs, et al (1974): Patterns of reproductive health care among the poor of San Antonio, Texas. *American Journal of Public Health 64*, 37–40.

Gordon, M. (1979): The concept of nursing diagnosis. In The Nursing Clinics of North America. Philadelphia: W. B. Saunders.

Gortner, S. (1975): Research for a practice profession. *Nursing Research 24*, 193–197.

Goslin, D. (ed.) (1969): Handbook of Socialization Theory and Research. Chicago: Rand McNally.

Grant, E. (1971): Facial expression and gesture. *Journal of Psychosomatic Research 15*.

Gray, B. (1976): Health needs of the elderly. *Nursing Research 25*, 433–438.

Grosieki, J. (1968): Effects of operant conditioning on modification of incontinence in neuropsychiatric geriatric patients. *Nursing Research 17,* 304–311.

Gunning, S. and Holmes, T. (1973): Dance therapy with psychotic children. *Archives of General Psychiatry 28.*

Habenstein, R. (ed.) (1970): Pathways to Data. Chicago: Aldine.

Hampe, S. (1974): Needs of the grieving spouse in the hospital setting. *Nursing Research 24,* 113–120.

Hanson, R. (1973): Effects of administering cold and warmed tube feedings. In Batey, M. (ed.), Communicating Nursing Research. Boulder, Colo.: WICHE.

Hain, M. and Chen S. (1976): Health needs of the elderly. *Nursing Research 25,* 433–439.

Hall, V. (1975): Statutory Regulation of the Scope of Nursing Practice—A Critical Survey. Chicago: National Joint Practice Commission.

Hardy, M. (ed.) (1975): Theoretical Foundations for Nursing. New York: MSS Information Corp.

Hardy, M. and Conway, M. (1978): Role Theory: Perspectives for Health Professionals. New York: Appleton.

Harrington, M. (1962): The Other America. New York: Macmillan.

Hasselmeyer, E. (1961): Behavior Patterns of Premature Infants. Washington, D.C.: Government Printing Office.

Highriter, M. (1977): The status of community health nursing research. *Nursing Research 26,* 183–238.

Hinsvark, I. (1974): Implications for action in the expanded role of the nurse. Nursing Clinics of North America.

Hodge, R., et al (1964): Occupational prestige in the United States 1925–1964. *American Journal of Sociology 70,* 286–302.

Hofling, C. et al (1967): Basic Psychiatric Concepts in Nursing (2nd ed.). Philadelphia: J. B. Lippincott.

Holaday, B. (1974): Achievement behavior in chronically ill children. *Nursing Research 23,* 25–30. (1980): Implementing the Johnson model for nursing practice. In Riehl, J. and Roy, C. (eds.), Conceptual Model for Nursing Practice. New York: Appleton.

Horn, B. (1978): Transcultural nursing and child-rearing of the Muckleshoot people. In Leininger, M. (ed.), Transcultural Nursing. New York: Wiley, pp. 286–302.

Huckaby, L. (1978): Cognitive and affective consequences of formative evaluation in graduate nursing students. *Nursing Research 27.*

Hughes, E., et al (1958): Twenty Thousand Nurses Tell Their Story. Philadelphia: J. B. Lippincott.

Hurwitz, F. and Eadie, F. (1977): Psychologic impact on nursing students of participation in abortion. *Nursing Research 26,* 112–120.

Jacobson, S. (1973): Ethical issues in experimentation with human subjects. *Nursing Forum 12,* 58–71.

Jacox, A. (1974): Theory construction in nursing: an overview. *Nursing Research 23,* 4–13.

Jacox, A. and Steward, M. (1973): Psychosocial Contingencies of the Pain Experience. Iowa City, Iowa: University of Iowa College of Nursing.

Johnson, A. (1977): Social Statistics Without Tears. New York: McGraw-Hill.

Johnson, D. (1959): The nature of a science of nursing. *Nursing Outlook.* (1968): Theory in nursing: borrowed and unique. *Nursing Research 17,* 206. (1980): The behavioral system model for nursing. In Riehl, J. and Roy, C. (eds.), Conceptual Models for Nursing Practice. New York: Appleton.

Johnson, J. et al (1977): Altering children's distress behavior during orthopedic cast removal. In Downs, F. and Newman, M., A Sourcebook of Nursing Research (2nd ed.). Philadelphia: F. A. Davis, pp. 33–45.

Johnson, M. (1975): Outcome criteria to evaluate postoperative respiratory status. *American Journal of Nursing 75,* 1474–1475.

Josten, L. (1979): Child abuse. In Jervik, D. and Martinson, I. (eds.), Women in Stress: A Nursing Perspective. New York: Appleton, pp. 218–236.

Kane, F. (1959): Clothing worn by out-patients to interviews. In *Psychiatric Communications.*

Kassenbaum, G. (1970): Strategies for the sociological study of criminal correctional systems. In Habenstein, R. (ed.), Pathways to Data. Chicago: Aldine.

Kendall, K. (1978): Maternal and child nursing in an Iranian village. In Leininger, M. (ed.), Transcultural Nursing. New York: Wiley, pp. 399–416.

Kerlinger, F. (1974): Foundations of Behavioral Research (2nd ed.). New York: Holt, Rinehart, and Winston.

King, I. (1971): Toward a Theory for Nursing. New York: Wiley.

Kjervik, D. and Martinson, I. (eds.) (1979): Women in Stress: A Nursing Perspective. New York: Appleton.

Klein, R. et al (1972): Psychiatric staff: uniforms or street clothes? *Archives of General Psychiatry 26* (Jan.).

Knapp, R. (1978): Social Statistics Without Tears. New York: McGraw-Hill.

Kohlenberg, R. (1973): Operant conditioning of human anal sphincter pressure. In *Journal of Applied Behavior Analysis 6,* 201–208.

Kuhn, T. (1962): The Structure of Scientific Revolutions. Chicago: University of Chicago Press.

La Rocco, S. and Polit, D. (1980): Women's knowledge about the menopause. *Nursing Research 29,* 10–13.

Leavitt, M. (1975): The discharge crisis: the experience of families of psychiatric patients. *Nursing Research 24,* 33–40.

Leininger, M. (1968): The research critique: nature, function and art. In Batey, M. (ed.), Communicating Nursing Research. Boulder, Colo.: WICHE. (1976): Doctoral programs for nurses: trends, questions and projected plans. *Nursing Research 24,* 434–441. (1978): Transcultural Nursing. New York: Wiley.

Leipold, W. (1963): Psychological distance in a dyadic interview as a function of introversion, extraversion, anxiety, social desirability and stress. Unpublished dissertation, University of North Dakota.

Leonard, R. et al (1975): The application of behavioral science to patient care as illustrated by the etiology and control of stress in clinical settings. In Verhonick, P. (ed.), Nursing Research I. Boston: Little, Brown, pp. 93–112 .

Levine, M. (1967): The four conservation principles of nursing. *Nursing Forum 6,* 45.

Lin, N. (1976): Foundations of Social Research. New York: McGraw-Hill.

Lindeman, C. (1975): Delphi survey of priorities in clinical nursing research. *Nursing Research 24*, 434–441.

Lindeman, C. and Van Aernam, B. (1977): Nursing intervention with the pre-surgical patient—the effects of structured and unstructured preoperative teaching. In Downs, F. and Newman, M. (eds.), A Sourcebook of Nursing Research. Philadelphia: F. A. Davis.

Lowery, B. and DuCette, J. (1976): Disease-related learning and disease control in diabetes as a function of the locus-of-control. *Nursing Research 25*, 358–362.

Mager, R. (1962): Preparing Instructional Objectives. Palo Alto, Calif.: Fearon.

Mahl, G. (1956): Disturbances and silences in the patient's speech in psycho-therapy. *Journal of Abnormal and Social Psychology 53*, 1–15.

Marshack, A. (1972): The Roots of Civilization. New York: McGraw-Hill.

Marshall, L. (1972): Patient reaction to sound in an intensive coronary care unit. In Batey, M. (ed.), Communicating Nursing Research. Boulder, Colo.: WICHE, pp. 81–97.

Mathwig, G. (1971): Nursing science—the theoretical core of nursing knowl-edge. *Image 4*, 20–23.

Maxwell, A. (1961): Analysing Qualitative Data. New York: Barnes & Noble.

McCorkle, R. (1981): Effects of touch on seriously ill patients. In Fox, D. and Leeser, I. (eds.), Readings on the Research Process in Nursing. New York: Appleton.

McGillicuddy, M. (1977): A study of the relationship between mothers' room-ing-in during their children's hospitalization and changes in selected areas of children's behavior. In Downs, F. and Newman, M. (eds), A Sourcebook of Nursing Research (2nd ed.). Philadelphia: F. A. Davis.

Mead, G. (1934): Mind, Self and Society. Chicago: University of Chicago.

Merton, R. (1968): Social Theory and Social Structure. New York: The Free Press.

Messick, D. (1968): Mathematical Thinking in Behavioral Sciences. San Fran-cisco: W. H. Freeman.

Mill, J. (1930): A System of Logic (8th ed.). New York: Longmans.

Miller, D. (ed.) (1970): Handbook of Research Design and Social Measurement (2nd ed.). New York: David McKay.

Mikaelian, H. (1972): A technique for measuring eye-foot coordination without visual guidance. *Behavior Research Methods and Instrumentation 4*, 17–18.

Mitchell, P. (ed.) (1973): Concepts Basic to Nursing. New York: McGraw-Hill.

Moore-Nunnally, D. and Aguiar, M. (1981): Patients' evaluation of their pre-natal and delivery care. In Fox, D. and Leeser, I. (eds.), Readings on the Research Process in Nursing. New York: Appleton.

Nakagawa, H. (1972): An epidemiological study of psychiatric symptom pattern change. In Batey, M. (ed.), Communicating Nursing Research. Boulder, Colo.: WICHE.

National Commission for the Study of Nursing and Nursing Education (1970): An Abstract for Action. New York: McGraw-Hill.

National Institute of Health (1974): Research projects involving human subjects.

National League for Nursing (1978): Characteristics of Baccalaureate Education in Nursing.

Nightingale, F. (1859): Notes on nursing (1970 ed.). London: Gerald Duckworth.

Neuman, G. (1980): The Betty Neuman health-care system model. In Riehl, J. and Roy, C. (eds.), Conceptual Models for Nursing Practice (2nd ed.). New York: Appleton.

Notter, L. (1963): Nursing research is every nurse's business. *Nursing Outlook 11*, 49–51.

Olgas, M. (1974): Relationship between parent's health status and body image of their children. *Nursing Research 23*, 319–324.

O'Neil, S. (1972): The application and methodological implication of behavior modification in nursing research. In Batey, M. (ed.), Communicating Nursing Research. Boulder, Colo.: WICHE.

Orem, D. (1971): Nursing: Concepts of Practice. New York: McGraw-Hill.

Orlando, I. (1961): The Dynamic Nurse–Patient Relationship. New York: G. P. Putnam's Sons.

Osgood, C. et al (1957): The Measurement of Meaning. Urbana: University of Illinois Press.

Parten, M. (1950): Surveys, Polls and Samples. New York: Harper and Brothers.

Pavlov, I. (1928): Lectures on Conditioned Reflex (trans. W. H. Gantt). New York: International Pub.

Peplau, H. (1952): Interpersonal Relations in Nursing. New York: G. P. Putnam's Sons.

Petrovich, D. et al (1968): Nursing apparel and pychiatric patients: a comparison of uniforms and street clothes. *Journal of Psychiatric Nursing 6*, 344.

Phillips, B. (1966): Social Research. New York: Macmillan.

Phillips, J. and Thompson, R. (1967): Statistics for Nurses. New York: Macmillan.

Polit, P. and Hungler, B. (1978): Nursing Research. New York: J. B. Lippincott.

Porter, C. (1974): Grade school children's perception of their internal body parts. *Nursing Research 23*, 384–391.

Puttock, D. (1972): Dance therapy. *Nursing Times 68*, 960–961.

Rathus, S. (1973): A thirty item schedule for assessing assertive behavior. *Behavior Therapy 4*, 398–406.

Reeder, L. et al. (1976): Handbook of Scales and Indices of Health Behavior. Pacific Palisade, Calif.: Goodyear Pub.

Resio, D. and Verhonick, P. (1973): On the measurement and analysis of clinical data in nursing. *Nursing Research 22*, 388–393.

Richardson, F. and Tasto, D. (1976): Development and factor analysis of a social anxiety inventory. *Behavior Therapy 7*, 453–462.

Riehl, J. and Roy, C. (1980): Conceptual Models for Nursing Practice (2nd ed). New York: Appleton.

Robinson, J. and Shaver, P.: Measures of Psychological Attitude (rev.). Ann Arbor: University of Michigan.

Robischon, P. (1971): Pica practice and other hand-mouth behavior and children's developmental level. *Nursing Research 20*, 4–16.

Rodgers, J. (1972): Relationship between sociability and personal space preference at two different times of day. *Perceptual and Motor Skills 35*, 519–526.

Rose, M. (1972): The effects of hospitalization on the coping behaviors of children. In Batey, M. (ed.), Communicating Nursing Research. Boulder, Colo.: WICHE.

Rottkamp, B. (1981): A behavior modification approach to nursing therapeutics in body positioning of spinal-cord-injured patients. In Fox, D. and Lesser, I. (eds.), Readings on the Research Process in Nursing. New York: Appleton.

Roy, C. (1980): The Roy adaptation model. In Riehl, J. and Roy, C. (eds.), Conceptual Models for Nursing Practice. New York: Appleton, pp. 179–188.

Rugh, J. and Schwitzgebel, R. (1977): Instrumentation for behavioral assessment. In Ciminero et al (eds.), Handbook of Behavioral Assessment. New York: Wiley, pp. 79–113.

Schlotfeldt, R. (1975): The need for a conceptual framework. In Verhonick, P. (ed.), Nursing Research II. Boston: Little, Brown.

Schmitt, F. and Wooldridge, P. (1981): Psychological preparation of surgical patients. In Fox, D. and Leeser, I. (eds.), Readings on the Research Process in Nursing. New York: Appleton.

Schulmann, J. and Reisman, J. (1959): An objective measurement of hyperactivity. *American Journal of Mental Deficiency 64*, 455–456.

Seaman, C. (1976): Elementary Research Methods. Charlottesville: University of Virginia Printing Press.

Selltiz, C. et al (1976): Research Methods in Social Relations. New York: Holt, Rinehart, and Winston.

Selye, H. (1965): The Stress of Life. New York: McGraw-Hill.

Shipley, R. and Harley, R. (1971): A device for estimating stability of stance in human subjects. *Psychophysiology 7*, 287–292.

Simon, J. (1978): Basic Research Methods in Social Science (2nd ed.). New York: Random House.

Skinner, B. (1953): Science and Human Behavior. New York: Macmillan.

Stetler, C. and Marram, G. (1976): Evaluating research findings for applicability in practice. *Nursing Outlook 24*, 559–563.

Stevens, B. (1979): Nursing Theory. Boston: Little, Brown.

Stillman, M. (1977): Women's health beliefs about breast cancer and breast self-examination. *Nursing Research 26*, 121–127.

Stouffer, S. (1950): Some observations on study design. *American Journal of Sociology 55*, 356–359.

Strunk, W. and White, E. (1972): The Elements of Style (2nd ed.). New York: Macmillan.

Swanson, A. (1977): Fearfulness of children in relation to maternal anxiety, self-differentiation and accuracy of perception. In Downs, F. and Newman, M. (eds.), A Sourcebook of Nursing Research (2nd ed.). Philadelphia: F. A. Davis.

Treece, E. and Treece, J. (1977): Elements of Research in Nursing (2nd ed.). St. Louis: C. V. Mosby.

Triplett, J. (1977): Characteristics and perceptions of low-income women and use of preventive health services: an exploratory study. In Downs, F. and Newman, M. (eds.), A Sourcebook of Nursing Research. Philadelphia: F. A. Davis.

Tripodi, T. et al (1969): The Assessment of Social Research. Itasca, Ill.: F. E. Peacock.

Turabian, K. (1973): A Manual for Writers of Term Papers, Theses, and Dissertations (4th ed.). Chicago: University of Chicago Press.

Valadez, A. and Anderson, E. (1972): Rehabilitation workshops: change in attitude of nurses. *Nursing Research 21,* 132–137.

Van Ort, S. and Gerber, R. (1976): Topical application of insulin in the treatment of decubitus ulcers. *Nursing Research 25,* 9–12.

Veatch, R. and Branson, R. (eds.) (1976): Ethics and Health Policy. Cambridge: Ballinger.

Verhonick, P. (ed.) (1975): Nursing Research I. Boston: Little, Brown. (1977): Nursing Research II. Boston: Little, Brown.

Vietze, P., et al (1974): A portable system for studying head movement in infants in relation to contingent and noncontingent sensory stimulation. *Behavior Research Methods and Instrumentation 6,* 338–340.

Wald, F. and Leonard, R. (1964): Toward development of nursing practice theory. *Nursing Reseach 13,* 309–313.

Walizer, M. and Wienir, P. (1978): Research Methods and Analysis. New York: Harper and Row.

Walk, R. (1956): Self-ratings of fear in a fear-invoking situation. *Journal of Abnormal and Social Psychology 52,* 171–178.

Wallace, W. (1971): The Logic of Science in Sociology. Chicago: Aldine.

Warner, W. et al (1949): Social Class in America. Chicago: Science Research Associates.

Webb, E. et al (1966): Unobtrusive Measures. Chicago: Rand McNally.

Williams, A. (1972): Study of factors contributing to skin breakdown. *Nursing Research 21,* 238–243.

Williams, M. (1972): A comparative study of postsurgical convalescence among women of two ethnic groups: Anglo and Mexican-American. In Batey, M. (ed.), Communicating Nursing Research. Boulder, Colo.: WICHE.

Windwer, C. (1977): Relationship among prospective parents' locus of control, social desirability, and choice of psychoprophylaxis. *Nursing Research 26,* 96–99.

Wolff, C. (1948): A psychology of gesture. London: Methuen.

Wooldridge, P. et al (1968): Behavioral Science, Social Practice, and the Nursing Profession. Cleveland: The Press of Case Western Reserve University.

Young, P. (1939): Scientific Social Surveys and Research. New York: Prentice Hall.

Zuckerman, M. (1960): The development of an affective adjective checklist for the measurement of anxiety. *Journal of Consulting and Clinical Psychology 24,* 457–462.

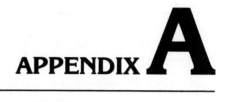

APPENDIX **A**

OBSERVATION AIDS

INSTRUCTIONS TO OBSERVERS

1. Check the Observer's Schedule daily to confirm hours of work.
2. Observations should cover two-hour periods (except for the night shift, which has fewer activities).
3. Every 10 (or 15) minutes, walk through the entire unit and record what each person (nursing personnel) in the unit is doing.
4. Whenever possible, observations of activities should be recorded in verb form. Example:
   a. Giving bath; not "bath"
   b. Taking TPR; not "TPR"
   c. Talking on telephone
   d. Is "off unit"
   e. Sitting; doing nothing
5. Activities of personnel need not be recorded in the order first observed. (The first person encountered may be a nursing student, and the second the head nurse; at the next observation, the first person encountered may be staff nurse No. 1.)
6. A code for persons observed is suggested to include:
   SU — Supervisor
   HN — Head nurse
   SN — Staff nurse

OBSERVATION RECORDING SHEET

Nursing Activity Study

Observer _____ *Date* _____ *Unit* _____ *Page* _____ *of* _____ *pages*

TIME	PERSONNEL OBSERVED	ACTIVITY	LEVEL	AREA

WEEKLY SCHEDULE FOR OBSERVER

Observer's Schedule*

DATES _____

UNIT _____

Hours of Observation	Mon.	Tues.	Wed.	Thurs.	Fri.
7:00–9:00 A.M.					
9:00–11:00 A.M.	name				
11:00 A.M.–1:00 P.M.					
1:00–3:00 P.M.	name				
3:00–5:00 P.M.	name				
5:00–7:00 P.M.					
7:00–9:00 P.M.	name				
9:00–11:00 P.M.	name				
11:00 P.M.–1:00 A.M.					
1:00–3:00 A.M.					
3:00–5:00 A.M.					
5:00–7:00 A.M.					

* Areas blocked out have been eliminated by means of random selection of periods of observation.

NST   —   Nursing student
PN   —   Practical nurse
CI   —   Clinical Instructor
PN-I   —   Practical-nurse instructor
NA   —   Nurse aide
O   —   Orderly

7. If a person is away from the unit at observation time, ask the person later where she or he was and record the response.
8. Record the time of observation, personnel, and the activity for each time period (10 or 15 minutes).

STUDY CODE

Classification of Activities by Level of Skill

Code

A = ADMINISTRATION ACTIVITIES (All coded as A in "Level Column"). Administration includes activities requiring nursing judgment. These involve responsibility for planning and providing effective patient care, for developing unit personnel, and for managing and operating the nursing unit.

  1. Patient care activities include:
    Assigning personnel to meet the individual needs of patients
    Planning and participating in unit education programs to ensure safe and effective nursing care
    Assisting the physician in the plan for patient care by directing the execution of orders and reporting to the physician the patient's symptoms, reactions, and progress
    Supervising and evaluating the effectiveness of patient care
    Giving nursing care for the purpose of observing a patient, establishing rapport with a patient, or teaching a member or members of the nursing staff
    Promoting, supervising, and evaluating the education and rehabilitation program for the patient and family
    Making nursing rounds to assess the patient's condition, progress, and immediate environment
  2. Development of unit personnel includes:
    Planning for the participation of nursing personnel in continuous learning experiences;
    Promoting personal growth and development of unit personnel;

Conducting written and oral evaluations of the performances of staff members.
   3. Unit management activities include:
Planning for and maintaining an environment conducive to the well-being of patients and personnel;
Promoting good interpersonal relationships;
Assisting in the development and implementation of nursing objectives and policies.

N = NURSING ACTIVITIES (all coded as N in "Level Column")
   Nursing activities include those involved directly and indirectly in giving nursing care to patients:
      Preparation of a nursing care plan for direct patient care
      Carrying out orders prescribed by the physician for individual
   patients
      Observing and reporting on a patient's symptoms, reactions,
   and progress
      Making out Rx sheet for direct patient care
      Recording intake and output.

C = CLERICAL ACTIVITIES (all coded as C in "Level Column")
   Clerical activities are those concerned with counting, copying, ordering, recording:
      Assembling chart forms for new patients
      Checking charts after discharge of patients
      Copying records, such as time sheets
      Transcribing orders, counting supplies or drugs
   Checking drugs from pharmacy
   Charting TPR on graph sheet

D = DIETARY ACTIVITIES (all coded as D in "Level Column")
   Dietary activities are those concerned with the routine serving of fluids, food, and nourishment:
      Caring for unit diet kitchen
      Carrying or picking up trays
      Cleaning water glasses and pitchers, and distributing fresh
   water and ice
      Preparing and serving nourishment between meals
      Setting up trays

H = HOUSEKEEPING ACTIVITIES (all coded as H in "Level Column").
Housekeeping activities are those concerned with the appearance
of the unit environment and the care of supplies and equipment:
    Making unoccupied beds
    Cleaning floors, windows, bathrooms, and service rooms
    Cleaning room after discharge of patient, including cleaning
and making up the bed
    Routine checking of the unit to maintain furnishings in good
order
    Dusting furniture, emptying wastebaskets, general cleaning
of the nursing station
    Distributing and collecting linens.

M = MESSENGER ACTIVITIES (all coded as M in "Level Column")
Messenger activities are those requiring absence from the unit for
transport services, escort service, and errands, such as:
    Accompanying patients to other parts of the hospital;
    Delivering requisitioned orders, both routine and emergency;
    Picking up drug and supply orders, both routine and emergency.

U = UNCLASSIFIED ACTIVITIES (all coded as U in "Level Column")
Unclassified activities are those that, by definition, are eliminated
from any of the preceding codes. Code U is used to identify those
activities that refer to the person as an individual (see Table A–1).
    The activity, not the person observed, is coded. The activity is
classified or coded in two dimensions—area and level—simultaneously. This means that each activity as entered on the Observation Recording Sheet will be coded in the same manner, regardless of who performs it, whether a nurse, clerk, or nurse aide (see
Table A–2).

TABLE A–1. OBSERVATION OF ACTIVITY CHECKLIST GUIDE

Time	Personnel Observed	Area	Level	Activity
10:00 A.M.	RN_1	2.1	U	Reading new pamphlet on diabetes.
10:30 A.M.	RN_2	0.1	U	Drinking chocolate milk.
11:00 A.M.	RN_3	0.2	U	Waiting to assist physician with a dressing.
11:30 A.M.	RN_4	0.1	U	Checking hour book for days off.

TABLE A–2

HN	1.4C	Copying medical order from order sheet to medicine
SN	1.4C	tickets.
NS	1.4C	
CI	1.4C	
HN	1.4A	Checking on orders as copied (by clerk).
SN	1.4A	
HN	2.1A	Showing nurse aide how to give a sitz bath.
SN	2.1A	
PN	2.1A	
SN	1.2A	Explaining intercom system to a new patient.
NA	1.2A	
HN	1.1N	Giving medicine to patient.
SN	1.1N	
PN	1.1N	
NST	1.1N	

Classification of Activities by Area of Nursing
Code   Subcode

1   PATIENT-CENTERED ACTIVITIES

These activities may occur in the patient's presence or away from the patient.

    1.1   *Direct Care*

Activities occurring in the presence of the patient that involve giving care, including:
Carrying out nursing procedures;
Assisting doctors with treatments or procedures;
Giving or assisting patients with personal hygiene.

    1.2   *Other Patient Activities Relating to Direct Care*

Conversing or exchanging pleasantries with the patients (talking with patients);
Evaluating the patients' need for care;
Escorting patients;
Interpreting procedures and practices to patients;
Observing the physical condition and behavior of patients;

Code   Subcode

1.2   *Other Patient Activities Relating to Direct Care* (Continued)

Teaching patients;
Making unoccupied beds, with patients at bedsides.

1.3   *Exchange of Information Concerning Patients*

This is mainly oral communication. These activities include:

Discussing an assignment of patient care;
Reading Kardex (nursing care plan);
Examining reports on the patient with other members of the unit or hospital staff, physicians, the patient's family and friends, or other interested persons or agencies;
Holding or attending demonstrations for teaching staff members individually or collectively;
Giving or receiving planned or impromptu instruction;
Observing and evaluating the quality of work performed;
Orienting new unit staff members;
Reading or questioning to gain more information about a drug, treatment, etc.;
Listening to or giving the morning, afternoon, or evening report;
Ordering specific drugs, diet, supplies, or equipment by telephone for a particular patient or for a few patients, but not unit supplies;
Participating in doctor's rounds;
Receiving or giving an assignment related to patient care.

1.4   *Indirect Care*

All patient-centered activities not classified under Code Numbers 1.1, 1.2, 1.3, including:

Maintaining patient's records;
Charting care given;
Checking physician's orders;
Completing form on patient's condition;

1.4   *Indirect Care* (Continued)

Making out written requisition for specific drugs, diet, supplies, or equipment for a particular patient;
Preparing medication and treatment trays;
Setting up and performing immediate aftercare of equipment;
Obtaining information from Kardex.

Code   *Subcode*

2   PERSONNEL-CENTERED ACTIVITIES

These activities are primarily concerned with professional growth and development of nursing service personnel and with personnel management.

2.1   *Professional Development of Staff*

Participation in all activities conducive to improved nursing service, as well as planned and unplanned events that increase the knowledge and skill of the staff.

2.2   *Personnel:* Other

Activities having to do with personnel management (personnel-centered activities), including:
Attending staff meetings;
Participating in individual conferences on personal matters related to work;
Maintaining personnel records and confering on personnel matters;
Obtaining physical examination on self by physician.

2.3   *Professional Nursing Student Program**

These activities include:
Discussing the nursing students' program with unit personnel, physicians, clinical instructors, and others;

---

*Activities in which nursing students are involved must be weighed carefully in terms of whether they are patient-centered or personnel-centered. If an activity is personnel-centered, a determination must be made as to whether it is for the student or for the unit staff of which the student is considered a part.

2.3   *Professional Nursing Student Program* (Continued)

Observing and evaluating the quality of work performed by nursing students;
Planning and selecting experience for nursing students;
Giving nursing students impromptu or planned instruction.

2.4   *Practical Nursing Student Program*

Activities concerned with the educational program or with experience for practical nursing students.

Code Subcode

3   UNIT-CENTERED ACTIVITIES

These activities are concerned primarily with the patient's environment and with equipment and supplies for the unit.

3.1   *Environment*

Cleaning and maintenance activities for the order and safety of the unit, including:
Cleaning patient's unit (patient not at bedside);
Making unoccupied bed (patient not at bedside);
Caring for unit after patient's discharge;
Cleaning of nurses' station, utility room, etc.

3.2   *Supplies and Equipment*

Activities concerned with obtaining, dispensing, or maintaining material for the unit, including:
Obtaining drug and linen supplies;
Checking drugs delivered by pharmacy;
Obtaining required supplies and equipment and conducting all discussions on this matter;
Obtaining and serving all foods and fluids;
Caring for supplies and equipment;
Maintaining the Kardex.

3.3   *Other Unit Activities:*

These include:
Performing work related to the activity analysis study;
Holding conversations to maintain rapport and good interpersonal relationships with unit and hospital staff, visitors, etc.;
Delivering mail to patients;
Holding discussions, compiling data, etc., in connection with any other studies;
Running errands on behalf of unit personnel;
Giving or receiving an interpretation of hospital policy as it affects the unit staff;
Maintaining unit records, such as time sheets, leave records, daily reports;
Reporting on or off duty;
Serving on committees for the purpose of discussing, revising, or formulating hospital and nursing policy and procedure.

Code	*Subcode*	

0   OTHER-CENTERED ACTIVITIES

0.1   *Personal*

These activities include all activities of a personal nature, e.g., coffee breaks, conversations about personal affairs.

0.2   *Standby Time*

Time spent waiting for the arrival of a person or thing prior to the start of an activity, including:
Waiting for a doctor to arrive, in order to assist with a spinal puncture;
Waiting for a sterile dressing tray to arrive, in order to change a patient's dressing.

APPENDIX B

SAMPLE QUESTIONNAIRE
AND INTERVIEW FORMS

SAMPLE QUESTIONNAIRE FORMAT

Directions

1. Please answer every question with a check mark (✔) or short response.
2. It should take approximately 45 minutes to complete the questionnaire.
3. Your signature is optional. You will not be identified individually, and your response will be treated in confidence.
4. Please return the completed questionnaire to _____ .
5. Thank you for your cooperation.

* * * * *

I. Background Information

	Code
1. Please check your age in the appropriate space.	
a. 20 years or less	a. ____
b. 21–25 years	b. ____
c. 26–30 years	c. ____
d. 31–35 years	d. ____
e. 36–40 years	e. ____
f. 41–45 years	f. ____

Continued

    g. 46–50 years   g. ____
    h. 51–55 years   h. ____
    i. More than 55 years   i. ____

2. From what type of basic educational program did you graduate? (Please check appropriate answer.)
    a. General nursing   a. ____
    b. Mental nursing   b. ____
    c. Other; specify _____   c. ____

3. What is your present position? (Please check appropriate answer.)
    a. Matron   a. ____
    b. Assistant matron   b. ____
    c. Departmental sister   c. ____
    d. Ward sister (Head nurse)   d. ____
    e. Staff nurse   e. ____
    f. Tutor (Instructor)   f. ____
    g. Other; specify _____   g. ____

4. How long have you worked in your present position? (Please check appropriate answer.)
    a. Less than 1 year   a. ____
    b. 1–3 years   b. ____
    c. 4–6 years   c. ____
    d. 7–9 years   d. ____
    e. 10–12 years   e. ____
    f. More than 12 years   f. ____

II. Patient Preference

1. What type of patients do you prefer to care for?

    _____

2. Please give the reason for your answer. _____

    _____
    _____
    _____

SAMPLE INTERVIEW SCHEDULE

1. a. Is this your first visit to the
      clinic?   Yes ____   No ____
   b. If the answer is "No,"
      when was the last time
      you visited the clinic?   _____
   c. Approximately how many
      times have you visited the
      clinic?   _____

2. For what reason did you come   a. Complaint of pain _____
   to the clinic today?   b. Complaint of other
                                       symptoms _____
                                   c. Wanted to see doctor _____
                                   d. Wanted laboratory test _____
                                   e. Wanted an examination _____
                                   f. Other reason; specify _____

                                      _____
                                      _____
                                      _____
                                      _____

3. How are you feeling now?   a. Sick (ill) _____
                                   b. Not sick but
                                      uncomfortable _____
                                   c. Healthy _____
                                   d. Other; specify _____

                                      _____
                                      _____

TABULATION SHEET FOR RECORD REVIEW

CLINIC REGISTER NUMBER	CLINIC VISIT NUMBER	SEX	RACE	AGE	MARITAL STATUS	HEIGHT	DIET	MEDICAL DIAGNOSIS	SIGNS AND SYMPTOMS	REMARKS

TABULATION SHEET FOR RECORD REVIEW

CLINIC REGISTER NUMBER	CLINIC VISIT NUMBER	SEX	RACE	AGE	MARITAL STATUS	HEIGHT	DIET	MEDICAL DIAGNOSIS	SIGNS AND SYMPTOMS	REMARKS

DUMMY TABLE: INITIAL ANALYSIS FOR IDENTIFYING PATTERNS OF SIMILARITY OR DIFFERENCE

LENGTH OF NURSING EXPERIENCE	TYPE OF PATIENT PREFERENCE												TOTAL
	Medical		*Surgical*		*Pediatric*		*Geriatric*						
	Acute	Chronic	Acute	Chronic	Acute	Chronic	Acute	Chronic					
Less than 6 months													
7 months to 5 years													
6–10 years													
11–15 years													
16–20 years													
21–25 years													
More than 25 years													
Total													

INDEX

Stability of reliability, 241
Standard deviation, 261–264
Standard scores, 264–265
Standardized questions, 207–208
Static group comparison design, 161 162f
Static studies, 163
Statistical guides, 103
Statistical inference. *See* Inferential
statistics
Statistical regression, 240
Stastical tests, 280
Statistics. *See* Descriptive statistics;
Inferential statistics
Stimulus-response, 109
Strata, 135
Stratified random sampling, 14
Stress, 114
Stress theories, 108, 114, 115
Structured interviews, 219
Structured observation, 184, 185
Subjective probability, 136–137
Summarizing, in review of literature,
91–93
Survey, 43, 47, 149, 151t, 163–165, 184
Syllogism, 26
Symbolic interaction, 108, 123–124
System, 116
Systematic errors, 279
Systematic sampling, 139–140
Systems theory, 108, 116–120

Tables, 47, 253–254
general purpose, 253
model of, 254t
special purpose, 253
Tabulation of data, 252–257
Target population. *See* Universe
Telephone interview, 222
Test-retest reliability, 241
Testing, internal validity jeopardized by,
240
Thematic Apperception Test, 221, 224
Theory, 22–26. *See also specific theory*
and abstract knowledge, 10
and classification, 188
comparison of, in review of literature,
93
definition of, 23, 27, 107
grand, 25
and measurement, 232
middle-range, 25
in nursing, 9, 23, 43, 63–64, 107–132
and observation, 185
in research project, 42–43
in research proposal, 66
as source of hypothesis, 27, 107
Theory construction, 20, 23, 24–26,
126–127, 153

Theory construction (*cont.*)
model of, 21f
Theory testing, 20, 23
model of, 21f
Thurstone scale, 235
Time
needed for research, 61–62
perception of, 187
and preliminary search of literature, 91
and surveys, 163–164
Time-movement studies, 187
Time series experimental design. 159–160
Total range, 259–260
Transvultural nursing, 124–125
Trend study, 164
True experimental design, 155–157
Two after-groups control design, 157
Type I error, 275, 278
Type II error, 275, 279

Unconscious person, as research subject,
80
Universe, 134
Unobtrusive observation, 185–187
Unstructured interview, 220–222
Unstructured observation, 184

Validity, 155, 237–240
concurrent, 238
construct, 238–239
content, 237
definition of, 236, 237
external, 239, 240
face, 238
internal, 239–240
in measurement, 236
predictive, 238
in scales, 236
Values, 73–74
Variables, 30–31
attribute, 31
definition of, 30
dependent, 31
extraneous, 31, 155
independent, 30–31
in research project, 41
Variance, measures of, 259–265
Verifier, 288
Vulnerable subjects, 78–80

Withdrawal from research, 77–78
Word association tests, 221
Working experiences, as source of
hypotheses, 28
Working hypotheses, 24–25, 28
Writing style, evaluation of, 99